A Guide to Humanistic Studies in Aging

A Guide to
Humanistic Studies in Aging

What Does It Mean to Grow Old?

Edited by

Thomas R. Cole

McGovern Chair in Medical Humanities,
Professor and Director
John P. McGovern, M.D. Center for Health,
Humanities, and the Human Spirit
The University of Texas Health Science Center at Houston
Houston, Texas

Ruth E. Ray

Professor of English and
Faculty Associate in Gerontology
English Department
Wayne State University
Detroit, Michigan

Robert Kastenbaum

Professor Emeritus of Gerontology
and Communications
Department of Communications
Arizona State University
Tempe, Arizona

The Johns Hopkins University Press
Baltimore

© 2010 The Johns Hopkins University Press
All rights reserved. Published 2010
Printed in the United States of America on acid-free paper

2 4 6 8 9 7 5 3 1

The Johns Hopkins University Press
2715 North Charles Street
Baltimore, Maryland 21218-4363
www.press.jhu.edu

Library of Congress Cataloging-in-Publication Data
A guide to humanistic studies in aging : what does it mean to grow old? /
edited by Thomas R. Cole, Ruth E. Ray, and Robert Kastenbaum.
p. ; cm.
Includes bibliographical references and index.
ISBN-13: 978-0-8018-9433-6 (hardcover : alk. paper)
ISBN-10: 0-8018-9433-6 (hardcover : alk. paper)
1. Aging. 2. Humanism. 3. Social perception. I. Cole, Thomas R., 1949–
II. Ray, Ruth E., 1954– III. Kastenbaum, Robert.
[DNLM: 1. Aging. 2. Humanism. 3. Social Perception. WT 104 G946 2010]
QP86.G85 2010
612.6′7—dc22   2009027106

A catalog record for this book is available from the British Library.

*Special discounts are available for bulk purchases of this book. For more information, please
contact Special Sales at 410-516-6936 or specialsales@press.jhu.edu.*

The Johns Hopkins University Press uses environmentally friendly book materials,
including recycled text paper that is composed of at least 30 percent post-consumer waste,
whenever possible. All of our book papers are acid-free, and our jackets and covers
are printed on paper with recycled content.

CONTENTS

JAN BAARS, Ph.D., Associate Professor, Department of Philosophy, Tilburg University, Tilburg, the Netherlands

GENE D. COHEN, M.D., Ph.D., Director, Center on Aging, Health, and Humanities, George Washington University, Kensington, Maryland

BRIAN DE VRIES, Ph.D., Professor of Gerontology, Department of Sexuality Studies, San Francisco State University, San Francisco, California

MARGARET M. GULLETTE, Ph.D., Resident Scholar, Women's Studies Research Center, Brandeis University, Waltham, Massachusetts

MARTHA B. HOLSTEIN, Ph.D., Teacher, Trainer, and Codirector, Center for Long-Term Care Reform, Health and Medicine Policy Research Group, Chicago, Illinois

STEPHEN KATZ, Ph.D., Professor, Department of Sociology, Trent University, Peterborough, Ontario, Canada

SHARON R. KAUFMAN, Ph.D., Professor of Medical Anthropology, UCSF Institute for Health and Aging, University of California, San Francisco, San Francisco, California

RÜDIGER KUNOW, Ph.D., Professor, Institute of English Studies and American Studies, Potsdam University, Potsdam, Germany

RONALD J. MANHEIMER, Ph.D., Executive Director, North Carolina Center for Creative Retirement, The University of North Carolina at Asheville, Asheville, North Carolina

SUSAN H. MCFADDEN, Ph.D., Professor, Department of Psychology, University of Wisconsin, Oshkosh, Wisconsin

KEVIN MCHUGH, Ph.D., Associate Professor of Geography, School of Geographical Sciences, Arizona State University, Tempe, Arizona

JANET L. RAMSEY, Ph.D., Associate Professor of Congregational Leadership, Luther Seminary, St. Paul, Minnesota

STEPHEN SAPP, Ph.D., Department Chair and Professor, Department of Religious Studies, College of Arts and Sciences, University of Miami, Coral Gables, Florida

PAT THANE, Ph.D., Leverhulme Professor of Contemporary British History and Director, Center for Contemporary British History, Institute of Historical Research, University of London, London, United Kingdom

BARBARA FREY WAXMAN, Ph.D., Professor, Department of English, University of North Carolina Wilmington, Wilmington, North Carolina

ANNE M. WYATT-BROWN, Ph.D., Emeritus Associate Professor, Program in Linguistics, University of Florida, Gainesville, Florida

ROBERT E. YAHNKE, Ph.D., Professor, College of Education and Human Development, University of Minnesota, Minneapolis, Minnesota

A Guide to Humanistic Studies in Aging

The Humanistic Study of Aging Past and Present, or Why Gerontology Still Needs Interpretive Inquiry

THOMAS R. COLE, PH.D., AND RUTH E. RAY, D.A.

This volume is the third in a series of books that began in 1992 under the title *Handbook of the Humanities and Aging* (Cole, Van Tassel, and Kastenbaum, 1992). Our original goal was to give formal shape to a new and inchoate field of knowledge—humanistic gerontology—that had recently emerged to address fundamental blind spots in scholarly knowledge about aging. As Tom Cole put it in the introduction to the first edition of the *Handbook,* "Over the past 20 years, many people have sensed that something important is missing in a purely scientific and professional gerontology. Mainstream gerontology—with its highly technical and instrumental, avowedly objective, value-neutral and specialized discourses—lacks an appropriate language for addressing basic moral and spiritual issues in our aging society. Researchers, teachers, students, professionals, patients, clients, administrators, and policymakers do not possess a ready way to speak to one another about fundamental questions of human existence" (p. xii). In this context, urgent existential, moral, and spiritual issues had no place on the map of gerontological knowledge. The basic question of humanistic gerontology—what does it mean to grow old?—had not been raised.

In the 1970s, professionally trained humanists in the United States—along with humanistically oriented social scientists and clinicians—awakened to these issues in the study of aging. Around 1975, various writings began to emerge, and over the next decade the implications of the humanities for gerontological research, education, public policy, and clinical practice became clearer. If we try to locate "the beginning" of humanistic gerontology, the best estimate is the year 1975, when historian David Van Tassel launched a two-year project, "Human Values and Aging," supported by the National Endowment for the Humanities (for earlier work, see Grmek, 1958; Gruman, 1966). At the time, a framework of "human values" had already been successfully developed by the Society for Health and Human Values, established in

1965 to challenge dehumanization in medicine and health care (Fox, 1985). Using the rhetoric of "human values," Van Tassel brought together senior and junior scholars in two interdisciplinary conferences to look at aging from various humanities disciplines. The best papers from these conferences were collected and edited in the first two volumes of humanistic gerontology (Spicker, Woodward, and Van Tassel, 1978; Van Tassel, 1979; see also Moss, 1976). Van Tassel was also a founding member of the Gerontological Society of America's Humanities and Arts Committee, created in 1976 at the request of former GSA president Joseph Freeman, a humanistically oriented physician and scholar (Achenbaum, 2007; Ansello, 2007).

Van Tassel's efforts opened up a steady stream of scholarship in the humanities and aging. By the mid-1980s more than 1,100 books and articles were cited in the annotated bibliography commissioned by the Humanities and Arts Committee of the Gerontological Society of America (Polisar et al., 1988). It was Bob Kastenbaum who saw the need to put fences around the "field" of humanistic gerontology and locate it on the map of gerontological knowledge. In 1984, on a yellow napkin at a Wendy's restaurant in New Orleans between Gerontological Society sessions, Bob, David Van Tassel, and Tom Cole sketched the topics and boundaries for an authoritative reference volume designed to conceptualize and introduce readers to humanistic gerontology—and to serve as a vehicle for its continued growth and maturation.

In 1990, the three major U.S. handbooks of aging (covering the fields of biology, psychology, and the social sciences) appeared in their third editions under the general editorship of James E. Birren. To legitimize humanities scholarship in the study of aging, Kastenbaum, Van Tassel, and Cole decided to publish the newly conceived reference volume as a "handbook." (We were not alone in this effort: handbooks of aging and geriatric psychiatry, mental health, nutrition, ethnicity, communication, family, and women also rolled off the presses between 1980 and 1997; see Katz, 2000, pp. 408ff.) At the same time, we self-consciously positioned our handbook against the grain of purely scientific and professional gerontological knowledge.

In 2000, after a substantial body of additional scholarship had appeared and new areas of interest emerged, Tom Cole and Robert Kastenbaum, now collaborating with English studies scholar Ruth Ray, produced the second edition of the *Handbook of the Humanities and Aging* (Cole, Kastenbaum, and Ray, 2000). Since 2000, the continuing pace and creativity of humanities and humanistic research in aging have reached a point that justifies another volume summarizing and configuring this work. (The recently launched [2007] *Journal of Humanities, Arts, and Aging,* edited by Dana Bradley and Anne Wyatt Brown, and the new [2009] series *Aging Studies in Europe,* edited by Heike Hartung and the Austrian scholar Roberta Maierhofer, indicate accelerating interest in the field.)

Although the 2000 edition of the *Handbook of the Humanities and Aging* featured primarily the work of American humanists and qualitative social scientists, in the 1990s a number of European social scientists and humanities scholars had also begun to address humanistic concerns, particularly the connection between aging and identity, and to rely on concepts from the humanities such as image and metaphor. British contributors to the interdisciplinary journal *Theory, Culture & Society* and authors of books that spun off from this journal were bringing the body and lived experience back into sociological scholarship. In *The Body: Social Process and Cultural Theory*, for example, editors Mike Featherstone, Mike Hepworth, and Bryan Turner (1991) argued that the body—including emotions, health, and fitness, as well as body metaphors and media images—is central to understanding the complex interrelationship of nature, culture, and society. In *Images of Aging: Cultural Representations of Later Life* Featherstone and Wernick (1995) critically examined cultural and historical representations of aging from midlife through old age, while Chris Gilleard and Paul Higgs argued in *Cultures of Aging: Self, Citizen and the Body* (2000) that identity in later life is based more on consumption than production, as reflected in lifestyle choices revolving around the body (choice of leisure activities, for example, or uses of technological innovations).

Featherstone and Hepworth (1989, 1995) use the metaphor of the mask to examine the connection between aging and identity, theorizing that the physical evidence of aging "masks" an inward self (or self-concept) that is typically much younger. The mask for these authors is a negative construct, as the youthful self (perceived as positive) becomes trapped or caged within an increasingly failing body. Alternatively, British scholar Simon Biggs used the metaphor of masquerade to suggest a more subtle and complex relationship between appearance and identity (1997, 1999, 2005). In Biggs's psychoanalytic formulation, the aging person engages in a "masquerade," altering physical appearance through makeup and hair dye, for example, as a "tactical manoeuvre to negotiate the contradiction between social ageism and the increased personal integration that accompanies adult ageing . . . Masking connects inner psychological and external social logic while affording an element of protection for parts of the self that cannot be easily expressed," thereby protecting the self from external attack and creating "a necessary inner space where one can build a stable identity" apart from appearance (Estes, Biggs, and Phillipson, 2003).

In the 1990s, other British social scientists were studying narrative and even literature in an effort to understand the experiences of aging. In *Images of Ageing*, for example, sociologist Mike Hepworth (2000) analyzed several fictional works from the theoretical perspective of symbolic interactionism. Gerontologist Bill Bytheway (1994) also looked to narrative, language, and cultural images in his research on ageism.

German and German-speaking scholars were also working this ground under the rubric of "cultural gerontology." Christoph Conrad and Hans-Joachim von Kondratowitz edited *Zur Kulturgeschichte des Alterns [Toward a Cultural History of Aging]* (1993), which contained chapters on issues of images of aging, retirement, medicine, the social contract, etc., in European history. Von Kondratowitz's early work (1991) included a study of the medicalization of aging in the eighteenth and nineteenth centuries. Thereafter he has been a leading force in organizing and editing a series of European international symposia under the rubric of cultural gerontology. These symposia have been held in Germany (1999), Sweden (2001), Finland (2003), England (2005), Denmark (1997), and Spain (2008). Volumes produced from these symposia include *Cultural Gerontology* (Anderson, 2002) and *Valuing Older People* (Edmondson and von Kondratowitz, 2009). Among German language scholars, the Austrian literary critic Roberta Maierhofer (1999, 2000) led the way in stimulating a strong interest in Age Studies, literature and narrative, especially in Departments of American Studies. Central to this effort today are Hartung and Maierhofer (2009) and Rüdiger Kunow (2009a, 2009b), author of chapter 13 in this volume.

In conceptualizing this third volume, we editors changed the genre from "handbook" to "guide," and we shifted the focus from "the humanities" to "humanistic inquiry." Choosing the term *guide* over *handbook* acknowledges something implicit from the beginning. In the introduction to the first edition, Tom Cole noted the irony of producing a "handbook" in the humanities. He might have gone further and said that the term was misleading and inaccurate.

Handbooks imply a kind of manual that distills bits of information for easy reference and problem solving. The introduction to the first edition made the point that knowledge in the humanities *is* sometimes directly useful for solving problems (e.g., applied ethics, public policy history). But knowledge in the humanities is more often *indirectly* useful "because it deepens understanding and enhances the opportunities for human flourishing" (Cole, Van Tassel, and Kastenbaum, 1992, p. xii). Our humanities handbook, we told readers of the first edition, would be "less scientific and instrumental, more historical, more concerned with the limits and conditions of its own knowledge, and more focused on questions of representation, meaning, and value than traditional handbooks in gerontology" (p. xii).

For the second edition of the *Handbook of the Humanities and Aging* (Cole, Kastenbaum, and Ray, 2000), Stephen Katz wrote a chapter that critiqued the handbook itself as a genre (Katz, 2000, chap. 20). Using Foucault's genealogical method of locating the historical links between knowledge and power, Katz revealed professionalized gerontology's tendency to "discipline" old people and to conceal its own self-interest in striving for scientific status. Katz's critical analysis of the handbook heightened our own awareness and made us, as editors of the current volume, wary of using the term. Because we do *not* mean for our volume to be read as an authoritative distillation of a body of systematic knowledge, we have chosen the more suggestive term *guide*. We also chose the word *humanistic* over *humanities* because the majority of scholarship on aging is produced not within traditional humanities disciplines but from the social sciences, clinical medicine, nursing, and social work, using qualitative methods rooted in the classical tradition of the humanities.

What Are the Humanities, and What Is Humanistic Inquiry?

The humanities, as a group of disciplines, were once narrowly construed but have become more encompassing over the past 30 years. In his nostalgic but useful review of the formation of the humanities in American universities, legal scholar Anthony T. Kronman identifies three historical phases: the first, and longest, began with the formation of Harvard College in the early seventeenth century and lasted until the Civil War; the second began with the establishment of the first universities after the Civil War and extended through the 1950s; and the third, our current phase, began in the 1960s. In the first two phases, the humanities included exclusively those disciplines that focused on the "organized study of the mysteries of life"—literature, philosophy, rhetoric, religion, history, the classics (Greek and Latin), and the fine arts (Kronman, 2007, pp. 45–46). Scholars in the first period taught and reinforced fixed systems of knowledge through a canon of classic texts and interpretations. For these early humanists, working in what Kronman calls the "age of piety," scholarship was conducted as an expression of religious beliefs and moral truths.

In the second phase, what Kronman (2007) calls the "age of secular humanism," piety gave way to moral relativism, and scholarship came to be characterized by a philosophy that "accepts the pluralistic belief in a variety of paths to fulfillment; assumes the number to be modest but remains agnostic as to how many there are; and acknowledges that some ways of life are likely to be incompatible with others" (p. 79).

Since the 1960s, secular humanism has been critiqued and largely overturned by the philosophical positions of poststructuralism and postmodernism, sometimes called "post-humanism" because of the cultural turn from the study of "humankind" as a coherent and fixed category toward the study of diverse peoples whose experiences are largely mediated by language, culture, and technology. In the current historical period, as Kirli and Yukseker (2004) note in discussing the development of cultural studies as a field, interaction between the humanities and the social sciences has become central, with each adopting the topics and methods of the other: "On the one hand, the humanities have started to utilize critical social scientific categories such as domination, class, hegemony, and resistance to investigate culture. On the other hand, the social sciences have begun to appropriate the epistemological concerns and the methodologies of the humanities such as ethnography, textual analysis, semiotics, deconstruction, and discourse analysis" (p. 141).

As a result of these post-1960 intellectual movements, the "humanities" in American universities are now much more inclusive. In their 2004 article "Engaging the Humanities," Cathy Davidson, vice provost of interdisciplinary studies at Duke University, and David Goldberg, director of the Humanities Research Institution at the University of California–Irvine, define the humanities "broadly and flexibly to include traditional humanities departments; crosscutting work in such interdisciplinary areas as ethnic studies, gender studies and new configurations in area studies or global studies; all aspects of the arts as well as narrative or theoretical social sciences; policy studies; legal theory; and science, technology, and information studies" (Davidson and Goldberg, 2004, p. 43).

Davidson and Goldberg, along with editors Richard Lee and Immanuel Wallerstein in *Overcoming the Two Cultures: Science versus the Humanities in the Modern World-System* (2004), attribute the expansion of the humanities to recent theoretical challenges to knowledge structures and disciplinary formations, as well as increasingly global interests and concerns that require a focus on social problems, rather than academic disciplines or institutions as the starting point for research and theorizing. This problem focus, evident in emerging areas such as science studies, complexity studies, cultural studies, medical humanities, and environmental studies, requires a shift from strictly disciplinary questions to interdisciplinary questions that explore overlaps and interconnections. Sunaryo, writing for the Lee and Wallerstein collection about the move toward interdisciplinarity in science studies, explains that "the ecological movement that emerged in the early 1960s has shifted from purely ecological or scientific concerns to philosophical ones, as in deep ecology, social ecology, ecofeminist, and ecological feminist movements, all of which brought social science [and humanities] into the picture. They examined the responsibility of science in the environmental crisis and questioned human domination of nature as well as human domination over other human beings in the form of oppression on the basis of generation, class, gender, race, or indigeneity" (Lee and Wallerstein, 2004, pp. 186–87).

Such changes in the intellectual environment of modern universities prompt Davidson and Goldberg to suggest a new term, *interdisciplinary humanities*, to reflect "a more productive model for reaching beyond the walls, inner and outer, of the academy." They describe interdisciplinary humanities as "more open to reading beyond the confines of values forged locally, whether the locale is temporal, spatial, or disciplinary"; interested in "objects of analysis that are more diffuse, more multiplicitous, and more fully prompted than those disciplinarily conceived"; and focused on "concerns identified as abundant in social and cultural life and in various geopolitical sites" (Davidson and Goldberg, 2004, pp. 48–50).

The interdisciplinary humanities share many characteristics with the disciplinary humanities. Michael Berube (2006), former director of the Illinois Program for Research in the Humanities at the University of Illinois at Urbana-Champaign, argues that today's interdisciplinary humanists are still creative and interpretive and are interested in expressing and understanding emotions, along with ideas. They differ from scholars in the hard sciences in studying objects and ideas "whose features are entirely a matter of collective human interpretation—such as, say, social justice," as opposed to objects that, although understandable through human interpretation, are themselves "untouched and indifferent to human interpretation," such as photons (p. 11). Put more simply, the arts and humanities are still concerned with mysteries— those things that have no definitive explanation—while the hard sciences are concerned with certitudes—those things that can be tested and verified.

The social sciences can go either way; some social scientists conduct creative, critical, and interpretive scholarship in the humanistic vein, while others strive for objective analysis in the search for empirical truth. Traditional methods that yet serve interdisciplinary humanists include close, critical reading and a regard for "truth" in the analysis of cultural texts. Such truth, as described by longtime literary critic Robert Scholes (1998), entails fairness, accuracy, and comprehensiveness, all of which require "scrupulous accuracy in citation, regard for what is already known about our subject, and rigor in situating and interrogating whatever material we are considering" (p. 57). Humanistic "truths" are often established through critical readings. Scholes (1998) describes the reading skills of the critic as twofold: an ability to read from "inside" the text—being sympathetic to the author's intentions—while also reading from "outside" the text—being critical of those intentions. The two strategies, in combination, demonstrate the critic's sensitivity to language and nuances of meaning, along with his or her ability to separate the self from the text. This distancing is necessary for gaining deeper insights and understandings and for creating new knowledge. As Scholes (1998) notes, "if we impose our own values on every text, we have nothing to criticize but ourselves" (p. 169). This is just as true of reading legal documents and social policies as it is of reading novels and life stories.

The interdisciplinary humanities also share a particular kind of questioning, along with certain objects of analysis, with the traditional humanities. Humanistic questions have always been, and still are, complex and difficult to answer: Why? What does it mean? For whom is it meaningful? To what can we compare it? How is it changing? Why does it matter? Our objects of analysis are "conceptual, linguistic, artifactual and textual" (Davidson and Goldberg, 2004, p. 47), although in the interdisciplinary humanities, these objects are much more broadly construed, as Scholes (1998) illustrates in describing the changes in his own scholarly interests over the years, which have extended from literary texts alone to "all the lively forms of expression and representation, verbal and visual, from epics and landscapes to cartoons and bumper stickers" (p. x). For today's humanists, "text" includes not just the "weaving of words," but the "fabrication of culture itself, in which we . . . find ourselves already woven" (Scholes, 1998, p. 73). In the medical humanities, patients have been described as "texts" for medical students and physicians to "read" (Jones, 1994). In Scholes's description, he demonstrates another characteristic of humanistic scholars—a preference for rich detail and the metaphorical use of language to express complex ideas.

New skills and abilities, too, are now required of interdisciplinary humanists. These include proficiency in reading across several areas of study; comfort in working at the intersections of multiple disciplines; an ability to talk and write for disciplinary scholars in ways they value, while also writing for interdisciplinary scholars; intellectual diversity and flexibility; an ability to use multiple methodologies and to ask a wider range of research questions; and, given the interest in the social problems addressed by today's scholars, an ability to speak to and write for a general audience outside of academe (Gonzalez, Niemeier, and Navrotsky, 2003; Davis and Goldberg, 2004). The latter ability is reflected in Part III of this collection—Age Studies in the Public Sphere—where contributors Stephen Katz and Kevin McHugh, Rüdiger Kunow, and Margaret Gullette discuss the general issues of ageism, globalization, and mobility by drawing examples from everyday life in the public sphere. Margaret Gullette, one of gerontology's few public intellectuals, also demonstrates how a scholar works to change the minds of general readers about aging and ageism.

The Humanistic Study of Aging
Postmodernism and the Interpretative Social Sciences

As we have noted, humanistic study comprises not only interdisciplinary humanities but also the recently developed human sciences or interpretive social sciences. These forms of inquiry within sociology, anthropology, and psychology draw on methods and questions rooted in the traditional humanities disciplines and have been influential in the development of humanistic gerontology.* Humanistic gerontology was born during a period of sweeping social and intellectual upheaval—just as the wave of postmodernism reached American shores (Harvey, 1989). It is important to remember that the term *postmodern* refers not only to a range of cultural and intellectual perspectives but also to a temporal watershed marking a new historical era. Observers such as Anthony Giddens (1991) use the label "late modern" rather than "postmodern," but no serious observer of contemporary culture doubts that the world has passed into a qualitatively new period of historical time. Think of the forces at play—the computer and the

*The following section was written collaboratively with Michelle Sierpina and originally published in Wilmoth and Ferraro (2006, chap. 12). Reproduced with the permission of Springer Publishing Company, LLC, New York, NY 10036.

digital revolution, which created an explosion of information and the speedup of almost everything, including the production of new scientific knowledge; the saturation of the self with images generated by all kinds of electronic media spurred by consumer culture; globalization, identity confusion, intensified status anxiety, and the rapid growth of immigration to the United States and Europe from Asia, the Middle East, Latin America, and, to a lesser extent, Africa. These forces burst old moral, intellectual, religious, and cultural boundaries; they have placed us in a period of the most extensive, frightening, and creative confusion since the Renaissance.

Under these historical conditions, previously accepted disciplinary boundaries and unifying ideas gave way to boundary crossings and "blurred genres"—forms of knowledge that accept (rather than erase) the inevitable contradiction, paradox, irony, and uncertainty in any explanation of human activity (Geertz, 1980). In 1998, the sociobiologist Edward Wilson predicted that the natural sciences and the humanities would continue as the "two great branches of learning in the 21st century"; the social sciences, he thought, would divide—"with one part folding into or becoming continuous with biology, and the other fusing with the humanities" (Manheimer, 2000, p. 89). Time has proven this prediction true.

Gerontology seems to be following this pattern, with the majority of social scientists leaning toward biology. An important minority, however, are pursuing qualitative methods, often under the rubric of the human sciences (as opposed to the natural sciences) (Thomas, 1988). The recent resurgence of the human sciences (Rabinow and Sullivan, 1987; Polkinghorne, 1988; Marcus, 1994) is fundamentally based on reappropriation of classic humanistic forms of knowing—in particular, *interpretation, rhetoric,* and *narrative.*

Interpretive inquiry, as Steven Weiland (2000) points out, acknowledges the perspective of the researcher while attempting "to reveal the meanings of human experience from the perspective of individuals, groups, institutions, and organizations being studied" (p. 240). It marks a radical departure from the hypothesis-driven, quantitative methods of modern science. As Bernice Neugarten, one of the founders of contemporary gerontology, announced when she embraced "the interpretive turn," "There are no immutable laws; no reductionist models that are securely based in logical self evidence; no 'received' truths; and surely no value free social science. Change is fundamental; change is dialectical; meanings are multiple and inexhaustible. The aim is understanding, within the limits of our cultural and historical present" (quoted in Weiland, 2000, p. 241).

The human (or interpretive) sciences insist that no knowledge of human beings is complete unless it does justice to the thoughts, feelings, and expressions of the people being studied (Taylor, 1979). In gerontology, the sociologist Jaber Gubrium has criticized the positivist methodology of his colleagues for neglecting subjectivity—that is, the lived experience of aging as expressed in the words, speech, stories, and writings of older people (see, e.g., Gubrium, 1993a, 1993b; Gubrium and Holstein, 1997). Gubrium's work, for example, on the experiences of nursing home residents involves extensive collection and interpretation of their spoken narratives (Gubrium, 1993b).

Contemporary philosophy of interpretation (hermeneutics) has made clear that every act of interpretation is itself a historically situated event. Understanding a story, a poem, a painting, or an action does not take place outside time but within it. Even the "best" interpretation is circumscribed by the interpreter's historical, social, and personal situation. Among psychologists of aging, Harry Berman (1994) effectively adopts this perspective in his work on autobiographical narratives of older writers—in particular, journals of the poet May Sarton. Among anthropologists of aging, Barbara Myerhoff and Sharon Kaufman rely heavily on humanistic concepts of interpretation and narrative (Kaufman, 1986; Kaminsky, 1992; Kaminsky and Weiss, 2007).

Rediscovery of narrative as an essential form of seeking and representing knowledge has profoundly shaped gerontology's understanding of the search for meaning and identity. Narrative's influence is pervasive—from psychiatrist Robert Butler's (1963) original formulation of the life review, to the revaluation of reminiscence in clinical work with elderly people (Kaminsky, 1984; Sherman, 1991; Webster and Haight, 2002), to the narrative study of development (Cohler, 1982; Randall and McKim, 2008), to the articulation of narrative gerontology (Kenyon, Clark, and de Vries, 2001), to the explosion of life story writing among elders (Kenyon and Randall, 1997; Ray, 2000; Birren and Cochran, 2001), to name just a few important areas. Ruth Ray (2000) articulates a basic concept underlying the narrative turn in gerontology: "There is a complex interrelationship between language and life. Language and symbol are constitutive of human belief and behavior, not mere reflections of underlying beliefs and behaviors. The life story in some sense constructs reality; interpretive or narrative change in a story provides the foundation for actual shifts in attitudes and behavior" (p. 27). Ray (2007) also points out that narrative approaches are often specifically used by humanists and interpretive social scientists as a "corrective gesture, countering previous tendencies to over-emphasize scientific knowing and to ignore or deny subjective knowing" in the field of gerontology (p. 63).

Along with interpretation and narrative, rhetoric has also emerged as a tool of gerontological study. As a style of inquiry, rhetoric attempts to understand how human beings use language to develop and sustain their social practices. As Stephen Weiland (2000) puts it, "Rhetoric of Inquiry focuses on science, scholarship, and the professions as social institutions with distinctive habits of communication." It explores, to quote Clifford Geertz, how a disciplinary discourse "gets its effects and what those are." Stephen Katz's *Disciplining Old Age: The Formation of Gerontological Knowledge* (1996) is an especially effective example of a "rhetoric of inquiry" in gerontology. Influenced by Foucault's emphasis on the link between power and knowledge, Katz alerts readers to the fact that gerontological knowledge can be used to "discipline" or control older people and the meanings they make of age.

The Practical Humanities: Bioethics and "Clinical" Creativity

Humanistic gerontology has enticed some academic humanists to "commute," so to speak, between theory and practice—between the library/classroom and the hospital, the nursing home, the congregation, or the community. The opportunity to "practice" (Carson, Burns and Cole, 2003) the humanities—either directly with older people themselves or indirectly with health care professionals—has borne special fruit in the areas of bioethics, spirituality, and creativity. As in other gerontological arenas, formally trained academic humanists are few in number compared to formally trained social scientists and health professionals. Such work is done at interstices of various disciplines, with all the excitement, messiness, and uncertainty that accompany new ventures.

Bioethics emerged in the early 1970s as a field of study and practice in the health care professions. As noted above, historical progress in medicine generated its own set of problems: the very technology that allowed people to live longer also gave rise to ethical dilemmas in death and dying. When was it permissible to terminate treatment or withdraw nutritional support? Who was authorized to make such decisions, and on what grounds? Although these problems can arise among patients of all ages, they occurred disproportionately with elderly patients, because more than two-thirds of all deaths occur at age 65 or older (Klatz, 2001; Moody, 2001).

By the late 1980s, significant literature on bioethics and aging had appeared. Scholars and researchers identified ethical problems distinctive to care of elderly people. Diminished mental capacity, for example, due to Alzheimer's disease or other forms of dementia, raised thorny questions about informed consent, autonomy, and proxy decision making. Other prominent issues included vulnerability to elder abuse, ethical problems in long-term care, and the just allocation of scarce medical resources (Callahan, 1987; Spicker, Ingman, and Lawson, 1987; Thornton, 1987).

Bioethics is itself a strikingly interdisciplinary field, drawing on the disciplines of philosophy, religious studies, law, qualitative and quantitative social sciences, and the basic and clinical sciences of the health care professions. Considered as a subfield of bioethics, "aging and bioethics" "undertakes the study of what morality ought to be for healthcare professionals responsible for the care of elderly patients and clients, for family members who participate in the care of elders in decisions about that care, for health institutions (broadly understood) responsible for the care of elderly patients and clients, and for society or guiding healthcare services for the elderly and their families" (McCullough, 2000, p. 94). Aging poses special problems for American bioethics, which has come to place so much emphasis on the principle of autonomy—the view that competent individuals have the right to make their own decisions about health care. Increasing disability due to progressive chronic disease gradually reduces an elderly individual's capacity for self-determination. Geriatricians have noted that the phenomenon of "fluctuating competence" challenges the traditional assumption that one is either autonomous or not. Advance directives—the Living Will and Durable Power of Attorney for Health Care—have attempted to extend the autonomy of patients beyond the point where they become incapacitated. Studies have shown, however, that patients rarely make use of these legal mechanisms and, when they do so, physicians often ignore them (The SUPPORT Investigators, 1996).

As Harry R. Moody (1992) has noted, the principle of autonomy was developed for and well suited to acute care and hospital settings, where a decision about treatment leads to a course of action followed by discharge. In the long-term care setting, however, decisions rarely take the form of "either/or" but tend to revolve around smaller, although no less important, decisions of everyday life: where to spend time, how to decorate one's room, when to eat, freedom to move around versus considerations of safety. Hence, a great deal of nursing home reform is based on attention to the personal daily needs of residents, in contrast to the bureaucratic needs of the nursing home (Thomas, 1999).

Ethical issues in health care policy for elderly people have occupied considerable attention since the 1980s. People over 65 enjoy excellent health care entitlements in the United States, and the growing cost of this care has generated a heated debate under the rubric of "justice between generations." Prominent philosophers have argued for restraining the growth of life-extending interventions among the very old in order to allocate health care resources more equitably to the young. Others have argued that such policies would constitute age discrimination. More enlightened policy makers would consider different needs for different periods in the life course; just as society spends more money on education for children, it is only fair to spend more money on health care for elderly people. These issues are likely to be decided by political negotiation rather than moral deliberation. But the problem of funding long-term care of the baby-boom generation may well prove to be the most intractable health care policy issue of all (The President's Council on Bioethics, 2005).

In addition to bioethics' contributions to patient care and public policy, the study and expression of creativity is a rapidly growing area of humanities practice in gerontology, sometimes in community settings and sometimes in clinical situations studied with scientific methods. "Creativity," says George Vaillant (2002), "can turn an old person into a young person." He believes that "creativity produces awe" and "provides a means of containing wonder" (p. 235). Perhaps Vaillant's observation helps account for the continuing productivity of great artists from Michelangelo to Picasso. But recent work in creativity and aging suggests that great artists may be exceptional only in the caliber of the works they produced. One can make a strong case that all people of all ages are creative to a greater or lesser degree. What is unique today about the intersection of aging and creativity is what Ronald J. Manheimer called in 1995 an "amazingly rich cultural milieu" that fosters opportunity for self-expression: "in the United States and other countries, many seniors have joined a class of mature citizens with unprecedented leisure time for pursuing recreation, entertainment, travel, knowledge of the arts and humanities, fellowship, civic duty, and physical fitness" (Manheimer, Snodgrass, and Moskow-McKenzie, 1995, p. xv). Manheimer's late twentieth-century portrait, of course, does not apply to poor and working-class elders. And the picture has been modified somewhat by rising rates of poverty, higher rates of labor force participation, and later ages of retirement brought on by the global economic downturn that began in 2008.

At about the time humanistic gerontology was taking root, pioneers such as Susan Perlstein and Bonnie L. Vorenberg were birthing their own approach to gerontology services. "In 1979, I founded Elders Share the Arts (ESTA) which focuses on living-history arts," says Perlstein (2004), "a way of synthesizing oral history and the creative arts." She continues, "In contrast to the apathy I encountered a quarter century ago, the recent growth of the field of creative aging thrills me" (p. 2). Two decades after the formation of ESTA, Perlstein partnered with the American Society on Aging to develop the National Center for Creative Aging (NCCA), an organization dedicated to supporting creative aging by maintaining a database of resources such as an e-mail newsletter, professional training, replication of best practices, and information exchanges. ESTA also supports research, policy and advocacy.

With beginnings in 1978, *Arts for Elders,* Vorenberg's arts academy and senior theater touring company, has provided leadership for others around the country, according to colleagues at the University of Nevada, Las Vegas, and has received funding from the National Endowment for the Arts (Senior Theater, 2004). Vorenberg's *Senior Theater Connections* (1999) is a compendium of resources, performing groups, and more, demonstrating how widespread this creative outlet for elders has become.

Another leader in the field of creativity for elders is Anne Davis Basting, founding director of the Center on Age and Community at the University of Wisconsin, Milwaukee. In her book *Stages of Age* (1998) Basting notes with surprise a "lack of recognition of aging in cross disciplinary explorations of cultural difference and social practice . . . Theories of social practice, including ground-breaking work of scholars such as historian Michel de Certeau and philosopher Judith Butler, tended to overlook physical and psychological changes inherent in the aging process" (p. 2). Basting developed the TimeSlips method of storytelling for people with dementia, including professional theater productions and a nationwide training network that have expanded her research far beyond the examination of senior performance (Basting, 2001, 2002). In *Forget Memory: Creating Better Lives for People with Dementia* (2009), Basting critiques the stories we tell about dementia in popular culture and offers an alternate approach to memory loss.

No less creative are the countless writers nationwide who express themselves by writing and sharing their life stories. Pioneers in this field include James Birren and Kathryn Cochran (2001), James Pennebaker (1990), Ronald Manheimer (1999), Ruth Ray (2000, 2008), and many others. Cole (2001) and colleagues have brought this process to national attention through the PBS film *Life Stories*. The evidence continues to mount that writing about life experiences has positive therapeutic effect (Pennebaker and Seagal, 1999; Smyth et al., 1999; Spiegel, 1999). Cohler and Cole (1996) suggest that "there can be no lifestory apart from the particular collaboration between narrator and listener, or [between] reader and text, apart from the matrix of their shared telling and listening" (pp. 61, 67). Thorsheim and Roberts (2004), researchers at St. Olaf College, may be taking the theory even further as they examine health outcomes, such as the lowering of blood pressure among story listeners. Their work suggests, for example, that listening to "remember when" stories, when they are particularly meaningful, significantly lowers blood pressure and heart rate.

Exercising creativity can be a healthy practice throughout life, but it may be particularly so in old age. Research points to positive health outcomes for those who practice even basic activities that exercise the mind. Studies mount in support of this concept. Scientists in Chicago saw that cognitive activity across the life span had positive effects (Wilson, Barnes, and Bennett, 2003). Not only quality of life but also length of life is expanded for those who exercise creativity. Such activities have been found to enhance survival in all causes of mortality (Glass et al., 1999). Recently, physicians at Albert Einstein College of Medicine in New York discovered that even reading, playing board games, or doing word games forestalled dementias in subjects 75 and older (Verghese et al., 2003).

Geriatrician Cohen (2000), author of chapter 8 in this volume, believes that opportunities for creative growth are often underappreciated. We are encouraged by the signs that the situation is changing. Robert Kastenbaum (2000) suggests that creativity is an essential ingredient for a healthy and meaningful old age. As he writes, "Those whose concerns center on mental health and illness might find valuable clues by exploring antecedents and consequences of thwarted creativity. People who do not have the opportunity to develop and express their sparks of creativity are apt to become deeply frustrated. This is a more stressful situation than is commonly realized, contributing to impaired relationships and deteriorated health. Viewed in this light, creativity is a central rather than a peripheral element in living a meaningful life through a great many years" (pp. 398–99).

The Humanities Disciplines:
History, Literature, Philosophy, and Religious Studies

American historians were the first in the humanities to ply their trade in the field of aging. Before the 1970s, the history of aging was written by sociologists and anthropologists (Haber, 2000). Working from large-scale models of social change (modernization theory), social scientists told a story of declining prestige, power, and income. According to this "grand narrative," older people enjoyed power and prestige before the coming of urban industrial society. They presided over three-generational patriarchal households, and their experience, knowledge, and control over property guaranteed a high social status. In the nineteenth century, as more people moved into cities and began working in factories, older people were separated from their families, forced out of the labor market, and relegated to the "scrap heap" of industrial society.

Historical research done by David Hackett Fischer, W. Andrew Achenbaum, Carole Haber (1983), Brian Gratton, and Thomas Cole, among others, revealed that this decline narrative was defective in several ways. Historians of colonial New England, for example, found that three-generational households were the exception rather than the norm. Most aging couples lived in two-generational households and were still responsible for the care of their adolescent children. When one spouse died or became incapacitated, the other spouse often moved into the household of a grown child. Whatever power they possessed came from control over resources or legal arrangements made in advance. Unlike immigrants from southern and eastern Europe, immigrants from northwestern Europe brought with them an ideal of independent households, which they pursued whenever resources allowed.

American historians also critiqued the large-scale quantitative generalizations sought by social science theories of modernization. They explored diaries, letters, and publications of the old. They probed the values and individual differences of older people, rather than treating them as a unified category. Rather than seeing old people as passive recipients of large-scale social forces, historians wanted to know how older people felt, what part they played in shaping their own history, and what views they had on the nature of a "good old age."

As Pat Thane (2000) pointed out, it is difficult to generalize about the history of aging in the West. "Historians of old-age in Britain have written primarily about demography and the material conditions of older people: the numbers of old people, their geographical distribution, their living arrangements; . . . household structures and family relationships: . . . welfare arrangements, medical provisions, property transactions, work and retirement" (p. 3). French historians have given attention not only to demography and welfare, but also to the history of medicine and to representations of old age. Work on old age in Germany, Canada, Australia, and New Zealand is fragmentary and still developing. Differences between social groups and different time periods, places, and national cultures create a patchwork of snapshots that defy generalizations.

In Europe, as in the United States, the long-standing belief that the status of older people is always declining is simply not supportable. Ironically, the history of old age in the twentieth century becomes less diverse and more uniform across national, cultural, and social boundaries, as the institutionalized life course and the welfare state become primary social institutions. Historians and social scientists have produced essential work for understanding the rise of the welfare state and American exceptionalism (Achenbaum, 1983; Myles, 1984).

After historians, literary scholars were the next academic humanists to explore aging through their own disciplinary lenses. Throughout the late 1970s and the 1980s, Kathleen Woodward was the most prolific writer and editor of work on aging, literature, and culture (Woodward, 1978, 1991; Woodward and Schwartz, 1986). In the 1990s, Woodward broadened her interests from literature to cultural studies, reflected in an edited collection on how women are "aged" by a visual culture of youth (Woodward, 1999). The task of literary criticism was twofold: to demonstrate literature's contribution to understanding aging and to demonstrate the impact of aging on the life and work of creative writers. Scholars argued convincingly that aging is an essential but missing element of literary criticism. They found little interest, however, in English departments or at the Modern Language Association. In traditional humanities departments—as in the culture at large—aging and old age were simply not welcome topics, although a 1999 collection on aging and identity in literature and the arts (Deats and Lenker, 1999) and a 2006 special issue of the *National Women's Studies Association Journal*, edited by a young literary scholar (Leni Marshall) and devoted to the subjects of aging, ageism, and old age, suggest that interest may be increasing.

In her survey of literary gerontology, Anne Wyatt Brown (1992)—herself an important contributor to this field—divided the scholarship at that time into five categories: (1) analyses of literary attitudes toward aging; (2) humanistic approaches to literature and aging; (3) psychoanalytic explorations of literary works and their authors; (4) applications of gerontological theories about autobiography, life review, and midlife transitions; and (5) psychoanalytically informed studies of the creative process.

One fascinating discovery of the 1980s was that older people were appearing as heroes and heroines in contemporary novels and short stories. In 1972, Simone de Beauvoir had confidently declared that an old person could not be a good hero for a novel; older people were "finished, set, with no hope, no developments to be looked for . . . nothing that can happen . . . that's of any importance" (de Beauvoir, 1972). Fifteen years later, however, Margaret Gullette was analyzing a new genre she called "midlife progress novels" (Gullette, 1988). Shortly thereafter, Constance Rooke (1992) identified the genre of "vollendungsroman" (story of completion)—novels presenting the struggle for affirmation in old age, offering a new paradigm of hope in contemporary fiction. Since the late 1990s Roberta Maierhofer has been studying women's search for identity in American literature, finding unusual heroines along the way (Maierhofer, 1999, 2000, 2004a, 2004b; Maierhofer and Hartung, 2007).

Throughout the 1990s and beyond, literary perspectives on aging were influenced by the cultural studies movement, the growth of narrative studies, and the proliferation of guided autobiography and life story programs for elders (Ray, 2000; Birren and Cochran, 2001). Margaret Gullette emerged as the primary theorist and practitioner of what she called "age studies"—modeled after studies of race, class, and gender (Gullette, 2000, 2004). During the same time period, Anne Basting and others were developing the field of performance studies and aging, which included both the theory and practice of theatrical work with elders (Basting, 1998).

Professional philosophers have contributed little to our knowledge of aging—with the exception of bioethics. Physiological, clinical, and behavioral criteria of "successful aging" have overshadowed philosophical inquiry into the meanings and purposes of old age, the rights and obligations of older people, etc. In 1982, however, Patrick McKee (1982) edited the first contemporary collection of ancient and modern philosophers on aging. More recently, philosopher Ronald Manheimer (2000) divided the study of philosophy and aging into four basic topics: (1) philosophers' depictions of the possibilities and limitations of later life; (2) ethical questions of meaning and purpose in old age; (3) the study of wisdom; and (4) the current relationship of academic philosophy to the study of aging.

The history of philosophy yields no single path as the way to a good old age or the role of older citizens. Plato, Aristotle, Cicero, Montaigne, and Schopenhauer—and more recently de Beauvoir, Norton, Moody, and Manheimer—all present ideals of old age that acknowledge its harsh reality and seek forms of adaptation, transformation, resignation, or engagement (de Beauvoir, 1972; Norton, 1976; Moody, 1988; Manheimer, 1999, 2000). Margaret Urban Walker's (2000) volume, *Mother Time,* is the first contemporary philosophical volume of feminist thought on aging, focusing primarily on ethical issues. Feminists remind us that questions about the meaning of aging are inseparable from race, gender, and class, as well as from the cultural, historical, and personal circumstances in which they arise.

Many traditional philosophical issues (the nature of time, identity of the self, wisdom, memory, and mortality) have been taken up by scholars in the social sciences and humanities (Birren and Clayton, 1980; Kaufman, 1986; Labouvie-Vief, 1990;

Tornstram, 1997). Gerontologists adopting methods of critical theory, phenomenology, and hermeneutics are making seminal qualitative and quantitative contributions. Perhaps the central limiting factor in this work is that few philosophers have made an effort to become knowledgeable in gerontology, and likewise, few gerontologists are philosophically trained or well read. An important exception is the Dutch philosopher and gerontologist Jan Baars, who has written extensively on issues of time and aging, as well as on critical gerontology and globalization (Baars et al., 2005; Baars and Visser, 2007). Baars continues his work in the philosophy of aging in chapter 4 of this volume.

A new and important figure in philosophy and literature is Helen Long. Her landmark, erudite book, *The Long Life* (2007), uses longevity as a lens through which to view central questions in moral philosophy: What is the relation between a long life and a good life? How long does identity persist? Do the changes that accompany aging alter the capacity for virtue? Long is less interested in the philosophy of aging than in how aging helps us understand philosophical problems. Her work has yet to be read by gerontological humanists or connected to humanistic gerontology.

As in philosophy, academic scholars in religious studies have had much less to say about aging than professors of pastoral care, ministers, rabbis, chaplains, and social scientists. A key exception here is Stephen Sapp, a religious studies scholar who formerly edited the *Journal of Religious Gerontology* and has written chapter 5 in this volume on aging in world religions. The classic text for addressing spiritual potential, aging in faith communities, pastoral care with older people, theological perspectives, and religious ethics is Kimble and McFadden's *Handbook of Aging, Spirituality and Religion* (1995). A second volume appeared in 2003. There is also a large body of religious research conducted by gerontologists (Levin, 1997). Studies of religion and health attest to the strong association between religion, health, and longevity (Koenig, McCullough, and Larson, 2001). But these studies do not probe the inner world of older congregants or the content of theologies and liturgies. The absence of humanistic inquiry in studies of religion, aging, and health reflects a fundamental flaw in such purely quantitative research. Health is assumed to be an end in itself, rather than a means to an end. In a secular society where life is no longer viewed as a spiritual journey, health in itself becomes a religion. Hence, the key cultural and personal question is left unasked: what does it mean to live a good life, to live well in religious terms?

Among the few religious studies scholars attempting to address these questions, Mel Kimble, Sheldon Isenberg, and Gene Thursby have looked, respectively, at aging in Judaism, Eastern Religions, and Christianity in the second edition of the *Handbook of the Humanities and Aging* (Cole, Kastenbaum, and Ray, 2000). In the *Guide to Humanistic Studies in Aging*, religious studies perspectives have been reduced to one chapter by Stephen Sapp, because there has not been a substantial body of new work in religious studies and aging since 2000.

The Chapters of This Volume

In their introduction to *Aging and Identity: A Humanities Perspective*, literary scholars Sara Deats and Lagretta Lenker (1999) argue that the dialectical tension between the positive and negative aspects of aging lends itself especially well to humanistic study. They suggest that, because of its traditional focus on the multiplicity of experience, humanistic inquiry offers valuable techniques for realizing the "interdisciplinary interaction" needed to understand the "Janus-face of age" in all its complexity (p. 8). In Ron Manheimer's words (chap. 9 of this volume), humanistic thinkers do not simplify in order to quantify, but insist on examining the *complexities* of aging, teaching us to "appreciate the multidimensional richness of older lives," both individual and collective. We offer this book to provoke and inspire scholars from many disciplines to consider new topics, follow new directions, and practice new methods in their own research on aging. We see the authors assembled here as seasoned guides to a new era of humanistic thinking about aging and old age.

Academic guides possess special knowledge that qualifies them to lead others through unknown territory. They establish points of interest and demonstrate how to navigate unknown areas. Each of the first three parts of this book might be read as a study guide written collaboratively by experienced travelers over humanistic terrain. The book overall provides insights into various topics of aging, as well as various methods of inquiry.

All of the authors, true to the interdisciplinary impulse, work from the premise that individuals and cultures are interrelated and co-constructed. To understand old people, one must understand the historical time, place, and culture in which they age; to understand the complex social phenomena of aging and old age, one must look closely at individuals as they age. Many of the authors make clear that the aging process is relational, that is, deeply imbedded in specific relationships among people, as well as specific relationships between people and places. Several humanistic methods, including close reading and interpretation, philosophical speculation, evocative description, critical analysis, narrative analysis, interview, and case study, are used to explore the complex issues of aging.

The contributors to Part I raise conceptual and philosophical issues from the perspective of the traditional humanistic disciplines—history, philosophy, literature, and religious studies. Pat Thane relies on close readings of historical texts to argue that cultural representations of old age have always shaped and still shape "individual imaginings of the life course and hence individual and collective action." More specifically, as Thane shows in her survey of the history of aging and old age in diverse Western cultures, "what takes shape in the political and economic spheres—for example, the provision of retirement pensions and their generosity or not—also helps shape private experiences and perceptions." She organizes her chapter around questions that can be answered through established historical methods—Did people in the past grow old? What was meant by "old age" in different places and at different times in history? How did the old survive?—and she helps us see how the answers are relevant today. Literary gerontologists Anne Wyatt-Brown and Barbara Waxman conduct close readings of selected literary texts to illustrate the relationship between cultural representations of old age and the lived experiences of aging. Wyatt-Brown reviews recent fiction and memoirs and finds that literary narratives create a vivid picture of aging that any reader can relate to, emotionally as well as intellectually, and that contemporary literature can teach us about the "varieties of the aging experience in our time." While Wyatt-Brown teaches us how to read for multiple representations of aging and old age, Waxman teaches us how to read critically for ageism and sexism—in both the text and ourselves. She offers a primer in feminist reader-response criticism as applied to fiction about old age. Her argument for the value of such criticism rests on the strong connection she sees between text and life: "literary texts have the potential to change readers' minds by humanizing elders and offering new versions of old age." This is especially true when readers have an age-sensitive critic like Waxman to show them how to interpret the visionary aspects of these texts.

Taking a more philosophical approach, Jan Baars and Stephen Sapp raise important existential questions about meaning in old age. Baars looks to ancient philosophical texts to understand the meaning of aging through time. He argues that gerontologists need to problematize their concept of time and address the mistaken reasoning that chronological time *causes* aging, a belief that does nothing to explain the multiple differences among people of the same age. Through close readings of philosophical texts, combined with the classic philosophical methods of rational speculation and problem posing, Baars comes to an understanding of old age that takes into account human vulnerability and the preciousness of time. His inquiry leads him to a deeper, more nuanced definition of aging as "living through unique situations with unique persons." Stephen Sapp, from the perspective of religious studies, raises the question, what does it mean to be human? He relies on close readings of texts and comparisons among the five major world religions (Hinduism, Buddhism, Christianity, Islam, and Judaism) to find his answer: the acceptance of mortality. Indeed, from all religious perspectives, human fulfillment depends on making the most of our allotted time in the face of death. Each of these religions provides specific teachings about how to treat those who are old and in close proximity to death.

In Part II, contributors demonstrate the possibilities of interdisciplinary humanities as applied to age studies. Scholars trained in the humanities and the social sciences take up several difficult questions: What is the connection between art and religion, and why is this relevant as we age? How is creativity related to health in old age? What does it mean to be "old" in a time of high-tech medicalization? What is our moral obligation to care for the old? What existential questions arise in the process of retirement, and to what end? Why are friendships especially important in old age—in some cases more important than family relationships? The authors in this section all work on the assumption that difficult questions require multiple research methods, rigorous questioning of assumptions and values, and a respect for emotions and experiential knowing in the study of old age. For example, Brian de Vries, a social scientist, combines his past quantitative research with his more recent interviews and narrative analyses to explore the multiple and complex meanings of friendship in old age. He draws on data he has collected over the past 17 years to make an empirical and conceptual case that researchers have been limited by their focus on friendship in a family-dominant context. He concludes that gerontologists can gain a "deeper and finer understanding of the *experience* of friendship" by studying individuals and groups living outside of this context, such as gay and lesbian elders.

Like de Vries, Susan McFadden and Jane Ramsey, Gene Cohen, Ron Manheimer, Sharon Kaufman, and Martha Holstein demonstrate the value of interviews, observations, and specific cases in developing a deeper understanding of the *experience* of old age. McFadden and Ramsey rely on "snapshots" of "imaginative moments" to show how specific elders are exploring the meaning of life and death through art. They draw parallels between art and religion, noting that both become more important in later life because they "illuminate the polarities and paradoxes of life"—the Janus face of old age.

Psychiatrist Gene Cohen describes the current interdisciplinary surge of interest in creativity and aging, noting that the interests of scholars and artists in this area range "from poetry to psychology, music to molecular biology, literary writing to life review, fine art to folk art." Cohen provides an overview of his own multisite research project, *The Impact of Professionally Conducted Cultural Programs on Older Adults*. He points to the linked capacities for creative expression and psychological growth throughout the life cycle and emphasizes the finding that healthy aging is best achieved when health promotion and prevention are accompanied by opportunities for creative engagement. Ron Manheimer, a philosopher by training and founding director of a center for creative aging, uses interviews and observations to create "miniature portraits" of five people and their "philosophical encounters" in retirement. Manheimer finds that the study of retirement is well suited to philosophical investigation because, like adolescence and other periods of life transition, it raises questions about identity, self in relation to others, mortality, and the meaning of life. Sharon Kaufman, a medical anthropologist, also draws from interviews with older adults to create three extended case studies that illustrate how medical technology is changing the experience of old age, giving rise to new qualities of life and expectations for the end of life. These changes call for a new way of thinking, what she calls "reflexive longevity," which involves reconsidering the meaning of "natural aging" in a society that is insatiable for medical intervention.

Like Kaufman, Martha Holstein is concerned about the ethics of care in contemporary culture, whether care by others or care of the self. She also claims the importance of experiential knowledge and argues for an intersubjective, interdisciplinary, and methodologically diverse approach to decision making that "takes emotions seriously as sources of moral knowledge and moral value" and that "embeds ethics in the everyday social worlds in which we live and work."

The contributors to Part III, all cultural studies scholars, employ the methods of semiotics (the study of signs and symbols), cultural analysis, and ideological critique to identify large-scale social issues and to argue the need for more critical scholarship on aging.

Stephen Katz and Kevin McHugh combine analysis and critique with narrative description to make their claim that specific retirement communities are "symbolic landscapes" that represent larger cultural narratives and ideologies about aging and identity. They focus on language that reflects these ideologies, such as the use of "snowbird" as a metaphor for sociability and mobility in later life. In presenting excerpts from interviews with elders in retirement communities and recreation vehicles, Katz and McHugh invite us to reconsider the meaning of "home" in a culture of speed and constant circulation. They also sketch the parameters of an emerging area of study called "spatial gerontology," an interdisciplinary collaboration that entails ethnographic microsociology, environmental gerontology, and migrational-global analysis.

Rüdiger Kunow works within this emerging area of spatial gerontology by examining some of the ways in which the experience and meaning of old age have been reconfigured under the aegis of capital-driven globalization. He complicates definitions of "age" and "globalization," argues for the need to develop a global perspective on individual and population aging, and analyzes specific cases of population aging in terms of the cultural discourses surrounding them. He argues that critical scholars need to "interrogate the statistical findings of demographic research and to view the field [of age studies] less as producer of knowledge on aging and more as a site of struggles over the presence of old age in the polity." Further, he finds that most research on aging is conducted exclusively from within the nation-state, even though "the production of demographical knowledge on the global distribution of aging bodies invites international and cross-cultural comparisons."

In her chapter, Margaret Gullette, who first developed the term "age studies" and linked it with cultural studies (see Gullette, 1997), shows that both ageism and sexism are alive and well in the United States in the cultural discourses of midlife job loss, hormone replacement therapy, and the duty-to-die arguments that construct old age as a "burden" on the individual and society. In her characteristically provocative call to social action, Gullette concludes that "although aging can't be fought (despite the promises of 'antiaging' products), agism can be. Americans need a vital multigenerational antiagist movement, the antidote to the perpetual drip-drip of cultural poison."

We present the final chapter, written by our coeditor Robert Kastenbaum, in a category of its own. In Part IV, Kastenbaum reflects on the *experience* of facing questions of meaning and mortality. He writes a personal account of his own efforts to regain his health after heart surgery in the company of several other "travelers" on the "dreadmill" at the rehabilitation center. The chapter is a kind of spiritual ethnography, filled with characters who are struggling to hold on to life while also learning to let go. Kastenbaum's fellow travelers have no energy to spare and no reason to fool themselves or anyone else. They escape efforts to place them into preestablished categories (pilgrims, saints, sages) and are "pragmatists by the inch." Describing these travelers and their existential grit, Kastenbaum helps us imagine our own future travels to an "authentic destination."

Finally, we provide an additional feature to this collection, an annotated filmography on American and foreign feature-length films that address issues of aging and old age. Robert Yahnke follows the themes of intergeneration and regeneration in 22 selected films that emphasize the affirming and redemptive aspects of old age. From the Japanese classic *Ikiru* to Bergman's *Wild Strawberries* and Peter Masterson's *The Trip to Bountiful*, Yahnke gives readers a tour of films that open viewers to the existential marrow of aging and dying.

REFERENCES

Achenbaum, W. A. 1983. *Shades of Gray.* Boston: Little Brown.
———. 2007. From building to dwelling: A liminal figure gazes at GSA's Humanities and Arts Committee. *Journal of Aging, Humanities, and the Arts* 1:259–66.
Anderson, L., ed. 2002. *Cultural Gerontology.* Westport, CT: Auburn House.
Ansello, E. F. 2007. In the beginning: On the 30th anniversary of the Committee on Humanities and Arts, the Gerontological Society of America. *Journal of Aging, Humanities, and the Arts* 1:267–76.
Baars, J., D. Dannefer, C. Phillipson, and A. Walker, eds. 2005. *Aging, Globalization and Inequality: The new critical gerontology.* Amityville, NY: Baywood Publishing Co.
Baars, J., and H. Visser, eds. 2007. *Aging and Time: Multidisciplinary perspectives.* Amityville, NY: Baywood Publishing Co.
Basting, A. 1998. *The Stages of Age: Performing age in contemporary American culture.* Ann Arbor: University of Michigan Press.
———. 2001. It's 1924 and somewhere in Texas, two nuns are driving a backwards Volkswagen: Storytelling with people with dementia. In *Aging and the Meaning of Time*, ed. S. H. McFadden and R. C. Atchley. New York: Springer.

——. 2002. *TimeSlips© Educational Guide*. Milwaukee: University of Wisconsin Press.

——. 2009. *Forget Memory: Creating better lives for people with dementia*. Baltimore: Johns Hopkins University Press.

Berman, H. 1994. *Interpreting the Aging Self: Personal journals of later life*. New York: Springer.

Berube, M. 2006. *Rhetorical Occasions*. Chapel Hill, NC: University of North Carolina Press.

Biggs, S. 1997. Choosing not to be old. Masks, bodies and identity management in later life. *Ageing and Society* 18:553–70.

——. 1999. The blurring of the life course: Narrative, memory and the question of authenticity. *Journal of Aging and Identity* 4:209–21.

——. 2005. Beyond appearances: Perspectives on identity in later life and some implications for method. *Journal of Gerontology: Social and Behavioral Sciences* 60B (3):113–25.

Birren, J., and V. Clayton. 1980. The development of wisdom across the lifespan: A reexamination of an ancient topic. In *Lifespan Development and Behavior*, vol. 3, ed. P. Baltes and O. Brim, Jr., 103–35. New York: Academic Press.

Birren, J. E., and K. N. Cochran. 2001. *Telling the Stories of Life through Guided Autobiography Groups*. Baltimore: Johns Hopkins University Press.

Brown, A. W. 1992. Literary gerontology comes of age. In *Handbook of the Humanities and Aging*, ed. T. R. Cole, D. D. Van Tassel, and R. Kastenbaum, 331–51. New York: Springer.

Butler, R. 1963. The life review: An interpretation of reminiscence in the aged. *Psychiatry* 26: 65–76.

Bytheway, W. 1994. *Ageism*. Buckingham: Open University Press.

Callahan, D. 1987. *Setting Limits: Medical goals in an aging society*. New York: Simon & Schuster.

Carson, R., C. R. Burns, and T. R. Cole, eds. 2003. *Practicing the Humanities: Engaging physicians and patients*. Hagerstown, MD: University Publishing Group.

Cohen, G. 2000. *The Creative Age*. New York: Avon Books.

Cohler, B. 1982. Personal narrative and life-course. In *Lifespan Development and Behavior*, vol. 4, ed. P. Baltes and O. Brim, Jr., 205–41. New York: Academic Press.

Cohler, B., and T. Cole. 1996. Studying older lives: Reciprocal acts of telling and listening. In *Aging and Biography: Explorations in adult development*, ed. J. Birren, G. Kenyon, J. Ruth, J. Schroots, and T. Svensson. New York: Springer.

Cole, T., producer 2001. *Life Stories*. [PBS Video]. Available from New River Media, 1219 Connecticut Ave. NW, Suite 200, Washington, DC 20036.

Cole, T. R., R. Kastenbaum, and R. Ray, eds. 2000. *Handbook of the Humanities and Aging*. 2nd ed. New York: Springer.

Cole, T. R., D. D. Van Tassel, and R. Kastenbaum, eds. 1992. *Handbook of the Humanities and Aging*. New York: Springer.

Conrad, C., and H.-J. von Kondratowitz. 1993. *Zur Kulturgeschichte des Alterns [Toward a Cultural History of Aging]*. Berlin: Deutsches Zentrum für Altersfragen.

Davidson, C. N., and D. T. Goldberg. 2004. Engaging the humanities. *Profession* 21:42–62.

Deats, S. M., and L. T. Lenker. 1999. *Aging and Identity: A humanities perspective*. Westport, CT: Praeger.

de Beauvoir, S. 1972. *The Coming-of-Age*. New York: W. W. Norton & Co.

Edmondson, R., and H.-J. von Kondratowitz. 2009. *Valuing Older People: A humanistic approach to ageing*. Bristol, UK: Policy Press.

Estes, C. L., S. Biggs, and C. Phillipson, eds. 2003. *Social Theory, Social Policy and Ageing: A critical introduction*. Buckingham: Open University Press.

Featherstone, M., and M. Hepworth. 1989. Ageing and old age: Reflections on the post-modern life course. In *Becoming and Being Old: Sociological approaches to later life*, ed. W. Bytheway. London: Sage.

———. 1995. Images of positive ageing. In *Ageing in Society*, ed. J. Bond and P. Coleman. London: Sage.

Featherstone, M., M. Hepworth, and B. Turner. 1991. *The Body: Social processes and cultural theory*. London: Sage.

Featherstone, M., and A. Wernick. 1995. *Images of Aging: Cultural representations of later life*. London: Routledge.

Fox, D. M. 1985. Who we are: The political origins of the medical humanities. *Theoretical Medicine* 6:327–41.

Geertz, C. 1980. Blurred genres: The refiguration of social thought. *American Scholar* 49: 165–79.

Giddens, A. 1991. *Modernity and Self-Identity*. Stanford: Stanford University Press.

Gilleard, C., and P. Higgs. 2000. *Cultures of Aging: Self, citizen and the body*. London: Prentice-Hall.

Glass, T. A., C. M. de Leon, R. A. Marotolli, and L. F. Berkman. 1999. Population based study of social and productive activities as predictors of survival among elderly Americans. *British Medical Journal* 319:478–83.

Gonzalez, C., D. A. Niemeier, and A. Navrotsky. 2003. The new generation of American scholars. *Academe*, July–August, 56–60.

Grmek, M. D. 1958. On ageing and old age: Basic problems and historic aspects of gerontology and geriatrics. *Monographia Biologicae* 5:57–162.

Gruman, G. J. 1966. A history of ideas about the prolongation of life. *Transactions of the American Philosophical Society* 56:3–102.

Gubrium, J. 1993a. *Gerontology and the Construction of Old Age: A study in discourse analysis*. New York: Aldine De Gruyter.

———. 1993b. *Speaking of Life: Horizons of meaning for nursing home residents*. Hawthorne, NY: Aldine De Gruyter.

Gubrium, J., and J. Holstein. 1997. *The New Language of Qualitative Methods*. New York: Oxford University Press.

Gullette, M. M. 1988. *Safe at Last in the Middle Years: The invention of the midlife progress novel*. Berkeley: University of California Press.

———. 1997. *Declining to Decline: Cultural combat and the politics of midlife*. London: University Press of Virginia.

———. 2000. Age studies as cultural studies. In *Handbook of the Humanities and Aging*, 2nd ed., ed. T. Cole, R. Kastenbaum, and R. Ray, 214–34. New York: Springer.

———. 2004. *Aged by Culture*. Chicago: University of Chicago Press.

Haber, C. 1983. *Beyond Sixty-five*. New York: Cambridge University Press.

———. 2000. Historians' approach to aging in America. In *Handbook of the Humanities and Aging*, 2nd ed., ed. T. Cole, R. Kastenbaum, and R. Ray, 25–40. New York: Springer.

Hartung, H., and R. Maierhofer, eds. 2009. *Narratives of Life: Mediating age*. Berlin: LIT Verlag (distributed by Transaction Publishers, Piscataway, NJ).

Harvey, D. 1989. *The Condition of Postmodernity.* Cambridge, MA: Blackwell.

Hepworth, M. 2000. *Images of Ageing.* Buckingham: Open University Press.

Jones, A. 1994. Reading patients—cautions and concerns. *Literature and Medicine* 13 (2):190–200.

Kaminsky, M., ed. 1984. *The Uses of Reminiscence.* New York: Haworth.

———, ed. 1992. *Remembered Lives: The work of ritual, storytelling, and growing older.* Ann Arbor: University of Michigan Press.

Kaminsky, M., and M. Weiss, eds. 2007. *Stories as Equipment for Living: Last talks and tales of Barbara Myerhoff.* Ann Arbor: University of Michigan Press.

Kastenbaum, R. 2000. Creativity and the arts. In *Handbook of the Humanities and Aging,* 2nd ed., ed. T. Cole, R. Kastenbaum, and R. Ray, 381–401. New York: Springer.

Katz, S. 1996. *Disciplining Old Age: The formation of gerontological knowledge.* Charlottesville: University Press of Virginia.

———. 2000. Reflections on the gerontological handbook. In *Handbook of the Humanities and Aging,* 2nd ed., ed. T. Cole, R. Kastenbaum, and R. Ray, 405–31. New York: Springer.

Kaufman, S. 1986. *The Ageless Self: Sources of meaning in late life.* Madison: University of Wisconsin Press.

Kenyon, G. M., P. G. Clark, and B. de Vries. 2001. *Narrative Gerontology: Theory, research, and practice.* New York: Springer.

Kenyon, G. M., and W. Randall. 1997. *Restorying Our Lives: Personal growth through autobiographical reflections.* Westport, CT: Praeger.

Kimble, M., and S. McFadden, eds. 1995. *Aging, Spirituality, and Religion: A handbook.* Minneapolis: Fortress Press.

Kirli, B. K., and D. Yukseker. 2004. The cultural turn in the social sciences and humanities. In *Overcoming the Two Cultures: Science versus the humanities in the modern world-system,* ed. R. E. Lee and I. Wallerstein, 128–43. Boulder, CO: Paradigm.

Klatz, R. 2001. Anti-aging medicine: Resounding, independent support for expansion of an innovative medical specialty. *Generations* 21:59–62.

Koenig, H., M. McCullough, and D. Larson, eds. 2001. *Handbook of Religion and Health.* New York: Oxford University Press.

Kronman, A. T. 2007. *Education's End: Why our colleges and universities have given up on the meaning of life.* New Haven, CT: Yale University Press.

Kunow, R. 2009a. *The Coming of Age—to American Studies.* Unpublished paper delivered at the "Workshop on Age Studies," University of Potsdam, July 16, 2009.

Kunow, R. 2009b. Narrative as intercultural drama: Life-writing by aged migrants. In *Narratives of Life: Mediating age,* ed. H. Hartung and R. Maierhofer. Berlin: LIT Verlag (distributed by Transaction Publishers, Piscataway, NJ).

Labouvie-Vief, G. 1990. Adaptive dimensions of adult cognition. In *Transitions of Aging,* ed. N. Datan and N. Logman, 3–26. New York: Academic Press.

Lee, R. E., and I. Wallerstein. 2004. *Overcoming the Two Cultures: Science versus the humanities in the modern world-system.* Boulder, CO: Paradigm.

Levin, J. 1997. Religious research in gerontology, 1980–1994: A systematic review. *Journal of Religious Gerontology* 10 (3):3–31.

Long, H. 2007. *The Long Life.* Oxford: Oxford University Press.

Maierhofer, R. 1999. Desperately seeking the self: Gender, age, and identity in Tillie Olsen's *Tell Me a Riddle. Educational Gerontology* 25 (2):129–41.

———. 2000. Simone de Beauvoir and the graying of American feminism. *Journal of Ageing and Identity* 5 (2):1087–2032.

———. 2004a. The old woman as the prototypical American—An anocritical approach to gender, age and identity. In *What Is American? New identities in US culture*, S. 319–36. Hg. Walter Hölbling, Klaus Rieser. Wien: LIT-Verlag.

———. 2004b. Third pregnancy: Women, ageing and identity in American culture. In *Old Age and Ageing in British and American Literature and Culture*, S. 155–71. Studien zur englischen Literatur. 16. Münster: LIT-Verlag.

Maierhofer, R., and H. Hartung, eds. 2007. Narratives of life: Aging and identity. *Journal of Aging, Humanities, and the Arts* (Special Issue) 1:3–4.

Manheimer, R. J. 1999. *A Map to the End of Time: Wayfarings with friends and philosophers.* New York: Norton Press.

———. 2000. Aging in the mirror of philosophy. In *Handbook of the Humanities and Aging*, 2nd ed., ed. T. R. Cole, R. Kastenbaum, and R. Ray, 77–92. New York: Springer.

Manheimer, R. J., D. D. Snodgrass, and D. Moskow-McKenzie. 1995. *Older Adult Education: A guide to research, programs, policies.* Westport, CT: Greenwood Press.

Marcus, G. 1994. On ideologies of reflexivity in contemporary efforts to remake the human sciences. *Poetics Today* 15:383–404.

McCullough, L. B. 2000. Bioethics and aging. In *Handbook of the Humanities and Aging*, 2nd ed., ed. T. R. Cole, R. Kastenbaum, and R. Ray, 93–113. New York: Springer.

McKee, P., ed. 1982. *Philosophical Foundations of Gerontology.* New York: Human Sciences Press.

Moody, H. R. 1988. A*bundance of Life: Human development policies for an aging society.* New York: Columbia University Press.

———. 1992. *Ethics in an Aging Society.* Baltimore: Johns Hopkins University Press.

———. 2001. Who's afraid of life extension? *Generations* 25:33–37.

Moss, W. 1976. *Humanistic Perspectives on Aging: An annotated bibliography and essay.* Ann Arbor: Institute of Gerontology, University of Michigan and Wayne State University.

Myles, J. 1984. *Old Age in the Welfare State.* Boston: Little Brown.

Norton, D. L. 1976. *Personal Destinies: A philosophy of ethical individualism.* Princeton: Princeton University Press.

Pennebaker, J. 1990. *Opening Up: The healing power of expressing emotions.* New York: Guilford Press.

Pennebaker, J., and J. Seagal. 1999. Forming a story: The health benefits of narrative. *Journal of Clinical Psychology* 55:1243–54.

Perlstein, S. 2004. Elder arts programs are thriving from California to the N.Y. Island. *Aging Today* 25:2. Retrieved July 8, 2004, from www.asaging.org/at/at-304/toc.cfm.

Polisar, D., L. Wygant, T. Cole, and C. Perdomo. 1988. *Where Do We Come From? What Are We? Where Are We Going? An annotated bibliography of aging and the humanities.* Washington, D.C.: Gerontological Society of America.

Polkinghorne, D. 1988. *Narrative Knowing and the Human Sciences.* Albany, NY: SUNY Press.

The President's Council on Bioethics. 2005. *Taking Care: Ethical caregiving in our aging society.* Washington, D.C.: Government Printing Office.

Rabinow, P., and W. Sullivan, eds. 1987. *Interpretive Social Science: A second look.* Berkeley: University of California Press.

Randall, W., and E. McKim. 2008. *Reading Our Lives: The poetics of growing old.* New York: Oxford University Press.

Ray, R. 2000. *Beyond Nostalgia: Aging and life story writing.* Charlottesville: University of Virginia Press.

——. 2007. Narratives as agents of social change: A new direction for narrative gerontologists. In *Critical Perspectives on Ageing Societies,* ed. M. Bernard and T. Scharf, 59–72. Bristol, UK: Policy Press.

——. 2008. *Endnotes: An intimate look at the end of life.* New York: Columbia University Press.

Rooke, C. 1992. Old age in contemporary fiction: A new paradigm of hope. In *Handbook of the Humanities and Aging,* ed. T. Cole, D. D. Van Tassel, and R. Kastenbaum, 241–57. New York: Springer.

Scholes, R. 1998. *The Rise and Fall of English.* New Haven, CT: Yale University Press.

Senior Theater. 2004. Retrieved July 9, 2004, from http://seniortheater.com.

Sherman, E. 1991. *Reminiscence and Self in Old Age.* New York: Springer.

Smyth, J. M., A. A. Stone, A. Hurewitz, and A. Kaell. 1999. Effects of writing about stressful experiences on symptom reduction in patients with asthma or rheumatoid arthritis. *Journal of the American Medical Association* 281:1304–9.

Spicker, S. F., S. R. Ingman, and I. Lawson, eds. 1987. *Ethical Dimensions of Geriatric Care.* Norwell, MA: Reidel.

Spicker, S., K. Woodward, and D. Van Tassel. 1978. *Aging and the Elderly: Humanistic perspectives in gerontology.* New York: Academic Press.

Spiegel, D. 1999. Healing words: Emotional expression and disease outcome. *Journal of the American Medical Association* 281:1328–29.

The SUPPORT Investigators. 1996. A controlled trial to improve care for the seriously ill hospitalized patients. *Journal of the American Medical Association* 274:1591–98.

Taylor, C. 1979. Interpretation and the sciences of man. In *Interpretive Social Science,* ed. R. Rabinow and W. Sullivan, 27–51. Berkeley: University of California Press.

Thane, P. 2000. The history of aging in the West. In *Handbook of the Humanities and Aging,* 2nd ed., ed. T. R. Cole, R. Kastenbaum, and R. Ray, 3–24. New York: Springer.

Thomas, L. E., ed. 1988. *Research on Adulthood and Aging: The human sciences approach.* Albany, NY: SUNY Press.

Thomas, W. H. 1999. *The Eden Alternative Handbook: The art of building human habitats.* Sherburne, NY: Summer Hill.

Thornton, J., ed. 1987. *Ethics and Aging.* Vancouver: University of British Columbia Press.

Thorsheim, H., and B. Roberts. 2004. *Reminiscing, Social Support, and Well Being.* Retrieved May 16, 2004, from www.stolaf.edu/people/thorshm/reminiscing-well-being.htm.

Tornstram, L. 1997. Gerotranscendence: A theory about maturing into old age. *Journal of Aging and Identity* 2:37–50.

Vaillant, G. 2002. *Aging Well: Surprising guideposts to a happier life from the landmark Harvard Study of Adult Development.* Boston: Little, Brown.

Van Tassel, D. D., ed. 1979. *Aging, Death, and the Completion of Being.* Philadelphia: University of Pennsylvania Press.

Verghese, J., et al. 2003. Leisure activities and the risk of dementia in the elderly. *New England Journal of Medicine* 25:2508–16.

von Kondratowitz, H.-J. 1991. The medicalization of old age: Continuity and change in Germany from the 18th to the early 19th century. In *Life, Death and the Elderly: Historical perspectives on Ageing*, ed. M. Pelling and R. M. Smith. London: Routledge.

Vorenberg, B. 1999. *Senior Theater Connections: The first directory of senior theater performing groups, professionals, and resources*. Portland, OR: ArtAge Publications.

Walker, M. U., ed. 2000. *Mother Time*. Lanham, MD: Rowman & Littlefield.

Webster, J., and B. Haight, eds. 2002. *Critical Advances in Reminiscence Work: From theory to application*. New York: Springer.

Weiland, S. 2000. Social sciences towards the humanities. In *Handbook of the Humanities and Aging*, 2nd ed., ed. T. Cole, R. Kastenbaum, and R. Ray, 235–57. New York: Springer.

Wilmoth, J., and K. Ferraro, eds. 2006. *Gerontology: Perspectives and issues*. 3rd ed. New York: Springer.

Wilson, R., L. Barnes, and D. Bennett. 2003. Assessment of lifetime participation in cognitively stimulating activities. *Journal of Clinical Experimental Neuropsychology* 25:634–42.

Woodward, K. 1978. *At Last, the Real Distinguished Thing: The late poems of Eliot, Pound, Stevens, and Williams*. Columbus: Ohio State University Press.

———. 1991. *Aging and Its Discontents: Freud and other fictions*. Bloomington: Indiana University Press.

———, ed. 1999. *Figuring Age: Women, bodies, generations*. Bloomington: Indiana University Press.

Woodward, K., and M. M. Schwartz, eds. 1986. *Memory and Desire: Aging literature psychoanalysis*. Bloomington: Indiana University Press.

DISCIPLINARY PERSPECTIVES

CHAPTER ONE

The History of Aging and Old Age in "Western" Cultures

PAT THANE, PH.D.

Old age has a history, despite the surprisingly resilient belief that in "the past" it was rare to grow old. Our understanding of this history is still incomplete, although it has been gradually growing in recent years. It is a complex history, as befits the stage of life that encompasses greater variety than any other. In any time period, especially the present, it has been represented as including people aged from their fifties to past 100; some of the richest and most powerful and the poorest and most excluded; those fit enough to run marathons in their eighties, as increasing numbers do all over the world, and the most frail.

Levels of knowledge and understanding of the histories of aging and old age are similarly diverse across different cultures and time periods. Among the European and predominantly English-speaking cultures, they have been relatively fully explored for Great Britain and the United States, mainly in relation to the numbers of older people, their geographical distribution, living arrangements, household structures and family relationships, welfare arrangements, medical provision, property transactions, work and retirement, social status, gender differences, and representations of older people (Haber, 1983; Thane, 2000; Botelho, 2004; Ottoway, 2004). France also has provided rich studies of the demography and medical provision for older people, with important work also on representations of old age and how the idea of old age was constructed in the past (Troyansky, 1989; Bourdelais, 1993, 1998). There are increasing but sparser studies of aspects of the history of aging in Germany (Borscheid, 1987; Kondratowitz, 1991; Conrad, 1994), Russia (Lovell, 2003), Spain, the Netherlands (Bulder, 1993), Canada (Montigny, 1997), Australia, and New Zealand. For many of these societies, however, distinctions between "Western" and "Eastern" cultures, which were always too crude, became less appropriate over the second half of the twentieth century, as increased international migration—of Turks to Germany, north Africans to France, south Asians to Britain and the Netherlands, Afro-Caribbean and African people to Britain, east Asians to Australia, people from everywhere to the United States, and much more in an increasingly disturbed and mobile world—made high-income countries more and more multicultural.

Important absences remain in our historical understanding that make it difficult to discuss similarities and differences across these diverse "Western" cultures or to compare them with other cultures. For example, awareness of gender is hardly a novelty in humanities scholarship, but it was slow to enter studies of old age. This was perhaps because historians shared the (mistaken) view of Georges Minois that, until relatively recently, the history of old age has been largely a history of men, because many women failed to survive the rigors of childbirth (Minois, 1989); or that of the medievalist, Joel Rosenthal, that "matriarchy and the culture of old women, whether on their own or in extended family households, is mostly a lost topic, worth investigation, but hard to treat other than anecdotally" (Rosenthal, 1996). Historians of women have shown both to be wrong, through the imaginative use of a wide range of sources (Stavenuiter, Jansens, and Bjisterfeld, 1995; Botelho and Thane, 1999; Ottoway, Botelho, and Kittredge, 2002; Ottoway, 2004).

If we are fully to understand the histories of aging and old age, we need to draw together many diverse forms of historical knowledge, of demographic and material experiences with cultural histories of the representation and self-representation of older people in different times and places, because these approaches to history can never be wholly separate from one another. Image is not distinct from experience, nor cultural history divorced from economic, social, and political history. Cultural representations of old age, whether drawn from philosophical or medical texts, literature, paintings, film, recorded expressions of everyday opinion, or any other source, shape individual imaginings of the life course and hence individual and collective action. If people are culturally conditioned to expect to be dependent and helpless past a certain age, they are more likely to become so, with consequences for their own lives and those of others, including those who care for them. What takes place in the political and economic spheres—for example, the provision of retirement pensions and their generosity, or not—also helps shape private experiences and perceptions.

If we are still far from achieving the "total" history of old age in "the West," how far are we along the way? Let us begin with the basic demographic picture.

Did People in "the Past" Grow Old?

People in "the past" did grow old, and in larger numbers than is often thought. However, the numbers surviving to what was defined in their times as "old age" varied from time to time, from country to country, and from place to place within nation-states. Even in ancient Rome it is calculated that about 6–8 percent of the population was aged over 60 (Parkin, 2003). Such estimates are insecure because they are based on scattered inscriptions on gravestones and rare documents, mainly referring to elite males. We know nothing about the life expectancy of slaves, although there are surviving images and literary accounts of aged slaves. In medieval Europe it is estimated that older people constituted not more than 8 percent of the population, and in some regions and periods it was "not above 5" (Shahar, 2005).

There are particularly detailed long-run studies of English population figures. Life expectancy at birth in England averaged around 35 years between the 1540s and 1800 (Wrigley and Schofield, 1981) and is unlikely to have been higher at any earlier time. But the high infant mortality rates at all times before the twentieth century, as in all countries, drastically pulled down such averages. Those who survived the hazardous first years of life had, even in the sixteenth century, a respectable chance of living at least into what would now be defined as middle age, and often longer, at least beyond 60 (Wrigley et al., 1997). It is estimated that the proportion of the English population aged over 60 fluctuated between 6 and 8 percent through the seventeenth century. In the late eighteenth century it was about 10 percent in France, Spain, and England.

But even within one country, the numbers varied from place to place. In the rapidly growing English city of Manchester, full of young migrants at the end of the eighteenth century during industrialization, only 3.4 percent of the population was over 60, 1.9 percent over 70. In depressed rural Sussex at the same time, which young people were fleeing in search of work in the towns, 19 percent were over 60, 7 percent over 70. Nationally the percentage fell to 6 in the nineteenth century, when high birthrates raised the percentage of the very young. Then from the late nineteenth century to the late twentieth, as birthrates and death rates in childhood, youth, and middle age fell, came the long climb in the proportion of the British population living past 60: 6 percent in 1911, 14 percent in 1951, and 18 percent in 1991. Most developed countries experienced this growth through the twentieth century.

France, by contrast, experienced falling rather than rising birthrates in the nineteenth century, which influenced the overall age structure. In the mid-eighteenth century 7 to 8 percent of the population was aged 60 or above. By 1860 the proportion was 10 percent; by the early twentieth century, 12 percent; by 1946, 14 percent (Bourdelais, 1998).

In Britain, there is clear evidence that women were a majority of those aged 60 or older from the time that vital statistics began to be officially and comprehensively recorded, in 1837. Women tended to live longer than men, on average, so far as we can tell, throughout Western history, although not always or everywhere. Childbirth, sadly, killed many women in the past, but it was never a mass killer in Western cultures (Schofield, 1986), and prime-age men often had higher death rates due to war, hazards at work, everyday violence, accidents, and disease. Medieval commentators noted that women seemed to live longer than men and wondered how that could be when it seemed natural that men were stronger and should live longer (Shahar, 1997). Physicians in eighteenth-century France were still puzzled by the consistency with which females "went against nature" and outlived men. In France in the mid-nineteenth century there were more old men than old women, but by the time of World War I women had gained the advantage in life expectancy, which they have never since relinquished (Bourdelais, 1998).

If there were divergent demographic experiences within the Old World of Europe, the New World of white-dominated colonies far from Europe was different again. Migrant countries disproportionately attracted males. In Australia and New Zealand by the later nineteenth century, most older white people were male. In Ontario, Canada, the balance among the incomers shifted from a majority of older men in 1851 to a female majority in 1901 (Montigny, 1997). In the United States the picture varied from place to place, according to length of settlement. Women in the United States are estimated, on average, to have had a lower life expectancy than men from the mid-seventeenth century to the 1890s (Haber and Gratton, 1994). The proportion of the U.S. white population aged 60 or older rose from 4 percent in 1830 to 6.4 percent in 1900 to 12.2 percent in 1950. The survival rates of black Americans were somewhat lower (Achenbaum, 1976); those of Native Americans (as of Australian aboriginals) may have been considerably so, but we do not know. Another important absence in historical work concerns such excluded and persecuted indigenous populations of lands settled by white migrants from Europe, whose births, deaths, and marriages were not deemed worthy of official registration until the recent past, making statistical calculation of age structure impossible.

The population of Ontario aged as the colony made the transition from migration to long-established settlement. Three percent of the population was aged over 60 in 1851, 4.6 percent in 1871, and 8.4 percent in 1901 (Montigny, 1997). Different Western societies "aged" at different paces and with different gender balances. It took France 140 years to double its percentage of the population of people over 60 from 9 percent to 18 percent (from 1836 to 1976); Sweden, 86 years (1876–1962); the United Kingdom, 45 years (1920–65); and the proportion over 60 had not reached 18 percent in the United States by the end of the twentieth century. Such varying paces of demographic change had probable cultural effects, but they have barely been explored.

The growing proportions of older people in Western societies over the twentieth century have, periodically, caused panics among politicians and intellectuals. This panic first became acute in Europe in the 1920s and 1930s because births were falling and life expectancy rising while outward migration of younger people to the New World continued (Thane, 1990; Bourdelais, 1993, 1998), although there were similar concerns in the United States (De Medeiros, 2008). It led right-wing authoritarian regimes to seek to bribe their people to have more children. Both the Hitler and

Mussolini regimes sought to increase birthrates by rewarding mothers of numerous children and taxing the childless. The USSR took a different route. Productive older people were praised, rewarded, and encouraged to stay at work. Stalin encouraged scientists to investigate methods of prolonging life (Lovell, 2003). There were fears of another world war and a perceived cultural threat to the dwindling populations of the West from the growth of nonwhite populations elsewhere (Thane, 1990).

The outcome in liberal France, Great Britain, and the United States, unlike the fascist and communist regimes, was doom-laden predictions from demographers and social scientists about the social conservatism and economic and military decline that would result from the advance of the "army of the aged." In France, such fears reinforced negative views of old age and stimulated efforts to increase the birthrate by improving child care and family allowances (Bourdelais, 1998). In Britain the initial negative assessment of an "aging society" led to research that demonstrated the under-estimated capabilities of many older people to work and to contribute to their families and communities, as well as to government-led attempts to improve their social conditions and diminish prejudice against them in the workplace and in society, although with limited success (Thane, 1990). There were similar developments in the United States (De Medeiros, 2008).

The panic about aging in the mid-twentieth century, which revived internationally from the 1980s, suggests a close link between the changing age structure of the population and cultural change: that changing proportions of old people in a society may influence attitudes toward them and affect their own behavior. But the different responses in Great Britain, France, the United States, Germany, Italy, and the USSR to similar demographic situations in the twentieth century suggest that the relationship between demography and culture is complex, variable, and, as yet, little understood.

A similar contrast can be found in studies of eighteenth-century France and Britain, when the proportions of older people and average expectancy of living to later ages were rising in both countries. In France this has been seen as a period when older people came into favor and acquired a positive image, in contrast to previous denigration: "This major [demographic] change in humanity's history was accompanied by a mutation in sensitivities, in perceptions of life and its different ages that transformed the conception of the older generation's role and position in society" (Bourdelais, 1998). Older people in France "began to be actively esteemed" as they had not before. One sign of this esteem was the establishment of pensions for public servants for the first time (Troyansky, 1989). No parallel change in esteem has been detected in Britain. Rather, by the end of the century, impoverished old people were less rather than more likely to receive poor relief (Ottoway, 2004). Pensions for public servants were also introduced for the first time, but, rather than signs of esteem, these were due to the professionalization of government: pensions explicitly provided an acceptable means to rid the public service of those thought to have aged past their usefulness (Raphael, 1964). Similar demographic regimes may have different cultural outcomes in different social, economic, and political contexts.

What Is "Old Age"?

But do statistics of the numbers of people above a certain age tell us everything about age structure or the meaning of "old age"? Conventionally, gerontologists and demographers choose 60 or 65 as the lower age limit of "old age." It is essential to choose a fixed age threshold to make statistical comparisons of age structure over time. But have these ages always had the same meanings in Western culture? Sixty and 65 are the most frequent threshold ages for payment of state or private pensions in present-day Western societies, and they have become common ages of retirement from paid work. These ages were generally fixed earlier in the twentieth century when both pensions and retirement gradually became normal features of aging in most Western countries, although nowhere were they universal before the 1940s. At that time they were thought to approximate to the ages at which most people were no longer fit for full-time paid work. Standards of physical fitness of people in their sixties rose in most Western countries over the course of the twentieth century. In some countries and some occupations (e.g., academic positions in the United States, public sector occupations in Australia), ages of retirement were raised or abolished in the later twentieth century and the first years of the twenty-first, when raising state pension ages became an important political issue in many European countries, as governments became concerned about the costs of pensioning aging populations. This followed a period from the 1980s to the late 1990s when retirement ages in many European countries fell for reasons connected with the state of national and international economies and the shakeout of expensive senior employees at a time of economic recession, or with personal preference, at a time when many managerial and professional employees had generous pensions (Kohli and Rein, 1991). This fall in retirement ages came at a time when physical fitness at later ages was increasing and was not consistently related to individual capacity for work. In the late twentieth century, for the first time, physical condition was detached from social and bureaucratic markers of "old age" and recently established age boundaries were destabilized. Were they more stable in the more distant past? How has old age been defined historically? Were people defined and perceived as "old" at earlier ages in previous centuries when living standards were lower?

The concept of old age was firmly present in all known past cultures, and it had multiple meanings and uses. Ages 60 and 70 have been used to signify the onset of old age in laws and institutions in Europe at least since medieval times. Age 60 was long the age at which law or custom permitted withdrawal from public activities on grounds of old age (Shahar, 1997). Even in ancient Greece the formal obligation to perform military service did not end until age 60, and men in their fifties were conscripted (Finley, 1983). In medieval England, in a succession of enactments from the Ordinance of Labourers of 1349 onward, men and women ceased at age 60 to be liable for compulsory service under the labor laws, to prosecution for vagrancy, or (in the case of men) to perform military service. From the thirteenth century, age 70 was set as the upper limit for jury service. Similar regulations held elsewhere in Europe. Exemption from military service in Castile and Leon in modern Spain, and in Modena and Florence in modern Italy, came only at age 70 (Shahar, 1997, 2005). Arguably, governments generally had an incentive to set such ages as high as possible when they frequently had the capacity to exact taxation in lieu of service. However, it is unlikely that such ages could credibly be set at levels far removed from popular perceptions of the threshold of old age and the capacities of older people. Furthermore, in medieval and early modern Europe (and in many societies in the twentieth century), there was no fixed retirement age for many elite positions, and appointments could be made at advanced ages. In England the average age at death of the nine seventeenth-century archbishops of Canterbury was 73, and the average age of appointment was 60. Between 1400 and 1600, the average age of election of the doges who ruled Venice was 72. Some were in their eighties when elected (Shahar, 2005). All of this suggests that, at all levels of society, even in the distant past it was not thought surprising that people remained active and mentally capable to late ages.

On the other hand, it was long assumed that most manual workers could not remain fully active at their trades much past age 50, especially when performance depended on such physical attributes as good eyesight. Literary evidence from the sixteenth century suggests that the fifties were regarded as the declining side of working maturity, the beginning of old age, as is still sometimes assumed. For women, old age was often thought to start earlier, in the late forties or about 50, at menopause, when women were thought to lose their central purpose in life: childbearing (Botelho and Thane, 1999). For men, the defining characteristic of the onset of old age was perceived as declining capacity for full-time work. For both men and women in preindustrial Europe, in everyday life, old age was defined primarily by appearance and capacities rather than by age-specific rules about pensions and retirement. Hence, people could be defined as "old" at variable ages. For example, English poor relief records in the eighteenth century first describe some people as "old" in their fifties, others not until their seventies. Supplicants for public service pensions in eighteenth-century France ranged in age from 54 to 80 (Troyansky, 1993).

This suggests that over many centuries old age has been defined in different ways in different contexts and for different social groups. It can be defined chronologically, functionally, or culturally. A fixed age threshold has long been a bureaucratic convenience for establishing age limits for rights and duties, such as access to pensions, or eligibility for public service, which would be more complex to administer if each case had to be judged individually. Fixed age boundaries became more pervasive in the twentieth century, and societies became more rigidly stratified by age as ages of entry to and exit from school and of retirement and receipt of pensions became fixed.

"Functional" old age is defined by capacity to perform the tasks expected of a self-sufficient adult male or female, such as paid or unpaid domestic work. "Cultural" old age means that an individual is said to "look old," according to the norms of the community, and is treated by others as "old." This expresses the value system of the community and may define individuals as "old" according to codes of dress or other commonly accepted signifiers.

Despite continuities over long time periods in both official and popular age definitions of the onset of old age, a high proportion of survivors in medieval and early modern society felt and looked "old" at earlier ages than in the recent past, due to poverty, harder lives, and lack of access to the means to disguise aging. The number of people who appeared to be "old" in past communities might have been greater, and they would have been a more visible presence, than is revealed simply by calculation of the number aged 60 or older.

It has long been recognized that there is immense variety in the pace and timing of human aging, that people do not age at the same speed or in the same ways. Since antiquity (Parkin, 1998), old age has been divided into stages in literary and visual representations. Some of these were elaborate, such as medieval "ages of man" schema, which divided life into three, four, seven, or twelve ages (Burrow, 1986; Sears, 1986). From at least the fourteenth century until the nineteenth, with echoes (mainly humorous) in the twentieth and twenty-first, images of the "Stages of Life" of Man, or more occasionally Woman, or still more occasionally both, were popular. They represented life experience as a series of steps ascending to a peak at about age 30 for women, at 40 or 50 for men, then declining to end at 90 or even 100, suggesting, again, that extreme old age was not unthinkable even in the distant past and could be represented as a normal feature of the narrative of life.

In everyday discourse, old age has been more commonly divided into what in early modern England was described as "green" old age, a time of fitness and activity, with perhaps some failing powers, and the later or last phase of decrepitude, a division that from the later twentieth century was less imaginatively labeled "young" and "old" old age, or the "Third" and "Fourth" ages, the latter labels originating in France. All of this suggests that it has long been recognized that "old age" is a category embracing great diversity of capacity and experience.

Modes of Survival: Work

Historians have discovered much about the ways in which older people supported themselves and were supported through time and how they lived and perceived their lives. Such public documents as wills, legal records, inventories, poor relief records, census statistics, and records of pension funds and such private sources as diaries, letters, biographies, and autobiographies can help us to understand the lives of older people in the past. Again, the picture is one of diversity, among social groups and across space and time (Troyansky, 1989; Pelling and Smith, 1991; Shahar, 1997; Botelho and Thane, 1999; Thane, 2000, 2005; Ottoway, Botelho, and Kittredge, 2002; Parkin, 2003; Ottoway, 2004).

Some older people have always possessed property, often in substantial amounts, with which they could support themselves to the end of life, employing others to care for them, if necessary, either in institutions or in their own households. In Europe, from medieval times until the nineteenth and twentieth centuries, particularly in rural regions of Ireland, parts of France, and eastern Europe, aging individuals could legally assign their property to relatives or nonrelatives in return for guaranteed support until death, and they could invoke the protection of the law if the agreement was not honored. Older people determinedly sought, whenever possible and for as long as possible, to control their own lives and retain their independence throughout much of Western culture throughout recorded history. This was, of course, easiest for those with property. For the propertyless and impoverished there was, through most of recorded time and in all places, little choice but to work for as long as they were able, whereas the propertied could always afford to retire from work when they chose (Smith, 1991; Harvey, 1993; Shahar, 1997). Then, as states and later business enterprises bureaucratized, from the eighteenth century, and became concerned about the efficiency of their officials, pensions were introduced to encourage retirement when aging impaired performance (Raphael, 1964; Thuillier, 1994; Troyansky, 1998).

Always, the poorest men and women expected, and were expected, to work to late ages, often excluded from, or refusing to accept, stigmatizing poor relief although living in pitiable conditions. For example, in a census of the poor taken in Norwich, England, in 1570, three widows, aged 74, 79, and 82, were described only as "*almost past work*" (my italics), and they were still earning small sums at spinning woolen cloth (Pelling, 1991). This remained so in most Western countries until the twentieth century. Poor relief systems encouraged older men and women to work, supplementing but not replacing meager incomes. In early modern Europe, most communities provided specified tasks for older people. Such activities as road mending, caring for the churchyard, fetching and carrying, and caring for horses on market days were tasks for old men. It was often easier for women to support themselves at later ages, caring for children, performing casual domestic labor such as cleaning or laundry, taking in lodgers, or running small shops or alehouses (Jutte, 1994).

This lifetime of toil was relieved for the poorest people by the emergence of retirement as a normal phase of life only in the mid-twentieth century. Retirement with pensions became established in white-collar occupations, in the public and private sectors, in most Western countries from the later nineteenth through the first half of the twentieth century. Retirement from blue-collar occupations did not increase significantly in North America, Europe, or Australasia until the 1940s and beyond (Ransom and Sutch, 1986; Johnson, 1994).

Why did retirement become a mass phenomenon at this time? Attempts to explain it as a feature of capitalist manipulation of a reserve army of labor (Phillipson, 1982; Macnicol, 1998) are unconvincing. The fastest spread of retirement coincided with the post–World War II labor shortage in most Western countries, when older people were needed in the labor force rather than in reserve. Similarly unconvincing are representations of retirement as marking the cultural marginalization of older people by exclusion from the supposed dignity of paid work. The work engaged in by poor older people throughout history was rarely dignified or respected. The main driver for retirement as a normal stage of life, normally occurring at around the minimum state pension age, seems to have been the introduction of improved pensions, provided by most Western states, and increasingly, in western Europe, by employers. These promised for most people, for the first time in history, at least tolerable incomes in later life, which made retirement before the onset of serious physical decline a realistic possibility. This coincided with increased capacity of younger relatives to assist older people in a period of generally rising living standards and full employment.

This transition to retirement as a normal phase of life occurred gradually. Many of the first generation of manual workers who experienced retirement found it difficult and were uncertain how to spend the unaccustomed leisure for which they had no opportunity to prepare themselves. Later generations could foresee retirement and could prepare a script for later life (Hannah, 1986; Thane, 2000). In the later twentieth century, the mass of workers experienced at the end of life the leisure previously available only to the better-off. This changed the structure and expectations of the life course.

However, especially in western Europe, in the 1980s and 1990s increasing numbers of people retired in their fifties, sometimes willingly but often under pressure from management engaged in "downsizing" their operations by removing expensive older workers at a time when economies were struggling (Kohli and Rein, 1991). From the later 1990s the pattern shifted again, when employers and governments became anxious to keep employees at work to later ages as they became aware of falling birthrates, the aging of populations, and the dwindling numbers of prime-age workers. This time, however, they faced resistance from workers who had come to look forward to retirement.

Older People and Their Families

Older people who had little or no savings or property, and who could not earn a living from a single source of employment, lived in what historians of early modern Europe call an "economy of makeshifts" and twentieth-century economists less picturesquely labeled "income packaging": pulling together a shifting variety of resources to survive.

It used to be assumed by social scientists that in preindustrial societies older people lived with and were supported by their children and other close relatives. Historians then established that, for as far back in time as can be traced, it has not been the norm in all Western societies for older people to share households with their married children (Laslett and Wall, 1972). Coresidence was conventional into the twentieth century in many Mediterranean societies and some north European peasant cultures, such as those of Ireland and parts of France, where land was the family's only asset and the heir shared land and household with the elders until their deaths (Kennedy, 1991; Troyansky, 1993). In much of northwestern Europe, however, elders retained control of their own households for as long as they were able, rarely sharing them with adult married children, although they might move to the home of a relative when they were no longer capable of independence, perhaps for just a short time before death.

Deep-rooted north European cultural traditions are expressed in the folklore of many countries, which, even in medieval times, expressed few illusions about the support that aging people could expect from close relatives, but conveyed warnings of the danger to older people of placing themselves and their possessions under the control of their children. Such stories achieved their most sublime expression in William Shakespeare's *King Lear,* in which the vain old king is betrayed by two of his daughters, once he has placed himself and his possessions in their care. *King Lear* was a reworking of a number of medieval folktales. Another warning to older people in the eighteenth century appeared on the gates of some towns in Brandenburg, which were hung with large clubs bearing the inscription "He who made himself dependent on his children for bread and suffers from want, he shall be knocked dead by this club" (Gaunt, 1983).

Most countries in medieval and early modern Europe incorporated into law some obligation on adult children and sometimes other close relatives to support their elders (for example, the English Poor Law from the late sixteenth century). This was the practice, if not the law, in parts of early modern Germany (Jutte, 1994). How frequently such practices were implemented was variable, not least because the close relatives of the aged poor were often very poor themselves and could not realistically be expected to give support (Thomson, 1991; Thane, 1996, 2000; Montigny, 1997). The customs and practice of the Old World were transported to the New, with adaptations to new circumstances. Migrants from Europe to North America, Australasia, and elsewhere took even more seriously independence and self-help, which was necessary for survival in sometimes inhospitable environments, and immigrant societies took time to build the communal, often faith-based, institutions that supplemented self- and family support in much of Europe (Montigny, 1997; Thomson, 1998).

But the fact that older people in many Western societies did not conventionally share a home with close relatives and determinedly retained their independence for as long as they were able does not mean that there were no close emotional ties and exchanges of support between the generations. There was a great deal of diversity in family forms and relationships (Laslett and Wall, 1972; Laslett, 1995). Parents and adult offspring might not share a household, but they often lived in close proximity, even in such a highly mobile society as England was for centuries before industrialization (Thane, 2000). Generally "kinship did not stop at the front door" (Anderson, 1971; Jutte, 1994): some close relatives, at least, often lived close enough to aging people to help them when needed. The Austrian sociologists Rosenmayr and Kockeis described the north European family as characterized by "intimacy at a distance" (Rosenmayr and Kockeis, 1963, pp. 418–19), the "intimacy" being as important as the "distance."

"In early modern Europe, old people could, in general, expect help from their children based on the sustenance and protection provided by parents during the childhood period" (Jutte, 1994, p. 85). Family members, at all social levels, exchanged support and services due to a mixture of material, calculative, and emotional motives. It was often an *exchange* relationship. Older people in the past, as now, were rarely simply dependent on others, unless they were in severe physical decline. They cared for grandchildren and sick people, supported younger people financially when they could afford it, and performed myriad other services for others. In a reversal of the older sociological orthodoxy that the generations lived together in preindustrial societies but were scattered by industrialization, research in Europe and the United States found that older people were more likely to share a household with their adult children in the growing industrial towns of the nineteenth century than in rural communities. This was due to a shortage of housing and the need of the younger generation for help, for example, with child care, in establishing themselves in the new environment. As industrial societies became more prosperous in the twentieth century, more older people could again live independently.

With lengthening life expectancy, over the past 100 (particularly the past 50) years, it has become more common for three or more generations to be alive together, and the opportunity for exchange has become more frequent (Bourdelais, 1998). Although over the past century, until today, increasing numbers of old people have lived alone, they were, and are, relatively rarely isolated or neglected by younger relatives (Rein and Salzman, 1995; Thane, 1998; *Ageing and Society*, 2006). Rather, more older people can seize the opportunity of greater affluence to keep the independent control of their own lives to which they have long aspired.

The importance of mutual support and exchange between the generations in the past has often been underestimated because it took the form of services or gifts in kind, which are difficult to trace historically because there was no reason for systematic records of such private, nonmonetary transactions to be made or to survive. It was a taken-for-granted activity of everyday life of the kind that is most difficult to reconstruct in the past. Even the participants might take such transfers so for granted that they denied their significance, as when a 67-year-old retired market gardener gave evidence to a British Royal Commission of Enquiry into the Condition of the Aged Poor in 1895. He lived alone in a country village, in a cottage and garden, rented an allotment, and kept a pig or two; both were useful sources of food and of earnings and/or exchange. He had occasional earnings from road mending. When asked if his five surviving children gave him help, he replied, "No, I have had to help them when I can. They have got large families most of them. I do what I can in that sense. I do not get anything from them in any way. The daughter that I have lives the length of this room perhaps from me and she looks after my house" (Thane, 2000). His daughter's housework was a service that must have contributed greatly to his comfort, but he so took it for granted that he did not define it as "help." In other respects, this man's story exemplifies family relations and the survival strategies of older people, which were not peculiar to England or to the later nineteenth century. His children were too poor and too burdened with children to given him financial support; instead, he helped them when he could. He was no longer in regular paid work but packaged together a living from the produce of his garden and occasional earnings. It would be surprising if he did not sometimes share meals with his daughter's family and give them some produce from his garden, both common forms of exchange within the families of those too poor to offer cash, part of the network of transactions that held together poor communities through the centuries, enabling survival in conditions of poverty (Jutte, 1994; Thane, 1996; Montigny, 1997).

However, not all older people had children or other close relatives to support them, especially in earlier centuries when high death rates meant that parents might outlive children. It has been estimated that up to one-third of women living to age 65 in seventeenth- and eighteenth-century England had no surviving children. By the mid-nineteenth century, perhaps two-thirds of 65-year-olds had surviving children (Pelling and Smith, 1991). In eighteenth-century France the average age at which a person became both fatherless and motherless was 29.5; in the 1970s it was 55 (Bourdelais,

1998). Also, geographical mobility, through centuries when transport was slow and many people were illiterate, might break contacts even with surviving children. Younger people were more likely than the older to migrate, in search of land or work. In the seventeenth century and before, such migration might predominantly occur within countries; in the nineteenth century, millions of (mainly younger) migrants moved from Europe to North and South America, Australia, New Zealand, and elsewhere, far from their elders. Although they often strove to keep in touch with them at a distance, close support was impossible. In the recent past it has become easier for relatives to keep in close touch even when they live far apart. Modern forms of communication—telephones, the internet, motor and air transport—facilitate contact even over long distances in ways unimaginable in past centuries.

Through the twentieth century, birthrates fell in most Western countries, although unevenly, and more slowly in the United States than in Europe. But death and marriage rates fell, including infant death rates. Consequently, in the early twenty-first century a higher proportion of older people than ever before have at least one surviving child, although the exceptionally low birthrates from the 1980s may mean that this ceases to be so for later cohorts of aging people. Most older people who have surviving children are in close contact with some or all of them. At all times, recipients of welfare relief have been more likely to lack surviving children, which further suggests the historical importance of family support. Also, modern "welfare states" seem not to have displaced family support for older people, as some social scientists once feared, because it remains strong; rather, welfare can facilitate family support, enabling relationships between generations to be easier and less tension-ridden by removing some of the economic and emotional costs from the family.

Even those who had no surviving blood relatives could form a supportive "family." Throughout history older men have married younger women able to look after them; rich older women have, more rarely, married younger men; widowers with children married women to care for them. For centuries, orphan children, or those whose parents were too poor to support them, were adopted by older people, gaining a home in return for assistance. Unrelated older people shared households for mutual support or assisted one another across household boundaries. Examples can be found as far apart as Norwich, England, in the sixteenth century and Ontario, Canada, in the mid-nineteenth century, and throughout early modern Europe (Jutte, 1994).

Aging and Social Welfare Services

When families have not been able, willing, or available to help, many older people have needed the support of welfare services, provided either by central or local government or by charity. In most past, and present, societies, older people have been more likely than the young to be very poor, especially if they were female. However, focusing on the aged poor risks suggesting that most older people in the past were both poor and dependent, when many were not. It diverts attention from those who were independent and sometimes wealthy. There is a danger of overestimating the importance of poor relief in the lives of older people because poor relief systems have left records whereas other, perhaps equally important sources of support, such as that within families, have not.

Nevertheless, poor relief and welfare have been important in the lives of many impoverished older people. Most modern states, to some degree, in the twentieth century became "welfare states," although the meaning of this term varies from place to place and over time. In Europe, modern welfare states are profoundly marked by each country's long tradition of poor relief. These traditions were transported by migrants to "new" countries and, once there, transformed.

All European countries for centuries had some system of provision for aged and other poor, who could not help themselves and had no family or other source of support. This was financed in diverse ways but generally by a combination of public taxation—probably most extensively in England, through the national Poor Law, which was in place from 1597 to 1948, although it had still earlier antecedents (Slack, 1990)—and voluntary charity, often religious in motivation and institutionalization. "Relief" of the poor could be payments in cash or kind (food, clothing, medical care) or shelter in a hospital or workhouse. It was of variable quality, within each country as well as over time, and was guided by varied principles: it might aim to support those whose poverty was deemed not to be their own fault, to rehabilitate those thought capable of being self-supporting, or to punish those thought responsible for their own indigence.

Everywhere, older people were a high proportion of recipients of relief, along with widows and children, but nowhere did reaching a defined age automatically qualify anyone for relief. The essential qualification was destitution (Jutte, 1994). Even where the poor relief system was relatively generous, relief could be refused even to the very old if they were judged capable of earning some income. This is an important contrast with modern state pension systems, which, whatever their inadequacies, normally provide for most of the population on attaining a certain age.

Countries of the New World tended to reject publicly funded welfare systems because, initially, they lacked both an established, substantial wealthy class capable of funding them and also the mass of miserable poverty that required them. Migrants traveled to new countries often to escape from poverty. Migrants in the nineteenth century, when "new" countries grew fastest, were often fleeing from punitive relief systems in Europe and had no desire to replicate them. Ideologically they placed a premium on independence and self-help. Australia and New Zealand, for example, never introduced publicly funded poor relief systems, relying instead on voluntary charity, sometimes (and increasingly over time) subsidized from public funds (Dickey, 1980; Thomson, 1998). The picture was similar in nineteenth-century Canada (Montigny, 1997).

In parts of the United States, the extent of unmet need required the introduction of poor relief, but "welfare" early acquired, and retained, more stigmatizing associations than elsewhere in Western countries. Most nation-states, at least by the eighteenth century, and commonly in the nineteenth and twentieth centuries, provided publicly funded pensions for public servants, for the disabled veterans of war, and sometimes for their families (Skocpol, 1992). Older people were, in most countries, the first to benefit from the transition, between the late nineteenth and the mid-twentieth centuries, from residual and often punitive poor relief systems to generally more comprehensive and generous state welfare systems. This was because, being mostly marginal to the labor and capital markets, they were generally the last substantial social group to gain from the general improvement in living standards that took place in the West during the nineteenth century. In addition, the "deservingness" and respectability of older people were more obvious to reluctant taxpayers, who had to pay the bill, than the needs of other impoverished groups such as the unemployed.

Old-age pensions were introduced throughout the West from the 1880s, but on different principles and for different reasons in various countries. Where the main motivation was mass poverty among older people due to the absence, or the deterrent and stigmatizing effects of, poor relief, pensions were noncontributory and targeted on the very poor, often mainly providing for women because they were poorest in old age, as in Denmark in 1891, New Zealand in 1898, most of the Australian states by the time of Federation in 1901, and Great Britain in 1908. Where the main motive was pressure from, and/or the desire of politicians to undermine, a growing labor movement, as well as to stimulate economic growth, as in Germany in 1889, they tended to be insurance based and target primarily the securely employed, generally male, worker (Baldwin, 1990; Hennock, 2007). Different cultural and political contexts produced different pension systems in different countries throughout the twentieth century (World Bank, 1994).

Older people have also gained from increasing medical knowledge over time, especially in the twentieth century. Knowledge of the history of geriatric medicine is sparse but growing (Stearns, 1977, pp. 80–118; Haber, 1983; Kondratowitz, 1991; Cole, 1992, pp. 92–109, 191–211). There has been continuous interest in the physical condition of aging people among medical specialists since Ancient Greece and Rome, although always as a minority medical interest. For centuries it was uncertain, and debated, whether old age as such should be defined as a disease, and little could be done to alleviate the diseases accompanying older, or indeed younger, ages other than to counsel temperance, good diet, and exercise, as specialists still do (Thane, 1993). Investigation and understanding of the pathology of physical deterioration with aging developed especially in nineteenth-century France, spurred on partly by the increasing numbers of older people in the French population (Bourdelais, 1993, 1998). Only in the twentieth century did medicine acquire the capacity to diagnose and cure extensively, and only in the mid-twentieth century were medical services sufficiently democratized in most Western countries to allow most older people access to medical treatment. Even so, all too often they tended to be at the end of the line for such treatment, their lives deemed less valuable than those of younger people.

The specialty of geriatrics developed in most Western countries from the early twentieth century. The name was invented in New York by an Austrian immigrant doctor, Ignatz Nascher, who developed methods of rehabilitation of older patients, determined to protect older people from neglect by the medical profession, who, he perceived, thought them uninteresting or unworthy of effort because they would soon die (Thane, 1993). Geriatrics developed from the 1930s, as concern grew about keeping fit the aging populations of most Western countries. However, geriatrics remains in most countries a low-status medical specialty. Research into the conditions that most affect older people, the means of treating them, and the specific impacts of drug therapies on older bodies all too often have lower priority for research than the needs of younger people. If they lack wealth and personal power, older people—even in their sixties with the potential for years of active life ahead—can still suffer from lower priority for treatment in favor of the young, although in most countries discrimination has become less overt, and more subject to protest by older people and their friends and families, than in the past.

Older people have gained greatly from the expansion of free or low-cost health care in most Western countries and from medical techniques designed for all age groups, such as coronary bypass surgery, organ transplants, and joint replacements. Understanding has grown of the potential of exercise and diet to extend the years of active life, and even to reverse neurological decline. At the same time many people have suffered at the end of life from developments in medical technology that can keep people "alive" while barely capable of experiencing a good quality of life. Medical developments have created, for some, exaggerated hopes that decline and death can be averted almost indefinitely. These appear to be more widespread in the United States, in some circles at least, than elsewhere and everywhere face some skepticism and challenges. They have created serious ethical and practical dilemmas for older people, their families, and their medical providers. When is it desirable, or not, to give a kidney transplant or a coronary bypass to someone in his or her eighties or nineties, who might as a result enjoy further years of active life? Or when is it preferable to ease the transition to death by provision of sensitive palliative care, knowledge of which also grew in the later twentieth century (Baltes and Baltes, 1990; Thane, 1993, 2000, pp. 436–57; Kirkwood, 1999)?

There are no simple, generalizable answers to these intensely difficult dilemmas, not least because the experience of later life continues to be diverse. By the early twenty-first century, on average, people in high-income countries were living to later ages, and appeared to be remaining fit to later ages, than was ever before imaginable. Some very old people can benefit from medical treatment that might cause misery for others. Research into levels of impairment in later life remains patchy but growing. In 1982, 20.4 percent of the U.S. over-65 population had impaired capacity for mobility and self-care; by 1998, the percentage had fallen to 16.6 (Manton and Gu, 2001; Fries, 2002). In the United Kingdom in 1980, 48 percent of people aged 85 or older could not walk out of doors unaided; by 2001, the percentage was 41 (Turner, 2004, p. 31). Many, although not all, older people have throughout history experienced a period of frailty and impairment before death. They now experience it at later ages and from different diseases than before. They may survive the pneumonia that would have killed them in the 1930s or before to experience dementia or other conditions, and modern medical treatment may prolong the period of dependency before death. Currently less than 1 in 100 of the population of the United States and Europe aged over 65 has various forms of dementia; by age 85, the number is 1 in 6 (Kirkwood, 1999, pp. 131–32).

Has the Social Status of Older People Declined?

Social scientists sometimes argue that the spread of pensions, retirement, and specialized medical care in the twentieth century increased the dependence and marginalization of older people, and that they have come to be less valued in modern society than in the past. The belief that the status of older people is declining has a long history. It is discussed, and dismissed, even in the opening pages of Plato's *Republic* (Plato, 1987, pp. 61–63; Parkin, 2005, pp. 31–70) and in a long succession of texts through the centuries. The longevity of this narrative trope suggests that it expresses persistent cultural fears of aging and neglect rather than representing transparent, dominant reality.

Early historical inquiry into old age tended to echo this narrative of decline. George Minois's history of old age in Western culture from antiquity to the Renaissance acknowledged variations and complexities in the experiences and perceptions of old age over this long time span: "not so much a continuous decline as a switchback evolution." But he concluded that "the general tendency however is towards degradation." He had no doubt that the "degradation" was greater still in modern society (Minois, 1989, pp. 6–7). An extensive body of work on old age in the United States since the eighteenth century finds the status of old people to be in decline over a variety of timescales: from the late eighteenth century to the early nineteenth and again in the mid-nineteenth century (Cole, 1992), and between the late nineteenth and twentieth centuries (Achenbaum, 1976; Haber, 1983). Historians have reconstructed the different experiences of the political elite of New England in the late eighteenth century (Fischer, 1978), attitudes to East Coast Protestant clergy in the late eighteenth century (Cole, 1992), studies of labor force participation and the antecedents of Social Security legislation (Achenbaum, 1976), and the emergence of geriatrics and the attitudes of social welfare professionals in the late nineteenth and twentieth centuries (Haber, 1983). These are mostly studies of white males. They have tended to cite the (scrupulously researched) experience of specific groups as representative of broader, even hegemonic, values, rather than as microstudies, valuable in themselves, contributing part, rather than the whole, of a complex total picture. The fact that some older men exerted power at a particular time is important, but it does not necessarily suggest that all old people at that time and place were highly regarded. In all times in Western culture, older people (female and male) who retained economic or any other form of power, along with their faculties, could command, or enforce, respect. At all times, also, powerless older people have (although not universally) been marginalized and denigrated.

More recent studies of old age in ancient (Parkin, 1998) and medieval Europe (Rosenthal, 1996; Shahar, 1997) and in France (Troyansky, 1989, 1998; Bourdelais, 1993, 1998), Germany (Borscheid, 1987; Kondratowitz, 1991; Conrad, 1994), and the United States (Haber and Gratton, 1994) between the eighteenth and twentieth centuries acknowledge the variety of experience in old age and abandon the pessimistic framework of decline. A richly textured history has emerged that makes clearer differences among social groups, as well as times and places, including among national cultures. For example, Troyansky describes the new confidence with which public servants requested pensions from the state in postrevolutionary France. They asserted a right to this reward and, in the process, self-consciously reviewed their lives and imagined a model of the life course that incorporated a period of pensioned retirement at its end. All of this appears to have been new in early-nineteenth-century France. In England, by contrast, aging small landowners, male and female, even in medieval times, vigorously pursued through the law-courts a period of retirement on their own terms, as they negotiated and defended contracts in which they transferred their lands to younger people (sometimes relatives, sometimes not) in return for care and material support (Clark, 1990; Smith, 1991). English men and women at all social levels from at least the twelfth century (Harvey, 1993; Rosenthal, 1996) wheedled pensions from monarchs, bishops, and other influential patrons, stressing the virtues of their past lives that merited support for a dignified old age. Even poor old people, in the nineteenth century and long before, asserted their right to poor relief in similar terms (Sokoll, 1997). The difference between the two countries may lie in the fact that formal equality before the law was long established in England, carrying with it a sense of equal rights that were strongly held even among poor people, however imperfect the reality, whereas in France such equality was the outcome, indeed the central objective, of the great Revolution of 1798. Such profound legal and political differences shaped different cultural experiences of old age.

The greatly enriched histories of old age of recent years have alerted us to the complexity of attitudes toward and experiences of older age in all times, as well as to the range of sources and methods through which historians can seek to reconstruct them. It can be tempting, for example, to conclude, as Minois (1989) does, that Shakespeare's dismal final age of the "seven ages of man," described by Jaques in *As You Like It*—"second childishness and mere oblivion; sans teeth, sans eyes, sans taste, sans everything"—is representative of sixteenth-century English perceptions of old age. However, you would have failed to note that Jaques is a relatively young man but is given the conventional literary attributes of an old man, such as melancholy, and that the dismal description of the "seventh age" is followed by the entrance on stage of an octogenarian, Adam, who has earlier described himself, and has been represented, as "strong and lusty." The pervasiveness in English popular drama and literature (for example, in the work of Chaucer) of irony and dialogue between conflicting—negative and positive—representations of old age, as well as its likely familiarity to medieval and early modern audiences, suggests the deep roots in English culture of an understanding of the diverse experiences of later life. Recent work suggests that this has been, and remains, the experience of many other cultures (Ottoway, Botelho, and Kittredge, 2002; Thane, 2005). Denial of old age, through such techniques as cosmetic surgery, and hostility to older people are pervasive in present-day Western culture, but so are strong challenges to such negative perceptions of aging from both older and younger people (*Ageing and Society*, 2004, 2006, 2007; Gullette, 2004; Chong et al., 2006; among many others).

Conclusion

In the twentieth century the experience of later life became more uniform across the national, cultural, and social boundaries of Western nations, but experience will always be diverse across such a large and varied age group, that is, if it makes any more sense to regard people aged 60 as more properly belonging to the same age group with those aged 100 than with those aged 40.

For the first time, it became normal in Western societies for almost everyone to grow old. For the first time in history, it became possible for everyone to imagine, and to plan, realistically, for a long life. Imaginings of the life course—philosophical, imaginative, or visual representations of the Stages of Life or the Journey of Life—had a long history, with roots in medieval and even ancient Europe, but these learned, often didactic, uses of the idea of the life course to convey a moral message (responsible, temperate behavior could increase one's chance of a long life) were quite different from the everyday practical expectation of long life that emerged in the later twentieth century (Cole, 1992). The cultural implications of this change are profound.

The characteristics of this later phase of life began to be universalized and democratized. Only from the mid-twentieth century did the mass of poorer people begin to share in old age what the better-off had always had: a regular income for which they did not need to work or degrade themselves by begging for poor relief or charity, and a period of leisured retirement between the end of paid work and the onset of physical decrepitude.

REFERENCES

Achenbaum, W. A. 1978. *Old Age in the New Land: The American experience since 1978*. Baltimore: Johns Hopkins University Press.

Ageing and Society. 2004. Special issue: Understanding quality of life in old age. *Ageing and Society* 24 (5).

———. 2006. Special issue: Family support for older people: Determinants and consequences. *Ageing and Society* 26 (5).

———. 2007. Special issue: Understanding vulnerabilities in old age. *Ageing and Society* 26 (1).

Anderson, M. 1971. *Family Structure in Nineteenth Century Lancashire*. Cambridge: Cambridge University Press.

Baldwin, P. 1990. *The Politics of Social Solidarity: Class bases of the European welfare states, 1875–1975*. Cambridge: Cambridge University Press.

Baltes, P., and M. Baltes. 1990. *Successful Aging: Perspectives from the behavioral sciences*. Cambridge: Cambridge University Press.

Borscheid, P. 1987. *Geschichte des Alters 16.–18. Jahrhundert*. Munster: F. Coppenrath.

Botelho, L. 2004. *Old Age and the English Poor Law, 1500–1700*. Woodbridge: Boydell Press.

Botelho, L., and P. Thane. 1999. *Women and Ageing in Britain since 1500*. London: Routledge.

Bourdelais, P. 1993. *Le Nouvel Age de la Vieillesse: Histoire du vieillissement de la population*. Paris: Editions Odile Jacob.

———. 1998. The ageing of the population: Relevant question or obsolete notions. In *Old Age from Antiquity to Post-modernity*, ed. P. Johnson and P. Thane. London: Routledge.

Bulder, E. 1993. *The Social Economics of Old Age: Strategies to maintain income in later life in the Netherlands, 1880–1940*. Amsterdam: Thesis Publishers.

Burrow, J. A. 1986. *The Ages of Man: A study in medieval writing and thought*. Oxford: Oxford University Press.

Chong, A., S. Ng, J. Woo, and A. Kwan. 2006. Positive ageing: The views of middle-aged and older adults in Hong Kong. *Ageing and Society* 26 (2):243–66.

Clark, E. 1990. The quest for security in medieval England. In *Aging and the Aged in Medieval Europe*, ed. M. M. Sheehan. Toronto: Pontifical Institute of Mediaeval Studies.

Cole, T. R. 1992. *The Journey of Life: A cultural history of aging in America.* Cambridge: Cambridge University Press.

Conrad, C. 1994. *Vom Greis zum Rentner: Der strukturwandel des alters in Dentschland zwischen 1830 und 1930.* Gottingen: Vandenhoeck and Ruprecht.

De Medeiros, K. 2008. From reproduction to new production: The shift in focus on older women's bodies in gerontological discourse after World War Two. Paper read at European Social Science History Conference, in Lisbon.

Dickey, B. 1980. *No Charity There: A short history of social welfare in Australia.* Melbourne: Thomas Nelson.

Finley, M. 1983. Old age in ancient Rome. *Ageing and Society* 3:391–408.

Fischer, D. H. 1978. *Growing Old in America.* New York: Oxford University Press.

Fries, J. 2002. Reducing disability in older age. *Journal of the American Medical Association* 288 (24):3164–66.

Gaunt, D. 1983. The property and kin relationships of retired farmers in northern and central Europe. In *Family Forms in Historic Europe.* Cambridge: Cambridge University Press.

Gullette, M. M. 2004. *Aged by Culture.* Chicago: University of Chicago Press.

Haber, C. 1983. *Beyond Sixty-five: The dilemma of old age in America's past.* New York: Cambridge University Press.

Haber, C., and B. Gratton. 1994. *Old Age and the Search for Security: An American social history.* Bloomington: Indiana University Press.

Hannah, L. 1986. *Inventing Retirement: The development of occupational pensions in Britain.* Cambridge: Cambridge University Press.

Harvey, B. 1993. *Living and Dying in England, 1100–1540.* Oxford: Oxford University Press.

Hennock, E. P. 2007. *The Origin of the Welfare State in England and Germany, 1850–1914.* Cambridge: Cambridge University Press.

Johnson, P. 1994. The employment and retirement of older men in England and Wales, 1881–1981. *Economic History Review* 47:106–28.

Jutte, R. 1994. *Poverty and Deviance in Early Modern Europe.* Cambridge: Cambridge University Press.

Kennedy, L. 1991. Farm succession in modern Ireland: Elements of a theory of inheritance. *Economic History Review* 3:478–96.

Kirkwood, T. 1999. *Time of Our Lives: Why ageing is neither inevitable nor necessary.* London: Phoenix.

Kohli, M., and M. Rein. 1991. The changing balance of work and retirement. In *Time for Retirement: Comparative studies of the labour force,* ed. M. Kohli, M. Rein, A.-M. Guillemard, and H. van Gunsteren. Cambridge: Cambridge University Press.

Laslett, P. 1995. Necessary knowledge: Age and aging in the societies of the past. In *The Politics of Retirement in Britain, 1878–1948,* ed. D. I. Kertzner and P. Laslett. Cambridge: Cambridge University Press.

Laslett, P., and R. Wall, eds. 1972. *Household and Family in Past Time.* Cambridge: Cambridge University Press.

Lovell, S. 2003. Soviet socialism and the construction of old age. *Jahrbucher für Geschichte Osteuroopas* 51:564–85.

Macnicol, J. 1998. *The Politics of Retirement in Britain, 1878–1948.* Cambridge: Cambridge University Press.

Manton, K. G., and X. Gu. 2001. Changes in the prevalence of chronic disability in the United States black and non-black population above age 65 from 1982 to 1999. *Proceedings of the National Academy of Sciences of the United States of America* 98 (11):6354–59.

Minois, G. 1989. *History of Old Age from Antiquity to Renaissance.* Trans. S. Hanbury-Tenison. Oxford: Polity.

Montigny, E.-A. 1997. *Foisted upon the Government: State responsibilities, family obligations and the care of the dependent aged in late nineteenth century Ontario.* Montreal: McGill-Queen's University Press.

Ottoway, S. 2004. *The Decline of Life: Old age in eighteenth century England.* Cambridge: Cambridge University Press.

Ottoway, S., L. Botelho, and K. Kittredge, eds. 2002. *Power and Poverty: Old age in the pre-industrial past.* Westport, London: Greenwood Press.

Parkin, T. 1998. Ageing in antiquity: Status and participation. In *Old Age from Antiquity to Post-modernity,* ed. P. Johnson and P. Thane. London: Routledge.

———. 2003. *Old Age in the Roman World: A cultural and social history.* Baltimore: Johns Hopkins University Press.

———. 2005. The ancient Greek and Roman worlds. In *The Long History of Old Age,* ed. P. Thane. London: Thames and Hudson.

Pelling, M. 1991. Old age, poverty and disability in Norwich. In *Life, Death and the Elderly: Historical perspectives on ageing,* ed. M. Pelling and R. M. Smith. London: Routledge.

Pelling, M., and R. M. Smith, eds. 1991. *Life, Death and the Elderly: Historical perspectives on ageing.* London: Routledge.

Phillipson, C. 1982. *Capitalism and the Construction of Old Age.* London: Macmillan.

Plato. 1987. *The Republic.* Trans. Desmond Lee. London: Penguin.

Ransom, R. L., and R. Sutch. 1986. The labor of older Americans: Retirement of man on and off the job, 1870–1937. *Journal of Economic History* 46:1–30.

Raphael, M. 1964. *Pension and Public Servants: A study of the origins of the British system.* Paris: Mouton.

Rein, M., and H. Salzman. 1995. Social integration, participation and exchange in five industrial countries. In *Older and Active: How Americans over 55 contribute to society,* ed. S. A. Bass. New Haven: Yale University Press.

Rosenmayr, L., and E. Kockeis. 1963. Proposition for a sociological theory of aging and the family. *International Social Science Journal* 3:418–19.

Rosenthal, J. T. 1996. *Old Age in Late Medieval England.* Philadelphia: University of Pennsylvania Press.

Schofield, R. S. 1986. Did the mothers really die? Three centuries of maternal mortality in "The World We Have Lost." In *The World We Have Gained,* ed. L. Bonfield et al. Oxford: Blackwell.

Sears, E. 1986. *The Ages of Man: Medieval interpretations of the life cycle.* Princeton: Princeton University Press.

Shahar, S. 1997. *Growing Old in the Middle Ages.* London: Routledge.

———. 2005. The Middle Ages and Renaissance. In *The Long History of Old Age,* ed. P. Thane. London: Thames and Hudson.

Skocpol, T. 1992. *Protecting Soldiers and Mothers: The political origins of social policy in the United States.* Cambridge: Harvard University Press.

Slack, P. 1990. *The English Poor Law, 1531–1782.* Cambridge: Cambridge University Press.

Smith, R. M. 1991. The manorial court and the elderly tenant in late medieval England. In *Life, Death and the Elderly: Historical perspectives on ageing,* ed. M. Pelling and R. M. Smith. London: Routledge.

Sokoll, T. 1997. Old age in poverty: The record of Essex Pauper letters, 1780–1834. In *Chronicling Poverty: The voices and strategies of the English poor, 1640–1840,* ed. T. Hitchcock et al. New York: St. Martin's Press.

Stavenuiter, M., S. Jansens, and K. Bjisterveld. 1995. *Lange Levens. stille getuigen. Oudere Vrowen in het verladen.* Zutpen: Walburg Pers.

Stearns, P. 1977. *Old Age in European Society.* London: Croom Helm.

Thane, P. 1990. The debate on the declining birth-rate in Britain: The "menace" of an ageing population, 1920s–1950s. *Continuity and Change* 5 (2):283–305.

———. 1993. Geriatrics. In *Companion Encyclopaedia to the History of Medicine,* ed. W. F. Bynum and R. Porter. London: Routledge.

———. 1996. Old people and their families in the English past. In *Charity: Self-interest and welfare in the English past,* ed. M. Daunton. London: UCL Press.

———. 1998. The family lives of old people. In *Old Age from Antiquity to Post-modernity,* ed. P. Johnson and P. Thane. London: Routledge.

———. 2000. *Old Age in English History: Past experiences, present issues.* Oxford: Oxford University Press.

———, ed. 2005. *The Long History of Old Age.* London: Thames and Hudson.

Thomson, D. 1991. The welfare of the elderly in the past: A family or community responsibility? In *Life, Death and the Elderly: Historical perspectives on ageing,* ed. M. Pelling and R. M. Smith. London: Routledge.

———. 1998. Old age in the New World: New Zealand's colonial welfare experiment. In *Old Age from Antiquity to Post-modernity,* ed. P. Johnson and P. Thane. London: Routledge.

Thuillier, G. 1994. *Les pensions de retraite des fonctionnaires au XIXeme siecle.* Paris: CHSS.

Troyansky, D. G. 1989. *Old Age in the Old Regime: Image and experience in eighteenth century France.* Ithaca: Cornell University Press.

———. 1993. Old age, retirement and the social contract in 18th and 19th century France. In *Zur Kulturgeschichte des Alterns* [*Toward a Cultural History of Aging*], ed. C. Conrad and H. J. Kondratowitz. Berlin: Deutsches Zentrum für Altersfragen.

———. 1998. Balancing social and cultural approaches to the history of old age and ageing in Europe: A review and an example from post-revolutionary France. In *Old Age from Antiquity to Post-modernity,* ed. P. Johnson and P. Thane. London: Routledge.

Turner, A. 2004. *Pensions, Challenges and Choices: The first report of the Pensions Commission.* London: UK Government, Stationery Office.

von Kondratowitz, H.-J. 1991. The medicalization of old age: Continuity and change in Germany from the 18th to the early 19th century. In *Life, Death and the Elderly: Historical perspective on ageing,* ed. M. Pelling and R. M. Smith. London: Routledge.

World Bank. 1994. *Averting the Old Age Crisis.* Washington: World Bank.

Wrigley, E. A., R. S. Davies, J. E. Oeppen, and R. S. Schofield. 1997. *English Population History from Family Reconstitutions, 1580–1837.* Cambridge: Cambridge University Press.

Wrigley, E. A., and R. S. Schofield. 1981. *The Population History of England, 1541–1871: A reconstruction.* London: Edward Arnold.

CHAPTER TWO

Resilience and Creativity in Aging

The Realms of Silver

ANNE M. WYATT-BROWN, PH.D.

In 1992, Canadian gerontologist Constance Rooke pointed out that "fiction concerned with old age" was growing "for both literary and sociological reasons" (1992, p. 242). As the aging population increased, writers and readers, she argued, were eager to explore what it felt like to be old. As a result, elderly characters were less likely to be what the English novelist E. M. Forster (1927) called "flat characters" and instead became fully round. Indeed, by the 1970s some were transformed into central figures.

In the past few years, many novels and memoirs have been written by older authors. They reveal the diversity of the aging experience. Of course, race and gender play important roles, but so do creativity and resilience, all qualities recognized by gerontological theorist Margaret Cruikshank (2003). Authors are just as vulnerable to physical decline and the loss of important people in their lives as are the rest of us. Being able to write about disability, loss, and mourning, however, allows them to share their experiences with a wide audience. Readers can take comfort in the knowledge that others have experienced the struggles that feel so threatening, painful, and never-ending.

This chapter examines recent literary works in conjunction with research questions that characterize age studies. One might wonder what fiction and life stories tell about the nature of aging today. Narratives have the capacity to create a picture of aging, one that most readers can easily understand and appreciate. Without literary gerontology, however, the representation might be one-sided, the view of the author and few others. Only by combining research with novels and memoirs can we begin to comprehend the varieties of aging experience in our time. The areas that will be explored include the following: late style, life review, midlife investigation and swan song, resilience, disability and retirement, caregiving, death, mourning, and medical reeducation.

Late Style

In a 1986 presentation, the late Samuel Atkin, training and supervising analyst of the New York Psychoanalytic Institute, reported that becoming old reminded him of his immigration to the United States from Russia at the age of 10. At 88, nine months before his death he declared, "Now I have entered a second new country . . . I feel the excitement of an explorer" (Atkin and Atkin, 1992, p. 10). Although he had Parkinson's disease and impotence caused by prostate surgery, he celebrated his continuing ability to have erotic thoughts and feelings. He welcomed the challenge of exploring this new stage of life. Only poets and novelists, he notes, have written about the excitement of aging, not doctors and analysts. Two other aging analysts, Virginia Clowser (1992) and Mervin Hurwitz (1992), compare old age to adolescence. They report that elderly people need a stable environment in order that they may adapt to new circumstances, both external and internal.

A major cause of these unsettled feelings is the challenge of bodily changes and the death of significant relatives and friends. Not surprisingly, literary work changes as writers age. The cultural critic Edward Said defined late style as "a new idiom" that artists develop in "their work and thoughts" toward the end of their lives. He recognized that late style cannot be encapsulated in one single notion although theorists may attempt to do so.[1] Instead, "late works," he notes, may "crown a lifetime of aesthetic endeavor" or, like the late plays of Ibsen, be a kind of creativity used "to stir up more anxiety, tamper irrevocably with the possibility of closure, and leave the audience more perplexed and unsettled than before" (Said, 2006, pp. 6–7). Said's comments help explain why late style varies so much from artist to artist and why realistic work can end ambiguously. Another difference is that some authors include life review in their late style work while others do not. Moreover, although elements of mourning appear in many late-life novels and memoirs, the nature of loss varies. Sometimes characters lose close friends and relatives; in other instances their sadness has to do with bodily changes or lost opportunities.

Two novels illustrate the ambiguity that late style sometimes creates: *The Sea Lady* (2006), by Margaret Drabble (b. June 5, 1939), and *Digging to America* (2006), by Anne Tyler (b. October 25, 1941). The nature of Drabble's late style becomes apparent when one compares *The Sea Lady* to *The Realms of Gold* (1975), published when she was 36. The heroine in the earlier novel, Frances Wingate, is an archeologist in her mid-thirties who falls in love with an older man, Karel, who is unhappily married. They separate for some time, but ultimately they are reunited in a happy marriage. Although her nephew commits suicide, taking his baby with him, and other characters die, at the end Frances and Karel comfort each other through these trials. Thus, they fulfill what Brian Morton (b. 1955), the author of *Starting Out in the Evening*

(1998),[2] a prize-winning intergenerational novel, says is the work of midlife. The task consists of "accompanying your beloved through life's disasters" (1998, p. 263). In a sentence or two Drabble contemplates what life might be like for Frances later on, gray-haired with grown children. "But further forward one cannot look. Or not yet" (Drabble, 1975, p. 345). More than 30 years later, Drabble contemplates the lives of older protagonists in quite a different fashion.

The Sea Lady features two characters in their sixties who need to reconsider earlier choices. Unlike Frances Wingate and Karel, whose separation was relatively short, Humphrey Clark and Ailsa Kelman have not seen each other since their abortive and damaging love affair, marriage, and divorce took place. Time has not been kind to Humphrey. He needs a professional assistant and minder to get through life. In contrast, Ailsa revels in her notoriety as an outspoken feminist, but even she is subject to nostalgia. The two meet again when they receive honorary degrees. This novel has much in common with *The Realms of Gold.* Drabble includes the details of place, of books, of games, and of food that evoke childhood memories. Unlike the earlier novel, more attention is paid to the past than to the present. The narration includes a Public Orator who asks whether Humphrey has a chance at "redemption" (Drabble, 2006, p. 135). Although he is declared too old to expect a second chance, surprisingly his reunion with Ailsa gives both of them a glimpse of a new lease on life. The ending, however, is more ambiguous than the happy marriage of Frances Wingate and Karel. "The journey draws to its end," Humphrey thinks at the novel's close, "but it is not over yet" (p. 345). A second marriage is possible, but it is by no means a foregone conclusion. Humphrey contemplates issuing a possible dinner invitation, yet the liveliness of the novel's style counters his passivity.

In *Digging to America*, Anne Tyler handles life review, a major aspect of her late style, more tangentially than Drabble. Her novel, however, represents what psycho-analyst George Pollock calls "the mourning-liberation process," a proceeding that may have "a creative outcome" (Pollock, 1998, p. 67). He says that therapy can help people complete their mourning and find new "creative freedoms, further develop-ment, joy, and the ability to embrace life" (p. 71). Most of the action in Tyler's novel takes place in the present rather than the past. Nonetheless, reconsidering past actions and thoughts turns out to be crucial. The novel combines the experience of two middle-aged couples who adopt Korean babies, along with the fate of the babies' new grandparents. The adopted infants give their families and friends great pleasure, but grandfather Dave's beloved wife dies of cancer. Tyler writes poignantly about the feelings of the recently bereaved, having lost her own husband in 1997 (Schillinger, 2006). After retiring from teaching, memories of his dead wife haunt Dave. He feels drawn to Iranian-born Maryam, whose own spouse died when she was 40, leaving her to confront her exile alone. Gradually the two grandparents, now in their mid-sixties, discover that their common plight unites them. Dave begins to equate abandoning one's home and language with "a permanent bereavement" (Tyler, 2006, p. 116). As his empathy expands, he discovers love for Maryam. Accepting the seriousness of her new attachment, however, is not as easy for Maryam.

In Tyler's novel, the capacity to review the past turns out to be crucial. For many years isolation has caused Maryam to suppress her feelings. She needs to recall both her love for her dead husband and his difficult temperament. Until she completes these psychic tasks, she cannot begin to acknowledge her feelings about Dave. Like the aging psychoanalysts who found old age to be as challenging and upsetting as adolescence, the two elders need the support of the two families. Although starting over feels like emigrating again, Tyler hints that these characters may have the necessary stamina.

Life Review

Two novels, *Exit Ghost* (2007), by Philip Roth (b. March 19, 1933), and *Old Filth* (2005), by Jane Gardam (b. July 11, 1928), demonstrate how crucial life review can be. *Exit Ghost* reverses the pattern of emotional growth, depicting the protagonist at the end as a diminished and frightened individual, who shuffles off the stage. Nathan Zuckerman, a writer who has appeared in earlier Roth novels, is now 71. He suffers from impotence and incontinence caused by prostate surgery. At the novel's beginning, however, he seems optimistic and open to new experiences. Contemplating an extended stay in New York, he tries to exchange dwellings with a young couple. In no time Zuckerman falls for the young shiksa wife, Jamie Logan, despite his infirmities and the yawning age gap. He also meets Richard Kliman, Jamie's ex-lover and the would-be biographer of the novelist E. I. Lonoff, years ago a hero of Zuckerman. Kliman believes that Lonoff's unfinished manuscript proves that he had an incestuous affair with his half-sister. At first Zuckerman feels confident that he can stop Kliman's exposé but gradually loses heart. Unlike the younger man, whom he believes feels "indestructible" and "not in the hands of his cells," Zuckerman is obsessed with his physical decline. At his stage of life, he believes that he is "experiencing the organic rebellion staged by the body against the elderly" (Roth, 2007, pp. 256–57). Frustrated by his inability to talk sense to Kliman, Zuckerman begs Jamie Logan to come to his hotel. When she refuses, he decamps for the Berkshires. There he completes the story "He and She," which he began in New York. In its final section He rejects She, a reversal of the author's own fate. Ironically, Zuckerman's narrative demonstrates the dangers of assuming that novels or manuscripts reveal their author's hidden past.[3]

Because little life review appears in *Exit Ghost*, except for a few fleeting memories of Lonoff, redemption for Zuckerman is clearly out of the question. The same is not necessarily true for Roth, who continues to produce remarkable novels on a regular basis. He had published a short fiction, *Everyman,* in 2006; it is even grimmer than *Exit Ghost.* It begins with the protagonist's funeral and ends with a long conversation with a grave digger at the cemetery where his parents lay and where he was to be buried shortly after the conversation. Most of the plot consists of the protagonist's lifelong health problems and his unhappy relationships with three wives and several lovers. Like Zuckerman, he finds a young woman, whom he calls the "childlike Varga girl in running shorts," attractive, but she is not tempted by the older man (Roth, 2006, pp. 130–34). This novel has the bleakness of the fifteenth-century *Everyman* with little of its religious overtones. *Exit Ghost* does not represent a swan song. Unlike Zuckerman, who suffers from prostate cancer and depression, Roth learned about the disease's horrors from his friends, not from his own experience (Weitzmann, 2007). Rather than despairing like his characters, Roth tells Hermione Lee in an interview that he has discarded Zuckerman and looks forward to finding out what character will next take his place (Lee, 2007). Perhaps writing about older men whose health problems are worse than his own keeps Roth cheerfully productive.

In contrast, Jane Gardam's *Old Filth* (2005) contains an extensive life review that heals an old wound. Sir Edward Feathers, known by colleagues as Old Filth, is a retired QC (Queen's Counsel) and a judge. He has spent most of his legal career in Hong Kong, where he was "said to have invented FILTH—Failed in London Try Hong Kong" (Gardam, 2005, p. 3). His legal colleagues describe him as a coelacanth, a prehistoric fish that was mistakenly thought to be extinct. To his surprise, Sir Edward's last years provide him with a complete reeducation.

Fortunately, the author's ironic sense of humor saves the novel from sentimentality or preachiness. Thanks to Feathers's ability to play a role, everyone misjudges the judge. In fact, Feathers, like Maryam, feels like an unwilling immigrant, still longing for British Malaya, his birthplace. Like most children of the Raj, Feathers was sent to London to be educated. Unfortunately, the household to which he was sent in Wales, along with two girl cousins, was ruled by a sadistic Welsh woman, Ma Didds. His situation is similar to Rudyard Kipling's childhood trauma, Gardam's inspiration for *Old Filth* (2005). A tragedy occurred about which nobody speaks, and Eddie is packed off to a boarding school to be educated. For many years Eddie appears to be cheerful, but after his wife dies, he visits his aging cousins.

The ideal life review that geriatric psychiatrist Robert Butler describes in *The Longevity Revolution* (2008) sounds like the one Sir Edward Feathers experiences. Reviewing one's life may be painful, Butler remarks, if one feels isolated. Many unhappy memories from childhood return to haunt people, but if they are lucky enough to find a way of resolving these old conflicts, they may be able to experience forgiveness and acquire a new sense of tranquility (Butler, 2008). Toward the novel's end, Sir Edward's cousin Babs, with her vicar in tow, visits Eddie, who is ailing. The vicar realizes that the two old people need to share their memories of Wales. Babs discovers that Eddie has blamed himself for Ma Didds's death, not knowing about her fatal cancer. Realizing that the two old people have carried the burden of pain and guilt for their murderous desires in silence for more than 70 years, Bab's vicar prays that God should comfort and heal the two sad cousins, whose lives have been so warped. Eddie feels so relieved to learn the truth that he is able to forgive the dead woman for her cruelty to the children. The serenity that Butler predicts allows Sir Edward to draw up a codicil to his will and depart for Malaysia, the place from which he had been so untimely ripped as a small child. Upon arrival, he dies suddenly and happily, having at last returned home. The lawyers in the Temple Garden hear the bell tolling for Sir Edward's death. Despite a monument inscribed with "*Lawyers, I suppose, were children once*" (Gardam, 2005, p. 257), they have no idea of the burden from which he had been relieved so soon before his death.

A Midlife Investigation and a Swan Song

Wish I Could Be There (2007), by Allen Shawn (b. 1948), and *All Will Be Well* (2006), by John McGahern (b. November 12, 1934), illustrate the difference between an account written in late middle age and a swan song. Sometime in his thirties, Shawn realized that he was agoraphobic. A friend encouraged him to write about phobia from the perspective of someone with the condition. Initially he felt shame "at the prospect of writing," but he also believed "it was a fear worth conquering." He did not attempt a memoir but limits himself "to the possible sources of my own psychological handicaps" (Shawn, 2007, p. xi). This restriction explains the parsimonious details about his emotions and his family life, even though he recognizes the importance of environment and heredity. He does discuss the trauma of having his retarded twin sister institutionalized (p. 97). Each time Shawn ventures into family history, he quickly turns the discussion to something in the medical literature. It is hard to avoid the thought that his discomfort might reflect the constrained environment in which he grew up. His father, who for many years was the editor of the *New Yorker*, conducted a long-term affair with Lillian Ross, a staff writer at the same magazine, but the world found out only some years after his death when Ross wrote about it. Mrs. Shawn knew of the relationship from the beginning, but her son was "almost thirty" before he learned of it (p. 36). Perhaps the etiology of Shawn's phobias is unknowable. At any rate, rather than blaming his upbringing or exploring his psyche, he diverts attention with stories of phobic individuals.

In contrast, John McGahern, who composed his memoir after receiving a diagnosis of cancer (Schudel, 2006), reveals how his upbringing shaped his adult life.

McGahern's mother tried hard to protect the children from the erratic behavior of her overbearing husband. Unfortunately, she died when McGahern was 9, leaving him and the other children at their father's mercy. Young Sean was devastated by his mother's death, but within a few weeks his father sought a replacement wife. It took him several years to find a willing woman, and in the meantime he continued his unpredictable ways, beating and berating the children at will. Education luckily provided Sean with an escape route. Less than one-third of the memoir covers the family's life after the children leave home. It ends abruptly with his father's death. McGahern sums up his mixed feelings about his father in a paragraph and then devotes the final page and a half to memories of his mother. The memoir ends there, having explained why he broke with the church and wrote novels that the clerics banned. He died March 20, 2006, a few months after the book appeared in the United States.

Some of the differences between Shawn's and McGahern's writing clearly have to do with the life stage that each had reached. Shawn was 59 when *Wish I Could Be There* was published. He has every reason to expect to live for many more years, too many to think of unburdening himself of his innermost thoughts and feelings. Moreover, his phobic temperament would make such revelations uncomfortable. On the other hand, McGahern began to compose his memoir knowing that he would die soon of cancer (Schudel, 2006). This memoir represents a leave taking, a last chance to memorialize his dead mother. He gave few interviews during his life, saying "Each of us has a private world, and the only difference between the reader and the writer is that the writer has the ability to describe and dramatize that private world. As a writer, I write to see. If I knew how it would end, I wouldn't write. It's a process of discovery" (Clarity, 2006). Because for the first time he knew how "it would end," he used his final work to reflect on his childhood and adolescence and to depict the influence of his mother and father on all the children in his family of origin as fairly as he could.

Resilience in Late-Life Memoirs

Three well-known authors, Aharon Appelfeld (b. February 16, 1932), Günter Grass (b. October 16, 1927), and John Hope Franklin (b. January 2, 1915), discovered early in life that writing provided a means of reinvention, "a strategy for maintaining self-respect" according to Cruikshank (2003, p. 22). All of them faced hardships, but creativity allowed them to transcend their struggles.

Holocaust survivor Aharon Appelfeld lost his parents at the age of 8. He managed to escape from a concentration camp and live in the forest by himself for several years, subsisting on water from streams and fruits that he picked. Talking put him at risk, for local people wanted to turn Jews in to the authorities. Unfortunately, his isolated wartime experiences made his postwar adjustment to life in Israel difficult. In the 1950s he tried to write about the war but found that his soul was caught up in the silence. Words became nearly impossible. He longed not to use speech to express emotion but to have feeling emerge from action. Writing novels, such as *Tzili* (1983), allowed him to explore his past at a remove. Tzili is a young girl considered by her relatives to be almost retarded, yet she survives wartime hardships that the author endured. In contrast to the novel, the chapters of his autobiography, *The Story of a Life* (2004), seem disconnected. Each contains separate memories of the past, and, as Appelfeld himself says, they do not provide a coherent narrative. Instead, the book represents an attempt to recapture memories, many of which Appelfeld had already used in his transcendent fiction.

Even after beginning to transform his life story into fiction, Appelfeld has continued to find it difficult to talk about the past without sounding banal. Words failed him, he thinks, because the past was recorded in his body, not in his mind. Writing fiction, however, allows him to reconstruct the atmosphere that he had absorbed wordlessly. This explanation helps to illuminate why the stories of horror that some survivors tell can seem flat, lacking in passion. Appelfeld's memoir does not teach directly about old age, but like an anthropological dig it uncovers the hidden child within. Paradoxically, although an act of writing, it illustrates the limits of words in coming to terms with trauma.

Just before publishing his memoir, *Peeling the Onion* (2007), German author Günter Grass admitted in an interview that he had been drafted into the Waffen SS, not the Wehrmacht.[4] Immediately his confession stirred considerable comment, even outrage (Agee, 2007). Many felt betrayed by Grass's previous silence. He had received the Nobel Prize for Literature in 1999, summarizing his military service in his acceptance speech as follows: "at fifteen I donned a uniform, at sixteen I learned what fear was, at seventeen I landed in an American POW camp" (Grass, 1999). Moreover, Grass had positioned himself as the conscience of contemporary Germany. He had kept silent for 60 years, he reports, because he felt shamed by his failure in youth to ask questions or to learn from those who resisted Nazi propaganda. Believing his country to need protection, he attempted to enlist in the submarine corps when he was 15. When at 16 he was assigned to the Waffen SS, he was not perturbed. He had not joined the SS youth group, but by 1944 the German military was desperate for conscripts.

In retrospect, the sad part is that shame kept Grass from unburdening himself earlier. His desire to serve his country was hardly unusual. For example, Hans J. Massaquoi, the son of a German nurse's aide and a Liberian playboy, as well as the grandson of a Liberian diplomat, was delighted when he received notice of his physical exam for Labor Service. During the war all fit young men had to be part of this unit before they were drafted into the Wehrmacht, the German army. To his horror, Massaquoi was rejected for any military service because he was of African descent, a rejection that troubled the young man considerably (Massaquoi, 2001). Moreover, in *Peeling the Onion*, Grass claimed never to have fired a shot. He survived, he recalls, only because of the help of a private first class, who later lost his legs and probably his life.

The memoir moves into the postwar period, describing how Grass managed to obtain an artistic education despite having almost no money. From an early age he had been fascinated by art, spending hours pouring over paintings he found on cigarette cards that his mother collected for him. Like prisoners in concentration camps who learned to scrounge food and other necessities, Grass became a remarkable organizer. Throughout his youth before he took up smoking, he would trade cigarettes for food and other useful items. The rest of the book explains how details from Grass's life, including his short stint in the SS, were converted into fiction.

Historian John Hope Franklin published his autobiography, *Mirror to America* (2005), when he was 90. He sought to remind Americans that the struggle for equality is not over. "The African American elder in the 1990s is a survivor," psychiatrist F. M. Baker reminds us. Even if blacks were reared in middle-class households with professional parents, beginning in childhood they become aware "of a negative evaluation of persons of African origin." Fortunately, Baker continues, "the elders' family, community, and church modeled effective ways of coping with racism" (Baker, 1998, p. 277).

Franklin's life seesawed between moments of great success, with assistance from blacks and whites alike, and painful and unreasonable rejections. Most of the memoir describes his education at Fisk and Harvard, the books he wrote, the universities in which he taught, and the important fellowships that he obtained. His productivity was truly remarkable, especially when one considers how many different courses he taught in the early days at African-American universities. As he himself acknowledges, he could not have achieved all that he did without the loving and active support of his wife, Aurelia, to whom he was married for nearly 60 years. Unfortunately, in 1990 Aurelia developed Alzheimer's disease, and after five years she had to be moved to a nursing home. Like many people Franklin was outraged when things began to disappear out of her closet. He is convinced that most of the thefts came from the underpaid staff (Franklin, 2005; Franklin, 2007, personal communication). After four years in the home, she died in 1999.

Most recently Franklin gave a speech at the inauguration of Drew Gilpin Faust as the first woman president of Harvard University (John Harvard's Journal, 2007). Drew Faust paid tribute to Franklin and his memoir depicting both his triumphs and his hardships; in his turn Franklin extolled her scholarship. The event made quite a homecoming for the distinguished speaker, one well deserved. Yet Franklin has had to face moments of prejudice, even in later life. In 1995 when giving a dinner for friends at the Cosmos Club, a woman mistook him for a servant and "ordered me to bring her coat" (Franklin, 2005, p. 340). If he could not escape from racism after writing many important books; serving on advisory boards to Presidents Carter and Clinton; being made president of the American Historical Association, the Organization of American Historians, the Southern Historical Association, and Phi Beta Kappa; and having been hired at white universities such as Brooklyn College and the University of Chicago when few African-Americans could find jobs, imagine the problems, he implies, that less active and less talented African-Americans might encounter. When he died on March 25, 2009, major newspapers carried his obituary and praised his long, successful career.

These three autobiographies represent different levels of success that memoirists can experience in their efforts to restore lost self-esteem through writing. Ironically, the force of the original threat does not predict the outcome in old age, at least in these three examples. Thanks to Hitler's efforts of extermination, Appelfeld lived a lonely and dangerous life throughout his childhood. Yet, his autobiography, written in his later sixties, is the most poetic of the three. He may have found it difficult to find words for his wartime experiences, but he has given readers many insights into his life, including both the misery of the war and the flowering of creativity that emerged from it.

In contrast, Grass's life was less traumatic, but he sounds as if he has missed an important opportunity in youth that no amount of writing can restore. He expresses regret in his memoir. For many years he composed novels that used his past indirectly. Now in his late seventies, he reflects on the bravery of his Uncle Franz, who defended the Polish post office against the German army and paid with his life. His parents never spoke of the uncle again, and the boy failed to ask them why or to question the worthiness of the Nazi regime. Like his parents who thought dismissing Uncle Franz's memory would make him disappear, throughout his active career Grass disguised his unhappy thoughts in his writing. "And as I clumsily interrogate and thereby clearly overtax the twelve-year-old" (who failed to ask the necessary questions), "I weigh each step I take in this fast-fading present, hear myself breathing, hear myself coughing, and live my way, as cheerfully as possible, toward death" (2007, p. 10).

Finally, the stories Franklin tells demonstrate how long lasting episodes of humiliation can be. Writing in his late eighties, he has not forgotten the legacy of unjust and humiliating treatment, the burden many African-Americans carry. Even during World War II, white Americans refused to allow him to enlist as a naval clerk, despite his Ph.D. and typing skills, solely because of his color (Franklin, 2005, p. 105). Franklin used hard work and scholarship to overcome his disadvantages, but no amount of recognition can eliminate memories of past injustice. He called his memoir

Mirror to America, hoping thereby to confront white Americans with the injustice of our society and the pain they have caused African-Americans.

Disability and Retirement

Disability is featured in *Memory Book* (2006), by Howard Engel (b. April 2, 1931), a Canadian writer of detective fiction. Sometime in 2001 Engel had a stroke that left him with alexia sine agraphia, a condition that Oliver Sacks reports allows him to write but not to read. Needless to say, writing became arduous, for Engel could not reread his drafts. As Sacks describes the process Engel underwent, "he decoded English print as if it was hieroglyphic." He also traced "the shapes of letters on the roof of his mouth" (Sacks, 2006, pp. 244–45). Benny Cooperman, Engel's detective, also suffers from alexia in the novel, caused by a blow to the head. Fortunately, a kind nurse gives Benny a notebook. She calls it a memory book, saying, "Let it become your memory. Let it help you" (Engel, 2005, p. 60). Unlike people who have Alzheimer's disease, for whom "the provision of memory aids and orientation procedures . . . is of only modest benefit" (Butler, 2008, p. 140), the memory book allows Benny to begin the task of reacquainting himself with the world around him. His descriptions of the hospital and the behavior of doctors and nurses reveal, as Sacks pointed out, that Engel had made good use of his time in rehabilitation, collecting stories of the patients and observing many social and linguistic interactions. The novel is compelling on its own terms, but doubly so when one considers how much effort Engel had to expend in its composition.

Another remarkable novelist struggling with disability was Minnesota author Jon Hassler (b. March 30, 1933). During the last 13 years Hassler suffered from progressive supranuclear palsy, which produces symptoms like Parkinson's. He had vision and speech problems. According to his wife, he could see but not move his eyes. He was wheelchair bound at the end but managed to keep writing with her help. According to obituaries, he completed a novel just before his death on March 20, 2008 (Williams, 2008).

From a relatively early age, Hassler had shown understanding of the emotional issues of aging, in particular retirement and self-esteem. For example, retirement in everyday life is often treated as primarily a financial question, and of course money plays an important role (see chapters on retirement in Butler, 2008 and Cruikshank, 2003). People are encouraged to put aside funds for their later life and to make decisions about their wills, trusts, powers of attorney, and medical directives. In reality, however, the prospect of ceasing to be employed frightens many people. Cruikshank observes that many retired people introduce themselves by their former occupation. This habit suggests "that the retirement role has limited meaning for them" (Cruikshank, 2003, p. 45). They fear the loss of companionship, meaningful activity, and their place in the world. Some cling to their jobs long past their useful-ness just to avoid loss of self-esteem, a problem Ron Manheimer has explored (2008). Also, according to psychoanalyst George Pollock (1998), retirement can cause a list of symptoms, including depression, anxiety, alcoholism, and paranoia.

When one considers the insensitive story American political journalist Michael Kingsley (b. March 9, 1951) tells in the *New Yorker*, it makes good sense to fear that retirement will represent a loss of status. He describes a time when he met a 90-year-old swimmer, who made the mistake of telling him not only his age but also the proud statement, "I used to be a judge." The younger assumed that the elder was boasting. Feeling intruded on, Kingsley decided that when the elder "was a judge—if he had been a judge—he had not felt the need to accost strangers and tell them that he was a judge." Insensitive to the old man's feelings, Kingsley reports, "And finally (I imag-ined, observing his face) came sadness: he had bungled a simple social interchange. So it must be true: he was past it" (Kingsley, 2008, p. 38).

Three weeks later, the man's grandson, Christopher Karachale, published a letter in the *New Yorker*. He chided Kingsley, not for his unkindness, but for assuming that his grandfather, who "had served for twenty years as a Los Angeles County Superior Court judge," would have judged one's life by longevity alone. Instead, the grandson declared, "he took pride in the length of his life not merely because of its length but because he was passionate about life and desired to teach others about the value of their own lives" (Karachale, 2008, p. 5). After reading both accounts, I'm convinced that the face of the proud old man showed despair at the negative reactions of Kingsley, not a fear that he was "past it."

Hassler, who wrote sensitively about a retired English professor in *Simon's Night* (1979), returned to the subject somewhat indirectly in his last novel, *The New Woman* (2005), published three years before his death. This narrative concentrates on aging, retirement, and the emotions. For many years Agatha McGee, the central hero of several of his novels, was an esteemed sixth-grade teacher and later principal of St. Isidore's. After her school was closed by the Catholic diocese, she felt a loss of respect from the community. Years pass and when at 87 her physical strength diminishes, regretfully she leaves her house for a sheltered apartment. Feeling ambivalent about the move, she returns home a week later. When her best friend, Lillian Kite, dies, she realizes how dependent she has been on her friend's willingness to do her household tasks. Fortunately, when she returns to the Sunset Senior Apartments, she discovers that her skills are still important even though she had stopped teaching 15 years before. In response to her great-nephew's threatened depression, she starts to lead a new support group, and in no time hundreds of members of the community join in. The novel ends with her recognition that founding and running the group have expanded her "range of motion" and provided her with "psychological therapy" (Hassler, 2005, p. 214). As Cruikshank puts it, "the long-lived whose talents have fully flowered show the rest of us something about human potential" (2003, p. 170). Agatha is such a vital character that when I heard of Hassler's death, my first regret was that I would never learn more about her.

Tony Hillerman (May 27, 1925–October 26, 2008) published *The Shape Shifter* (2006) when he was 81. He had previously published *Skeleton Man* (2004), in which retired Navajo policeman, Joe Leaphorn, turns the day-to-day detective work over to Jim Chee and Bernie Manuelito, who are young enough to descend into a canyon to find a missing diamond. In the earlier novel, Leaphorn acts like a Greek chorus, telling his retired friends about what happened and ultimately how Jim and Bernie solve the case. In *The Shape Shifter*, Leaphorn is the primary figure. Recently retired, he is attracted by the chance to solve an old cold case that doesn't involve climbing down canyons. This case turns out to be sufficiently demanding and draws on Hillerman's knowledge of the Vietnam conflict, a war that occurred when he was middle-aged. The novels Hillerman wrote in his late seventies and early eighties confront the threats to self-esteem that retired people experience. Joe Leaphorn is by no means delighted with his new status. Upon returning to the police headquarters he once ran, he is not recognized by the receptionist, even though he has been retired for only one month (Hillerman, 2006, p. 10). Nonetheless, he manages to use his contacts from earlier days and his famous intuition to solve a case that no one else even thought needed a solution. Hillerman is unusual in his understanding of the feelings of bereavement that retired people sometimes experience when their work life ceases. Nonetheless, Leaphorn, his elderly protagonist, finds vital ways of contributing to police work thanks to his memory of past cases and his understanding of his people's culture. Hillerman's style of writing is less emotionally intuitive than Hassler's, but his retired characters are convincing in the ways that they cope with their new status.

Caregiving

When disability is extreme, the person often needs full-time caregiving. In some instances, individuals are kept at home and family members try to meet their needs. *An Uncertain Inheritance* (Casey, 2007) consists of nonfiction essays written by those who have given care and a few who received it. Neither situation turns out to be easy. Those who care for family members often feel stressed to their limit and beyond. Dementia makes life particularly difficult, but helping a mother who resents her loss of independence can also be stressful. Cruikshank comments that caregiving can increase the conflict between mothers and daughters and create a new tension between the daughter's needs and her responsibilities (2003, p. 126). In a few cases described in the essays, the dying person ended life in a hospice or an assisted living facility, a decision that lifted some of the burden from the family. Some who needed to receive care discuss how difficult accepting help was for them; others discuss the unusual relationships that sometimes develop between caregiver and recipient (Fortini, 2007; Solomon, 2007). These essays are of great value because of their searing honesty. Too often, caregiving and receiving are treated in the literature as if they were bearable or even uplifting. This is not always the case. These essays explore a range of reactions that should illuminate readers.

A more irenic memoir by feminist author Alix Kates Shulman (b. August 17, 1932), *To Love What Is* (2008), describes the sometimes difficult but ultimately rewarding process of caring for her husband Scott York (b. January 25, 1929). Scott began to experience some memory loss in the 1990s after spending seven hours on a heart-lung machine to replace a valve destroyed by an aortic aneurysm. His memory was somewhat impaired, a condition made dramatically worse by his 2004 fall from a sleeping loft in Maine. For a year, Shulman fought hard to restore him to his previous condition. She stayed by his side endlessly, overseeing his therapy and seeking out possible treatments. Eventually she realized that she had to accept his new condition. Luckily for her, Scott sounds like a remarkable person. He makes intelligent and appropriate responses when she reads him her work in progress. On the whole he sounds like a loving, charming person. His dependency on her, however, made it difficult for her to have any time alone to write. Eventually she has found "Scott Watchers," people with whom he enjoys spending time while she works (2008, p. 134). As long as one of the watchers gives her five hours a day to write, she finds caring for Scott fulfilling. He has maintained his social skills although his short-term memory is defective. Sometimes to her surprise a recent event transfers from short- to long-term memory, allowing Scott to recall past pleasure. On the whole, however, he forgets moments from the recent past no matter how much he has enjoyed them. Luckily Shulman's love for Scott continues to sustain her despite his occasional outbursts of temper and frustration. Unlike the unhappy caregivers in *An Uncertain Inheritance*, Shulman finds that loving Scott gives pleasure to both of them. Perhaps sometime in the future Scott will need some kind of institutional care, but if that time should come, a friend of hers has remarked, "the women residents will start lining up for him" (2008, p. 177). Writing this memoir has allowed Shulman to share her story and receive positive responses from readers. In return we learn much about the brain and about the problems and satisfactions of caring for someone we love.

Hospice

Fortunately, hospice caregiving, in one's home or in a facility, is available for many dying people. Two nonfictional accounts explain how hospice works and why its care can be so rewarding to family members as well as the patients. When German scholar Nicholas Eschenbruch (b. 1972) began his fieldwork at what he called Stadtwald Hospice, he expected to learn how people die. Instead, he discovered that hospice workers make every effort to delay social death until the person's body gives out. He points out that people experience social death when they are isolated from the important people in their lives or are talked over as if they were not present. Once that stage has occurred, the person often is unable to engage in any meaningful life review (Eschenbruch, 2007).

Some people fear entering a hospice because doing so admits that death is imminent. One memoir, *Too Soon to Say Goodbye* (Buchwald, 2006c), should cheer them up. Art Buchwald (October 20, 1925–January 17, 2007) moved into a Washington hospice on February 7, 2006. His doctors told him his kidneys were failing, but he decided to forgo dialysis. He expected to die fairly quickly, but to everyone's surprise he was still alive months later. His survival was especially remarkable given his history of severe depression, about which he wrote openly (Buchwald, 2006a). In honor of his reprieve, he decided to write a final memoir. Most of his doctors attributed his survival to the remarkable attention that he received from his friends. Buchwald had not been forgotten before his kidneys failed, but at a gala celebration three weeks before his 80th birthday he complained that the *New York Times* had dropped his 50-year-old column from the *International Herald Tribune* (Buchwald, 2006c, p. 11). He published his first new syndicated column January 3, 2006 and continued publishing from his hospice room beginning March 7, reworking some of the material for his final memoir (Buchwald, 2006b). Eventually he left hospice and moved back in with his son. This narrative suggests that in special circumstances a stream of visitors and being able to see one's writing in print can boost the morale of a hospice patient to such an extent that his life is extended. For those of us less famous and talented than Buchwald, his story suggests that entering hospice may in some instances prolong life. Their caregivers believe in allowing patients to continue their life work. They seek methods to help those in their care to be true to their core selves. For instance, the willingness of the hospice staff to allow Buchwald to hold court in the lounge demonstrates Eschenbruch's contention that a primary goal of hospice is to do everything possible to keep patients happy and connected to their environment.

Fear of Death

What can make caregiving especially arduous is that some dying relatives have a pathological fear of dying. Those who worry about leaving children behind (Picardie, 2007), however, are generally less wearing than those who feel that they should be able to master death. Ironically, people who have in the past struggled with success to overcome illness sometimes turn out to be disruptive and angry at the end of their lives when all efforts are in vain. For example, Helen Schulman describes the last 10 years of her father's life as difficult, and "the last five were horrific" (Schulman, 2007, p. 1). His fear was so great that he told his daughter, "you and your love don't help me" (p. 3). As she pointed out, his illnesses were so hard to bear because "his whole life had been about tenacity. But he couldn't conquer death, could he?" (p. 7). As a result of his difficult emotional state, she found that taking care of her father gave "no rewards. There was only my father's compelling need, and my useless love for him" (p. 8).

David Rieff (b. September 28, 1952) has also written in *Swimming in a Sea of Death* (2008) of his miserable experience trying to help his mother, Susan Sontag (January 16, 1933–December 28, 2004), die with some shred of dignity. His ordeal began March 28, 2004, when his mother told him that one of her blood tests had indicated that something was wrong. Sontag had been diagnosed with breast cancer in 1975 and with uterine sarcoma in 1998. She had survived both by courage and determination. From the start of this final disease, her physician, Dr. A., told her that the condition was untreatable. He advised her to do nothing until her myelodysplastic syndrome (MDS) " 'converted' . . . into 'full-blown' AML, acute myeloid leukemia." Palliative drugs might relieve some of the pain, but the doctor did not advise a bone marrow transplant (Rieff, 2008, p. 9). Unfortunately, Sontag insisted on trying everything, including a bone marrow transplant, which failed. After great suffering, she died, leaving her son to feel guilty about his inability to help his mother effectively.

Much of the book is concentrated on the son's unhappy feelings. Rieff was convinced that he had to encourage his mother, indeed to lie to her, lest she have a mental collapse from her overwhelming fear of death. Throughout Sontag's final illness he says, "I found *myself* to be on emotional life support" (2008, p. 101) and inadequate to the task of giving her emotional aid. He wrote the memoir to sort out and confess his reactions rather than attempt to memorialize his mother. Unfortunately, by concentrating on Sontag's fears at the end of life and her difficult behavior, Rieff risks diminishing her status and reputation. Those who read this memoir may find that his portrayal replaces their memories of her remarkable work and impressive persona.

Nonetheless, one cannot help but wish that Sontag had known Irvin Yalom (b. June 13, 1931), emeritus professor of psychiatry, whose *Staring at the Sun* (2008) describes his treatment efforts to help patients recognize and overcome their fear of death. Repeatedly he reminds readers that "although the *physicality of death destroys us, the idea of death saves us*" (Yalom, 2008, p. 33). The purpose of his therapeutic approach is to help patients confront their fears and discover compensating thoughts that help them minimize their despair. Yalom sounds like a compassionate and helpful therapist, but unlike most of his patients, Sontag was too ill to enter therapy. Moreover, Sontag believed that she had cheated death in the past by her own efforts. Like Helen Schulman's father, Sontag wanted to fight death despite the cost. Her efforts at self-reliance caused her to place an emotional demand on her son. As a result, a few years after she died, he still finds it difficult to mourn his mother.

Mourning and Memorializing the Dead

One novel and three memoirs provide good examples that reveal different ways of mourning and memorializing the dead. As psychoanalyst George Pollock says, "individuals may have different *significances* for each other at various periods of adult life" (1998, p. 44). Therefore, much depends on the relationship of the authors with the dead person, the ages of the writers, the length of time of the final illnesses, and the time elapsed since the death occurred. For example, *About Alice* (2006), Calvin Trillin's (b. December 5, 1935) account of his wife's death, is relatively positive when compared to Rieff's recollections. Of course, Rieff was 17 years younger than Trillin and full of ambivalent feelings about his mother.

In contrast, Trillin's marriage to Alice (May 8, 1938–September 11, 2001) had been happy, and he wrote the memoir as a tribute to his beloved so that readers would know what she was like. Alice died the evening that the World Trade Center was destroyed. Trillin, a journalist on the staff of the *New Yorker*, had consistently regarded her as his muse and editor. Alice's history of illness has much in common with Sontag's. Alice developed cancer at 38; Sontag was 42. Both were given little chance to beat the odds. The year Alice died, she underwent bypass surgery because the radiation she endured to cure the cancer had damaged her heart. Sontag developed myelodysplastic syndrome, "a lethal kind of blood cancer" in 2004, a few months before she died (Rieff, 2008, pp. 6–7). Alice, however, had set an achievable specific goal; she wanted to see both daughters married. Calvin Trillin thinks that she accepted "a deal that allowed her to see her girls grow up." He reports attempting to feel as lucky as Alice did. He concludes, "Some days I can and some days I can't." Unfortunately for Sontag and Rieff, Sontag was not "the incorrigible and ridiculous optimist" that Alice was (Trillin, 2006, p. 78). As a result of their different temperaments, their survivors are left in very different emotional states. In contrast to Rieff's portrait of his difficult mother, readers will find Trillin's portrayal of Alice to be touching.

English novelist Penelope Lively (b. March 17, 1933) used the conventions of the family saga in the novel *Consequences* (2007) as a means of memorializing her late husband. She describes three generations of an English family whose members experience love and loss. Because Lively herself has had considerable experiences with both conditions—she lost her husband of 41 years in 1998, but has two children and six grandchildren—it is not surprising that she sees family life as a continuum. The novel illustrates a pattern of contingencies, a combination of fortuitous events and tragedies with one event leading to another, much like her own life.

Lively's novel begins with an unexpected meeting of two young people from different social strata. Lively declares in an earlier memoir (2001) that meeting one's spouse depends on good fortune. She herself had grown up in Egypt in considerable comfort. After the war she was sent to England at 12, following her parents' divorce. The uprooting was traumatic partly because Lively's Egyptian upbringing had not prepared her for understanding the unwritten rules of British social mores. As a result she felt like an outsider in school, as if she were in permanent exile (Lively, 1994). She met her husband at Oxford but was aware how fortuitous their meeting was. Had it not been for the war, Jack Lively would not have attended Cambridge and Oxford, where he met Penelope. He was evacuated to a farm where the farmer's wife recognized his intelligence. She tutored him so that he was able to enter a grammar school, the only school that would prepare poor children for a university (Lively, 2001). In the prewar period the two would not have encountered each other because few women and few working-class men went to Oxford or Cambridge.

Given the dependence of the plot of *Consequences* on chance, what ties these episodes together is that the events are firmly rooted in places, primarily Somerset and London, the natal places of the author's mother and father (Lively, 1994). The first generation is the shortest lived, but what happens to them continues to influence their children and grandchildren for years to come. All of these female protagonists are single mothers for a time. Luckily the women are competent managers and are able to support their offspring until they are fortunate enough to find a new lover at midlife. Lively manages to balance the losses and grief, which are heartfelt, with unexpected moments of joy. Just when one thinks that the characters have passed their prime, they unexpectedly find someone to love who loves them. In this novel, resilience and remarkable creativity are family traits, ones that Lively's writing suggests characterize her own life.

The next two memoirs are written by daughters whose relatives have died. Haitian American novelist Edwidge Danticat's (b. January 19, 1969) memoir, *Brother, I'm Dying* (2007), describes the last days of her father and uncle. She was especially close to her uncle because her parents had been forced to leave their children behind for eight years in order to get visitor visas for their initial trip to the United States. They had no legal status until they had another child born there. Despite the traumatic separation, the children were well taken care of by their father's oldest brother, Joseph, and his wife. Luckily, they made loving parental substitutes, and the children did not suffer the kind of misery Eddie Feathers and his girl cousins had experienced at the hands of Ma Didds (Gardam, 2005).

The health of both father and uncle failed about the same time. At 69 her father suffered from idiopathic pulmonary fibrosis, an untreatable and incurable disease of the lungs. Her uncle, who had been operated on for cancer of the larynx, was forced to leave Haiti to escape marauding gangs. They held the old pastor responsible for some deaths that U.N. troops had inflicted on their members. Unfortunately, Uncle Joseph made the mistake of requesting temporary asylum of the U.S. customs agents, who promptly sent the 81-year-old man to Krome detention center, where he died after being treated incompetently and inhumanely. The memoir continues with the birth of Mira, Danticat's daughter, who was named for the author's dying father. It ends with his death. At its conclusion, Danticat imagines her father and uncle walking peacefully together in Haiti, having escaped from their shared grave site in Queens. It is an idyllic and peaceful scene, one that the two old men deserve after their ordeals. Not surprisingly the memoir won the 2007 National Book Critics Circle Award for autobiography. It was short-listed for the 2007 National Book Award for nonfiction.

Several things make this memoir outstanding. Besides the beauty of her writing, Danticat reveals a sensitive understanding of her elders, both her parents in New York and her uncle and aunt in Haiti. Although she had been left behind in Haiti for many years, she converted the painful separation into a source of creativity. She expresses affection and love for all her relatives, the uncle who protected and cared for her, and the parents who loved her deeply. Moreover, she reveals determination in her efforts to uncover the incompetent medical treatment her uncle received while in U.S. custody. Prying information out of the unwilling federal agency took a great deal of time. She was assisted by the Florida Immigrant Advocacy Center, whose "legal action and extremely persistent Freedom of Information Act requests" helped her find out under what circumstances her uncle died so soon after entering U.S. custody (Danticat, 2007, p. 271). She wrote about all this painful material in luminous prose, somehow keeping her justifiable anger under control. On May 5, 2008, about a year after her memoir was published, a front-page story in the *New York Times* revealed that 66 people had died "in immigration custody from January 2004 to November 2007" (Bernstein, 2008, p. A1). The *Times* listed the 66 names on a Web site,[5] and on page 2 of that list, Joseph Dantica's name appeared.[6] The other detainees had also received incompetent medical care, and their families were not adequately notified about their fate even after repeated questions. On May 11, 2008, the *Washington Post* started a series on the detainee deaths and also included Dantica's story (Priest and Goldstein, 2008).

American memorist and MacArthur Fellow Patricia Hampl's (b. 1946) *The Florist's*

Daughter (2007) describes the lives and deaths of her parents. Like Danticat's family, Hampl's parents were embedded in their place of birth, in their case St. Paul, Minnesota, a place much safer than Haiti and from which they were not exiled. In fact, Hampl feels that she must apologize for her decision to remain in St. Paul despite her adolescent desire to flee, following the example of the city's famous son, F. Scott Fitzgerald.

Hampl devotes attention to the differences between her parents' characters. Her Irish mother she calls both Leo the Lion, after her astrological sign, and the Archivist. Late in life her mother confides that she would have preferred to be a writer rather than a file clerk in a library, but she lacked her daughter's education. She had a critical eye and often was capable of fierce reactions. She encouraged her daughter's reading and studying, characteristics Hampl claims are Irish. In contrast, her Czech father, the florist, had an artistic temperament. Moreover, he insisted on believing that people were good at heart, a conviction that made him easy to cheat. Although he was a practicing Catholic, he permitted his male floral designers to wear eye shadow, angora sweaters, and make up. They were forgiven their louche ways for the sake of their art. As a young girl, Hampl spent much time in the shop her father managed and obviously enjoyed herself observing its denizens.

In old age Hampl's parents, like Danticat's father and uncle, had increasingly severe medical problems. Hampl's father had heart disease. Her mother had some small strokes and eventually developed dementia. The two of them reacted to their declining health in different ways. Hampl's gentle father was the ideal patient, one who never complained. In contrast, her mother fought bitterly against her decline and often against those who tried to assist her. For some time Hampl wondered which parent would go first, but ultimately her father died of a heart attack, leaving his ailing frail wife behind.

Hampl's parents could not feel like pioneers when they were old. They may have felt like adolescents, but according to their daughter old age had few positive features for them. On the other hand, Hampl herself drew closer to both parents as they became frailer. Her father discarded his submissive attitude near the end of his life. On the last visit, his cardiologist told him that he could obtain hospice care for the dying man. Instead of acquiescing, Hampl's father went out and bought a new Buick. This was surely rash, but it gave him a sense of control over what was left of his life. After her father's death, Hampl's mother went into a nursing home. Fortunately, Hampl found visiting her to be fascinating rather than a chore to be abhorred. Her mother chatted away cheerfully, making little sense, but smiling a sweet smile, one that the daughter found attractive. Because her mother remained a lively, unpredictable person, her last days resembled the shipboard trip she thought she was taking. Even though she was trapped in a declining body, for some reason her imagination was unleashed, making her last days a remarkable and timely adventure for her daughter and herself. Most remarkable is Hampl's portrayal of the last years of her parents as rewarding and often funny. Many daughters would resent the amount of time and attention that her parents needed so desperately. Instead, Hampl wrote about her caregiving with affection and humor, showing respect for and understanding of her frail and sometimes exasperating parents.

In contrast to the two memoirs written by daughters, American writer Joan Didion's (b. December 3, 1934) memoir, *The Year of Magical Thinking* (2005), covers the first year after the unexpected death of her husband, John Gregory Dunne (b. May 25, 1932), on December 30, 2003. Although a quick death can spare the dying person a long and painful illness, such a death is often hard on family members. Moreover, even though the individual may have an inkling of his or her demise, even those close to that person rarely do. Didion describes the day of her husband's death as "ordinary," but surely that is an exaggeration. Five days before, on Christmas Day, their daughter, Quintana Roo Dunne, fell ill with what seemed to be flu but quickly changed into a life-threatening illness. Didion and her husband had just returned from visiting their comatose daughter in her hospital room when he had a fatal heart attack.

Few people suffer at the same time the death of a husband and the serious illness of a child. Given Didion's career as an author, it is not surprising that she turned to writing about her husband, daughter, and herself, roughly 10 months after her child's hospitalization and her husband's death. The author's magical thinking consisted of refusing to admit that he was dead. As a result, Didion reports that she kept refusing to get rid of all of her husband's shoes, lest he need them upon return. In March, when her daughter went into a coma again in Los Angeles, Didion moved out there and visited every day. Like Edwidge Danticat, who managed to get all the details of her uncle's incarceration by repeatedly filing Freedom of Information Act requests, Joan Didion studied medical books in order to understand what was happening to her daughter and to reduce her grief. She hoped to understand all that the doctors said and implied by their jargon. This education helped her ward off memories of John and feelings of guilt, the "if only" syndrome that worries survivors who are suffering from traumatic events.

When Quintana appeared to be recovering and eventually went home to her husband, Didion began to mourn rather than grieve as she had done so far. Grief, she reports, is something that happens to the bereaved. Mourning occurs when the individual begins to react to grief. At the memoir's end her daughter appears to be doing well, but sadly not for long. The daughter died August 26, 2005, shortly before the book was published. When asked if she wanted to add a section on Quintana's death, Didion stoically refused to tamper with the ending (McKinley, 2005). Didion's writing offers insight into how we grieve, mourn, and survive, changed forever but still able to record these life events. It won the National Book Award for nonfiction, a well-deserved prize.

Medical Reeducation

In recent years, physicians such as Jerome Groopman (b. 1952) and Pauline Chen (b. 1964) have written several books about the necessity of recognizing in their practice human emotions, their own and that of their patients. In *The Measure of Our Days* (1997), Groopman describes how in 1979 his suffering from a severe back injury taught him how patients feel, a lesson that has stayed with him. Because of his religious beliefs, he does not hesitate to invoke concepts of the soul. In fact, he notes that his training, while technically useful, had failed to prepare him for understanding his patients' emotional states. In one important case, which Groopman describes in *The Anatomy of Hope* (2004), a young woman had ignored signs of breast cancer because she thought God was punishing her for having an affair. Ultimately, her attending physician convinced her to have chemotherapy, but it was too late. Unfortunately, the attending physician did not discuss how he convinced the recalcitrant patient to cooperate, but in retrospect Groopman claims that he was too young to have understood the case in all of its ramifications. In his most recent book, *How Doctors Think* (2007), Groopman writes to educate patients so that they can assist in caring for themselves.

Pauline Chen in *Final Exam* (2007) describes how medical training failed to prepare her for understanding her patients' emotions and needs. Like Groopman, as a young doctor she also lacked insight, partly because her surgical training emphasized techniques, not the need to be aware of the feelings of those on whom she operated. Chen recalls avoiding giving patients bad news. She became an expert on leaving the room quickly and busying herself with paperwork to avoid painful confrontations. Luckily, she learned new ways of behaving from one compassionate attending physician who stayed with a woman as her husband was nearing his end. His example did not keep her from avoiding dying people for many years, but in time her patients and taking a writing course taught her to be more helpful. Like Groopman, she hopes that her book will encourage physicians and programs to change.

Conclusion

These novels and memoirs reveal that, as the population ages and medical care improves, more people will continue writing into old age. In the future we can expect more authors to give us their views on aging from a variety of compelling perspectives.

Any of these works could become part of the training of gerontologists and geriatricians, depending on the needs of the courses in question. First, the novels present what could be case histories of elders. Many of their characters learn to use their later life to overcome earlier trauma or mistakes made when they were young. Second, the memoirs reveal how important being able to explain themselves to an audience can be for those facing death or mourning the loss of relatives. Finally, the secondary literature, the third element, allows students to compare the particulars of vibrant literature and personal recollections to the generalizations of research in the field. By combining these three sources, students can learn to empathize about situations they have not yet faced in their own lives.

NOTES

1. In an essay on the Brentano Quartet's concerts on late style, Alex Ross complains that Theodor Adorno's essay on late style in Beethoven cannot be applied to other compositions that are more radiant (Ross, 2008, p. 82).

2. Morton's novel features a 71-year-old novelist named Leonard Schiller, whose books are out of print and who has been attempting to complete another work for the past 10 years. Although Schiller is the lynchpin of the plot, much of Morton's attention is concentrated on Heather Wolfe, a young scholar, Ariel Schiller, his 40-year-old daughter, and her lover, Casey Davis. Although Morton shows respect for Schiller's urgent desire to complete his novel, his heart is with the attempts of Ariel and Casey to create a new life together.

3. Even some writers of comics realize how fanciful memoir writing can be. Wiley Miller (b. 1951) shows the difference between reality and memoir writing. An elderly wife with her hair in curlers brings a cup of coffee to her equally unattractive husband, who writes, "Then, out of the ugliness of war, a stunning vision of beauty stood before me" (Miller, 2008).

4. According to *Wikipedia* (accessed May 5, 2009; http://en.wikipedia.org/wiki/G%C3 %BCnter_Grass), reference to the interview appeared in *Zeit Online* (August 17, 2006). In November 2007, Grass instituted a lawsuit against Random House for a statement in a new biography in which Michael Jürgs claims that Grass "willingly joined the Waffen SS" (Edidin, 2007, p. A20).

5. Available at http://graphics8.nytimes.com/packages/pdf/nyregion/ICE_FOIA.pdf.

6. Nina Bernstein and Margot Williams (2008) discuss the detainee deaths and publish the Immigration and Customs Enforcement list (n.d.).

REFERENCES

Agee, J. 2007. The good German. Review of Günter Grass's "The Peeling Onion." *Washington Post, Book World*, July 8, BW04–05.

Appelfeld, A. 1983. *Tzili: The story of a life*. Trans. D. Bilu. New York: E. P. Dutton.

———. 2004. *The Story of a Life*. Trans. A. Halter. New York: Schocken Books.

Atkin, S., and A. Atkin. 1992. On being old (A psychoanalyst's new world). In *How Psychiatrists Look at Aging*, ed. G. H. Pollock. Madison: International Universities Press.

Baker, F. M. 1998. The African American elder. In *The Course of Life, Volume VII: Completing the journey*, ed. G. H. Pollock and S. I. Greenspan. Madison: International Universities Press.

Bernstein, N. 2008. Few details on immigrants who died in U.S. custody. *New York Times (Washington edition)*, May 5, pp. A1, A18.

Bernstein, N., and M. Williams. 2008. Immigration agency's list of deaths in custody. *New York Times*, www.nytimes.com/2008/05/05/nyregion/05detain-list.html?ref=nyregion.

Buchwald, A. 2006a. The art of darkness. *Washington Post (Maryland edition)*, January 3, p. C03.

———. 2006b. Having a high time where you'd least expect it. *Washington Post (Maryland edition)*, March 7, p. C03.

———. 2006c. *Too Soon to Say Goodbye*. New York: Random House.

Butler, R. N. 2008. *The Longevity Revolution: The benefits and challenges of living a long life*. New York: Public Affairs.

Casey, N., ed. 2007. *An Uncertain Inheritance: Writers on caring for family*. New York: William Morrow.

Chen, P. W. 2007. *Final Exam: A surgeon's reflections on mortality*. New York: Alfred A. Knopf.

Clarity, J. F. 2006. John McGahern, chronicler of Irish rural life, dies at 71. *New York Times*, www.nytimes.com/2006/03/31/books/31mcgahern.html?pagewanted=print.

Clowser, V. L. 1992. Aging in a mirror. In *How Psychiatrists Look at Aging*, ed. G. H. Pollock. Madison: International University Press.

Cruikshank, M. 2003. *Learning to Be Old: Gender, culture, and aging*. Lanham: Rowman & Littlefield Publishers.

Danticat, E. 2007. *Brother, I'm Dying*. New York: Alfred A. Knopf.

Didion, J. 2005. *The Year of Magical Thinking*. New York: Alfred A. Knopf.

Drabble, M. 1975. *The Realms of Gold*. New York: Popular Library.

———. 2006. *The Sea Lady: A late romance*. Orlando: Harcourt.

Edidin, P., compiler 2007. Nobel laureate sues publisher. *New York Times (national edition)*, November 24, p. A20.

Engel, H. 2005. *Memory Book*. New York: Carroll & Graf Publishers.

Eschenbruch, N. 2007. *Nursing Stories: Life and death in a German hospice*. New York: Berghahn Books.

Forster, E. M. 1927. *Aspects of the Novel*. London: Edward Arnold.

Fortini, A. 2007. The vital role. In *An Uncertain Inheritance: Writers on caring for family*, ed. N. Casey. New York: William Morrow.

Franklin, J. H. 2005. *Mirror to America: The autobiography of John Hope Franklin*. New York: Farrar, Straus, and Giroux.

Gardam, J. 2005. *Old Filth*. London: Abacus.

Grass, G. 1999. Nobel Lecture: "To Be Continued . . . ," http://nobelprize.org/nobel_prizes/literature/laureates/1999/lecture-e.html.

———. 2007. *Peeling the Onion*. Trans. M. H. Heim. Orlando: Harcourt.

Groopman, J. 1997. *The Measure of Our Days: A spiritual exploration of illness*. New York: Viking Penguin.

———. 2004. *The Anatomy of Hope: How people prevail in the face of illness*. New York: Random House.

———. 2007. *How Doctors Think*. Boston: Houghton Mifflin Company.

Hampl, P. 2007. *The Florist's Daughter*. Orlando: Harcourt.

Hassler, J. 1979. *Simon's Night*. New York: Atheneum.

———. 2005. *The New Woman*. New York: Viking.

Hillerman, T. 2004. *Skeleton Man*. New York: HarperCollins.

———. 2006. *The Shape Shifter*. New York: HarperCollins.

Hurwitz, M. H. 1992. A psychoanalyst retires. In *How Psychiatrists Look at Aging*, ed. G. H. Pollock. Madison: International Universities Press.

John Harvard's Journal. 2007. Twenty-eighth, and first. *Harvard Magazine*, November–December, pp. 54–59.

Karachale, C. A. 2008. A long life. *New Yorker*, April 28, p. 5.

Kingsley, M. 2008. Mine is longer than yours. *New Yorker*, April 7, pp. 38–42.

Lee, H. 2007. Age makes a difference. *New Yorker*, October 7, pp. 56–62.

Lively, P. 1994. *Oleander, Jacaranda: A childhood perceived: A memoir*. New York: HarperCollins.

———. 2001. *A House Unlocked*. New York: Grove Press.

———. 2007. *Consequences*. New York: Viking.

Manheimer, R. 2008. The paradox of beneficial retirement: A journey into the vortex of nothingness. *Journal of Aging, Humanities, and the Arts* 2 (2):84–98.

Massaquoi, H. J. 2001. *Destined to Witness: Growing up black in Nazi Germany*. New York: Perennial.

McGahern, J. 2005. *All Will Be Well: A memoir*. New York: Alfred A. Knopf.

McKinley, J. 2005. Joan Didion's new book faces tragedy. *New York Times*, www.nytimes.com/2005/08/29/books/29didi.html?pagewanted=print.

Miller, W. 2008. Non sequitur. *The Sun*, May 11.

Morton, B. 1998. *Starting Out in the Evening*. New York: Crown Publishers.

Picardie, J. 2007. Ruth. In *An Uncertain Inheritance: Writers on caring for family*, ed. N. Casey. New York: William Morrow.

Pollock, G. H. 1998. Aging or aged: Development or pathology. In *The Course of Life: Volume VII: Completing the journey*, ed. G. H. Pollock and S. I. Greenspan. Madison: International Universities Press.

Priest, D., and A. Goldstein. 2008. System of neglect. *Washington Post*, May 11, pp. A1, A8–A10.

Rieff, D. 2008. *Swimming in a Sea of Death: A son's memoir*. New York: Simon & Schuster.

Rooke, C. 1992. Old age in contemporary fiction: A new paradigm of hope. In *Handbook of the Humanities and Aging*, ed. T. R. Cole, D. D. Van Tassel, and R. Kastenbaum. New York: Springer.

Ross, A. 2008. End notes. *New Yorker*, May 5, pp. 82–83.

Roth, P. 2006. *Everyman*. Boston: Houghton Mifflin.

———. 2007. *Exit Ghost*. Boston: Houghton Mifflin.

Sacks, O. 2006. Afterword. In *Memory Book*. New York: Carroll & Graf Publishers.

Said, E. W. 2006. *On Late Style: Music and literature against the grain*. New York: Pantheon Books.

Schillinger, L. 2006. The accidental friendship. *New York Times Book Review*, May 21, p. 14.

Schudel, M. 2006. Celebrated Irish novelist John McGahern, 71. *Washington Post*, April 1, p. B06.

Schulman, H. 2007. My father the garbage head. In *An Uncertain Inheritance: Writers on caring for family*, ed. N. Casey. New York: William Morrow.

Shawn, A. 2007. *Wish I Could Be There: Notes from a phobic life*. New York: Viking.

Shulman, A. K. 2008. *To Love What Is: A marriage transformed*. New York: Farrar, Straus, and Giroux.

Solomon, A. 2007. Notes on accepting care. In *An Uncertain Inheritance: Writers on caring for family*, ed. N. Casey. New York: William Morrow.

Trillin, C. 2006. *About Alice*. New York: Random House.

Tyler, A. 2006. *Digging to America*. New York: Alfred A. Knopf.

Weitzmann, M. 2007. In conversation with . . . Phillip Roth. *Washington Post*, September 30, p. BW11.

Williams, S. T. 2008. Jon Hassler, beloved Minnesota novelist, dead at 74. *Star Tribune*, www.startribune.com/entertainment/books/16855736.html.

Yalom, I. D. 2008. *Staring at the Sun: Overcoming the terror of death*. San Francisco: Jossey-Bass.

CHAPTER THREE

Literary Texts and Literary Critics Team Up against Ageism

BARBARA FREY WAXMAN, PH.D.

Literary texts not only entertain, not only reflect the society in which they are produced, but also are capable of changing people's attitudes and politics, of influencing the world. Literature has this capacity because, as Steven Lynn explains, "Inhabiting a literary work, we can see how other people live; we can see, to a certain extent, through other people's eyes. We can momentarily transcend the boundaries of our lives" (Lynn, 2008, pp. 3–4). Literature can take us out of ourselves and our usual settings, making us more conscious of our unexamined beliefs and assumptions and giving us new food for thought. Literary criticism, also known as critical theory, guides less-experienced readers in how to inhabit a text more fully, how to interpret a text more deeply, and how to grasp the ways in which the meanings of a text are created. Hence, literary criticism is "concerned with those ideas that are essential to the process of making skilled judgments about literature" (p. 10); it is the activity of interpreting the meanings of a literary text while analyzing how the elements of that text work together to convey those meanings. As literary critics work to figure out and articulate a text's significance, often they consider how the author's biography influences our reading of a text, how the text's cultural and historical context helps to shape its meanings, particularly for readers of different time periods, and the ways in which all sorts of readers interact with texts to create their meanings.

Of great interest to many literary critics are the types of readers that the author probably had in mind when writing, readers whose identities and situations are, in turn, reflected in the language of the text itself. What educational background did the author expect the reader to have? Does the text assume some specialized knowledge among its readers, or does the text define terms and obscure references so that the text becomes readily accessible to the general reader? To what kinds of audiences, with what kinds of memberships in a particular age group, race, gender, ethnicity, or socioeconomic class, is the text addressed? How do specific textual elements shape readers' responses? These are the questions or issues literary critics usually grapple with in order to come up with a profile of the text's "implied reader"; the implied reader is defined by Steven Lynn as "a fiction, a composite of lots of real readers" (Lynn, 2008, p. 103). To anticipate and describe the response of this implied reader to a text is a significant part of the work of many literary critics, especially those known as "reader-response critics." Also among these critics are literary gerontologists, scholars who study aging through literary texts. Literary gerontologists seek and examine literature (fiction, nonfiction, poetry, and drama) that prominently depicts older characters and that develops themes, settings, and plots about later life. I write this chapter as both a literary gerontologist and a reader-response critic.

As a literary gerontologist, I take up the issue of the implied reader here because it is central to reader-response criticism and because this kind of literary criticism offers a useful way to expose and challenge the ageism in literary texts that reflect societal prejudices against the old; to make some readers aware of ambivalent attitudes they harbor toward elders and their own anxieties about later life, by anticipating and articulating these readers' complex reactions to literary elders; and to deepen readers' awareness of literary texts that portray alternative versions of old age or other ways of performing "elderhood." My role as a reader-response critic vis-à-vis literary gerontology is to show all kinds of readers the step-by-step process of their interaction with a literary text about later life, the process of making sense of the text, the process of anticipating meaning and noticing both where the text surprises and where the text fulfills readers' expectations, especially about older characters and events associated with later life. I do not assume that readers will know what makes them react to a text in a particular way because linguistic manipulations can be subtle, so I want to point out how passages in a text ordinarily will elicit reactions from readers, as, for example, when a literary old man falls in love with a literary old woman and the couple interact sexually; to name readers' reactions to this behavior; and to show readers how the text is manipulating them to think or feel a certain way about these elderly characters or to react with approval or disapproval to an event in these characters' lives.

Through the tools of reader-response criticism, then, I want to raise readers' consciousnesses not only about textual manipulation but also about the assumptions and cultural and personal baggage about old age that they bring to the process of reading these texts about aging; they need to know how this baggage shapes their interpretations. While it is true that literary critics may not always reach a wide readership, literary critics who are also examining pressing social issues embedded in literature, such as that of adult children caring for elderly parents, may be able to capture a wider audience and have more of an impact on how people read—and how they afterward might behave, thereby revealing how texts work to initiate cultural change.

But we still need to answer more specifically, who is the implied reader of these literary texts about elders and old age? Usually these literary works are accessible to general readers without expertise in issues of aging. The texts will supply background and explanation of gerontological issues. Additionally, some readers will bring experiences with elderly parents or other relatives to the reading of these literary texts. On the other hand, it is also likely that general readers will bring to their reading of these texts the ageist biases of our society: disgust for bodily deterioration associated with growing old, the tendency to treat elders as if they are invisible or less than human, the inclination to behave with comic derision toward elders who do not "act their age" or who are forgetful and disoriented. Readers unconsciously "armed" against old people might be less receptive to sympathetic portrayals of elderly bachelors and widows or of creative self-discoveries in later life. Both authors and reader-response literary critics will need to make readers aware of this potential hostility to literature about elders and old age. Stronger, more evocative language, more dramatic scenarios, and vivid, realistic dialogue between elders and others are required to break down these barriers to receptivity to literary elders and positive portrayals of later life.

Yet I also imagine that these texts are addressed to another sort of implied reader: one who has additional knowledge, experience, or curiosity about aging; that means readers who are older, readers who are closely involved with elderly parents or other older relatives (especially those who may act as their caregivers), readers who work with the old, gerontology students, gerontology professors, and gerontologists. These more specialized readers may still harbor ageist attitudes, but they are less likely to do so. They are more likely to be receptive to literature about aging because they are in tune with its goals to resist ageism, and they may be eager to embrace this literature as a learning tool for general readers and for students. Literary critics and literary gerontologists aim to assist these specialized readers—gerontologists and others—to appreciate the power of literary texts to raise important issues of aging, to humanize elders, and to envision new versions of old age. Readers who care about the literature of aging, who want to delve deeper into its subtler messages and to understand why or how particular texts create such an emotional response in them, will turn to literary critics to find out. Gerontologists familiar with the objective language of case studies about elderly people in the social sciences will inevitably contrast these to literary portrayals of elders; reader-response critics will show gerontologists how the language of literature, ordinarily more intimate and evocative, is capable of profoundly changing peoples' minds.

Founding mother of reader-response criticism Louise Rosenblatt expresses well how literature, by actively engaging readers' imaginations so that they will identify with characters from all walks of life, is a force for change in readers; literary critics can augment literature's power by modeling and encouraging this kind of active reading: "When there is active participation in literature . . . [we develop] the ability to escape from the limitations of time and place and environment, the capacity to envisage alternatives in ways of life and in moral and social choices, the sensitivity to thought and feeling and needs of other personalities" (Rosenblatt, 1983, pp. 290–91). Literary gerontologist Kathleen Woodward also has examined how reading literature may be "an act of imaginative identification which may lead to understanding of the experience of old age" (1991, p. 13). Woodward also cites the reading theories of Hans Robert Jauss, especially his notion of a reader's "horizon of expectations," in which the reader's previous experiences and memories, in this case concerning her own aging or that of parents and friends, may prompt her reconnection with texts of aging read in the past and may affect her current and future reactions to literary texts about later life (p. 14).

Raman Selden usefully sees a reader's "horizon of expectations" in terms of that reader's cultural and historical context, with the values, beliefs, and literary conventions of that era providing the framework for the reading response (1989, p. 122). Hence, if an old man portrayed in fiction is, for example, expected by contemporary readers to act like the conventional character known as the "dirty old man" who is motivated by uncontrolled and inappropriate desire, these readers will be surprised by a new literary version of the virile old man and react to textual cues in the character portrayal that deviate from the stereotype. In the process of figuring out the meanings of the text and identifying with the new kind of elder, the reader's horizon of expectations will be adjusted. The reader will be enabled to imagine a sexually vital and emotionally vibrant aged person. Thus, cultural work is being done by the negotiations between the reader and the text. In Rosenblatt's words, "The evocation of a work of art is itself a form of experience in the real world, one that can be related to the other forms of experience. Sometimes what has been lived through is felt to be a version of the real, as in naturalistic fiction. Sometimes it is felt as an escape from it, an experiencing of alternative possibilities" (Rosenblatt, 1994, p. 32). This is the sort of reading experience that does the cultural work of challenging ageism, and reader-response critics help to intensify such an experience for less-experienced readers.

Sometimes ageism is coupled with sexism in literary portrayals of elderly men and elderly women—portrayals of elderly women in particular, I would argue. Women in our youth-worshipping culture are often thought to age less gracefully than men, and literature frequently reflects (but sometimes challenges) such an assumption. To read a literary text for its representations of both age and gender, for its ageism and its sexism, the tools of feminist literary criticism can profitably be combined with those of reader-response criticism.

Feminist Literary Criticism *with* Reader-Response Criticism

For the enterprise of challenging ageism in this chapter, I use reader-response criticism in combination with feminist literary criticism. Feminist theorist Myra Jehlen's definition of feminist thinking is useful to begin with: "Feminist thinking is really re-thinking, an examination of the way certain assumptions about women and the fe-male character enter into fundamental assumptions that organize all our thinking . . . Such radical skepticism is an ideal intellectual stance that can generate genuinely new understandings" (Jehlen, 1983, p. 69). Feminist literary criticism approaches texts with radical skepticism, especially about received sexual categories: "Unsettling our various sexual categories has provided a rich opportunity in the arena of literary criticism for all kinds of redefinition and debate, about what it means to be a man [young and old] or a woman [young and old], about how one becomes such an entity . . . about what such processes reveal about our culture" (Lynn, 2008, p. 233). Feminist literary critics thus uncover, rethink, and challenge literary stereotypes, mainly those of gender, sexual orientation, race, class, and ethnicity. Most feminist critics read primarily to root out examples of gender, race, ethnic, and class oppression and hurtful assumptions of inequality represented in literary texts.

In many ways these emphases and these practitioners have been inspired by the Women's Movement (Second Wave) and the Civil Rights Movement born in the 1950s and 1960s. Feminist literary critics write with concern about how the voices of women, people of color, immigrants, and the poor have been silenced or margin-alized. They write about exploitation. They strive to empower the silenced by examin-ing them in texts and by recovering forgotten or suppressed texts written by women. Historically, however, few feminist literary critics have analyzed texts for age and ageism. This neglect is probably an indicator of how age factors have been silenced in the literary world and in academe. This gap in the practice of feminist literary criticism may also be due to the fact that feminist literary criticism at first was used by younger women involved in the Women's Movement who were less concerned with ageism than with other forms of oppression. Thus, reading for age and ageism is one kind of work that feminist literary gerontologists may contribute to both feminist literary criticism and gerontology.

Feminist literary criticism is compatible with reader-response criticism in that both methodologies look at the cultural assumptions that implied readers bring to the interpretation of texts, including those about gender and other factors that shape our identities. Both also are interested in exposing hurtful cultural assumptions embed-ded in texts (in stereotypes, for example) that trigger defensive or angry reactions in readers. It makes a difference to both feminist literary critics and reader-response critics, then, whether a reader is a female or a male; whether a text is written before, during, or after the Women's Movement and the Civil Rights Movement; what race and ethnic group the reader belongs to; whether that reader is working-class or affluent; and how old that reader is.

Both approaches to textual interpretation also have a tendency to make allowances for idiosyncratic readings of texts and not to overgeneralize that "all women" will respond in one way to, say, Hemingway, and "all men" will respond in another, different way. Finally, both reader-response criticism and feminist literary criticism are aware of and sympathetic to the thinking of the resisting reader, the one who resists stereotypical characterizations and received notions, the reader who questions and challenges texts that reinforce the hegemonic culture, affirm the patriarchy, assert racism, or raise up the American-born over the immigrant. That is why many literary critics, including myself, use methods from both of these forms of criticism. In this chapter I do foreground more than the typical feminist critic the factors of age and age oppression in literary texts, and I react more assiduously against ageist characterizations than some other reader-response critics, simply because I also select and interpret specific texts as a literary gerontologist.

The term "resisting reader," so useful to the literary gerontologist battling ageism, was coined by feminist literary critic Judith Fetterley in her book *The Resisting Reader: A Feminist Approach to American Fiction* (1978). The resisting feminist reader (or critic) challenges traditional cultural and literary depictions that stereotype women, people of color, older people, the poor, or gays, portrayals that dehumanize or oppress them or that perpetuate assumptions of a specific group's inferiority. Literary critic Gregory Jay gives high marks to Fetterley for helping to launch a movement in literary criticism that has augmented the powerful cultural work performed by literary texts; he says, "Fetterley's emphasis on the power of literary texts to shape the beliefs and actions of readers and whole societies helped start a wave of literary criticism now associated with the term 'cultural work' . . . This kind of analysis aims to produce an account of the cultural work done by texts as they make their way into the minds of readers and cultures" (Jay, 1998). I subscribe to Jay's and Fetterley's position that literary texts can affect whole societies and do important work for social betterment, even when they are presenting sexist or ageist notions in their characters and plots, precisely because resisting literary critics will interrogate and undermine these sexist or ageist notions in the texts and raise general readers' awareness of how these damaging notions operate both in texts and in society.

Feminist reader-response critics, moreover, might aim their resistance not only against ageist stereotypes in literature but also against prescriptive, narrow views of how to "age well." Pointing out our cultural assumptions, from TV commercials, films, pop novels, and magazines that picture the tanned, well-aged woman, still svelte and athletic and enjoying the good life, the feminist reader-response critic may react against such portrayals of aged-to-perfection women and make room for a multitude of elderly females (and males) in all shapes and sizes and degrees of vigor.

Finally, feminist reader-response critics will help less-experienced readers to notice textual differences between the depictions of old women and old men; that old women are often doubly stereotyped in a literary setting is seen as far back as the nineteenth century in the sexist and ageist characterization of Miss Havisham (Dickens's jilted bride and insanely vindictive old maid in *Great Expectations*). Older men are more often than older women depicted as dignified leaders or culture-tenders in society (think of the courageous and manly attorney Atticus Finch in *To Kill a Mockingbird*). The feminist reader-response critic will reveal how such literary texts manipulate readers to accept the assignment of the important culture-tender role to the male and the lesser role of the nasty old crone to the female—and will question that role assignment. Feminist reader-response critics who read for gender and sexism as well as age and ageism in literary texts can help to guide readers toward broader horizons of expectations and greater tolerance when they encounter all kinds of older characters in literary texts.

Reading M. F. K. Fisher's *Sister Age* for Age and Ageism

Let me now illustrate how a feminist reader-response critic might use these critical tools to examine narratives about older characters such as those portrayed in M. F. K. Fisher's *Sister Age* (1984). *Sister Age* is a collection of pieces about aging written over a period of 40 years, published between 1964 and 1983. In particular, I discuss Fisher's Foreword, "The Oldest Man," "The Reunion," and "A Question Answered," examining characters' ways of performing old age, the narrators' reflections on what a good old age is, and some of the varied challenges of later life depicted in the pieces. I also discuss Fisher's Afterword, written when she was in her seventies. Then I compare Fisher's characterizations to a portrait of an elder in an essay from Maya Angelou's collection *Wouldn't Take Nothing for My Journey Now*, "Living Well. Living Good." I choose Angelou's text for comparison because it was published in a later cultural moment than Fisher's essays and because it depicts the aging of a woman of color, a source for constructive contrast to "Sister Age" and Fisher's other elderly characters.

In her Foreword, Fisher introduces readers to her muses, the sources of inspiration for her writing on "the art of aging" (Fisher, 1984, p. 4). Some are characters she has encountered, "Sister Age's messengers," who are expert practitioners of aging, such as her paternal grandfather, possessor of "great strength and dignity that were mine for the taking" (p. 4). Literary critics, trained to explore the implications of figurative language, most likely notice that Fisher creates this personification of old age as a concerned female sibling and as an effective diplomatic figure who sends out emissaries to guide others through the "foreign territory" of later life. A feminist critic also probably notes the emphasis on "sister," or the feminine personification of age, as a way to make age seem less threatening, more gentle. Moving among both female and male emissaries of aging and those of all races and classes, the author introduces the idea that elders—including Fisher herself—can offer insights to younger people about the art of aging: "Certainly there were violent, flashlike meetings all my life, with people much older than I, of different colors and sexes and social positions, who left marks to be deciphered later . . . The art of aging is learned, subtly but firmly, this way" (pp. 4–5). As general readers negotiate the universal meanings of the language here—because aging happens to all people—reader-response criticism encourages us self-consciously to recognize the text's invitation to turn inward and recall the people in our own lives whose weight of years, experience, and wisdom marked us in some important way. The text prompts readers to wonder what particular people in the narrator's life taught her about the art of aging; we want to turn the pages and learn more about these people; the text prompts us to look on them as illuminating truths about old age. They are inspiring mentors. And readers' awareness is being heightened to notice when these mentors cross our own paths.

Besides the people in her life that guide her through the foreign country of old age, Fisher's narrator reflects in the Foreword on an art object that for her epitomizes old age and that becomes an important muse. It is a crumbling portrait that she finds in Zurich during her travels and christens "Sister Age." On it is depicted an unattractive old woman with sad eyes named Ursula von Ott, who is in mourning alongside a memorial bust of her son. The narrator speculates that it was painted that way by an "angry and impatient adolescent" male, her son, before his death (p. 10). The narrator's companion Tim is quoted as commenting snidely on Ursula's ugliness, and Fisher's reply is that she is "past vanity" (p. 8); I would take that reply as a feminist retort! The son, a soldier heading off to war, is not past vanity in imagining that, should he die on the battlefield, his mother would experience "the inevitable loneliness of a bereaved parent" (p. 10). His lack of respect for what bereavement and aging would do to her is recorded here. Readers could resist the egotistical son's view of the aged mother in a few ways.

A feminist reading of this passage might resist the characterization of the old woman's "ugliness," deeming it a sexist judgment by a male who only prizes females for their youthful beauty. On the other hand, readers might pause over the author's pronouncement that Ursula von Ott was past vanity, intrigued by the sense that she might have resisted societal norms about womanly appearance and that there were other things in later life more important to her than society's pronouncements about her appearance. This is an inchoate idea about later life for women that may be instructive to readers (those who, in Nora Ephron's words, "feel bad about [their] neck[s]," perhaps; Ephron, 2006). Negative epithets may be applied sneeringly to Ursula as a way for the narrator to point out the ageism rampant in the culture of the 1970s and 1980s: she is a "lorn crone" and "an old biddy" (p. 10). Yet the narrator moves beyond sneering later to accord her a new respect. Ursula kindles and sustains the author's imagination in subsequent years, so that Fisher is inspired by the "the implacable secret strength of the old" (p. 11).

The enduring strength is richly symbolized in the fate of the portrait, as Fisher reports it: it becomes prey to time in the form of predatory silverfish that eat most of the pigment on the portrait except that depicting Ursula herself. Of course, the narrative itself also survives the ravages of time and silverfish, giving Ursula an eternal life and readers a glimpse into Fisher's old age. It survives, the implication seems to be, to teach readers about the wider perspective of the old: "her eyes look with a supreme and confident detachment past all the nonsense of wars, insects, birth and death, love" (p. 12). There may be some feminist pride in the tone of this passage, as Ursula is able to construct this purview beyond the messes created by the men of the world. The narrator acknowledges that this portrait is teaching her to simplify her life and to clarify her priorities. She ends the Foreword by claiming Ursula as her teacher and sister. We are all kin to Sister Age, and Fisher would have readers acknowledge this kinship too.

Also depicted as no longer weighed down by the trivial and the quotidian is the 99-year-old Frenchman Pepe Connes in the chapter "The Oldest Man." The narrator represents his masculinity favorably, in comparison to "Sister Age's" femininity. Pepe is described by the narrator as a man of vigor, with strong hands and keen memory, possessing an "imperturbable" mind, a detachment from time and "human hungers" (pp. 162, 168). He seems to have passed some of this skill in detachment on to his 74-year-old son, Georges, the narrator's friend and former professor. Detachment may be a learned behavior, something for readers to learn too, if they want to. If Pepe is past human hungers, readers may pause and wonder how he has moved into other realms than those fleshly and material passions that tie humans in midlife to the quotidian; his suprahuman perspective may teach readers that we need not be so circumscribed by the everyday. Noting the setting for the chapter, where Pepe lives—in the town of Le Truel, 3,500 feet up in the Aveyron mountain range of France—symbolically we literary critics might sense that he breathes a rarified air, purified of the trivial struggles down below. That Pepe's eyes are "large and bright" (p. 156) may tell readers that he has keen vision, vision that sees beyond the trivia of daily life.

Of interest also is the narrator's sheepish confession that she is "shy of him," due not only to his reserve but also to his "great age" (p. 150). How many of us would connect with such a confession, would feel discomfort among the very old? It is well to bring such discomforts to consciousness as preamble to challenging our ageism. She also challenges ageism in other subtle ways, by, for example, noticing Pepe's "fresh and powdery" smell: nary an aura of decay about him (p. 150). His hands too belie the stereotyped view of an old man's hands; they are "not at all mottled or gnarled, with the loose papery skin one expects in old hands. They . . . [are] well-formed, firm and sturdy to the touch, and as steady as a healthy young man's" (p. 166). Another unpleasant stereotype is being undermined here.

Not so steady are his also-elderly son's hands. This raises another kind of issue for the implied reader who may already be familiar with some real-life issues of aging: the challenges to the adult caregiver of the elderly parent. Georges is nervous about the fragility and vulnerability of his old father and about his responsibility for Pepe's well-being, magnified by their isolation in the mountain village. Having a very old parent ages the son, in some emotional way beyond his years. He confesses to Fisher's narrator: "I live in constant apprehension—a fall, a chill. Each year I say that this is the last one" (p. 166); he may mean here the last year of Pepe's sojourn in the mountains (he lives there with his son only during the warmer months of the year) or his last on earth. In either sense, Georges is "quite nervous and shaky about being alone with his father" (p. 166). A subtext of this chapter, then, is that the also-aging adult child is a caregiver somewhat burdened emotionally by the fragility of the elderly parent and the inevitable approach of that parent's death. By delineating this relationship between adult child and aged parent, Fisher's narrator acknowledges, as much as a gerontological case study might, some of the conditions and stresses facing the caregiver, while reinforcing for many readers the expectation of fulfilling this responsibility and the essential humanness of both fragile parent and adult child taking on the parental role.

The story ends on a realistic note, as the narrator marks Pepe's demise at 101 years of age and observes with regret that his death by lung congestion was "painful, and even cruel"; his last few days are days of questioning why he is suffering and "why we are born," of complaining that Georges is physically hurting him. Still, the narrator notes a "generous" moment of acknowledgment by Pepe to his devoted caregiver son that "it is I who have hurt you" (p. 174). Readers will likely feel some relief at the inclusion of this sentence in the narrative's ending: the toils of the caregiver do not go unnoticed.

Some of Fisher's other literary elders, like the reclusive Professor Lucien Revenant, become tellers of a cautionary tale: we often delay, till it is too late, the deepening of our friendships, the pursuit of our social pleasures, the parties and good food shared. The narrator, allowing us access to the professor's inner thoughts, takes us through his day of planning, after "recovery" from a serious illness, for a reunion party to which he has invited five dear friends with whom he hasn't kept up contact. Readers see him interacting with employees at a bakery—chatting there about "geriatric gastronomy" (p. 145)—and making purchases at a liquor store; we observe his use of clothing to protect his health from a cold winter's day, his "dry cold skin," hands stiffened by the cold, and his tiredness. We anticipate with him, in his growing excitement, the arrival of his guests. As he prepares and waits, we learn through Lucien's reverie about the regrettable things left undone in his life: in particular, his life-changing decision (or suspension of active decision?) to pursue work on his thesis and to put off till too late the gratification of marrying his friend Rachel: "if he had only had enough money and had managed to finish the thesis, he might well have asked her to . . . share her life with him. Even before it could be, it had seemed too late" (p. 146). The money issue and the work issue are mere rationalizations for the professor's procrastination and ultimate rejection of love and companionship. His life had become "a long dull dropping away" from the relationships that humanize and warm us (p. 148), that make our lives pleasantly spicy and intoxicating instead of ploddingly routine.

The reader-response critic will help readers to see that it is not till the final paragraph of the story that we will recognize, with a jolt to our expectations, the context of the professor's reunion and Fisher's use of magical realism. The magical realism (a term for a literary merging of realistically depicted people, places, and events with supernatural happenings or settings that may contribute a symbolic, psychological, or metaphysical significance to the literary work) is signaled at the end of the story when the narrator tersely informs us that the professor's not-well-attended funeral had been that morning and that the five friends had died well before he had (p. 148). Hence, readers have been witnessing a reunion beyond the grave of the newly dead man, seeing his attempt to compensate for a life not fully lived.

A feminist critic might consider whether this depiction of a male bachelor character who is unsociable is stereotypical and reflective of the culture of the 1970s, when men were less oriented toward participation in domestic life. Might other male bachelors, especially in the twenty-first century, have sought friendships and cultivated fuller lives that involved women and children, even without benefit of marriage—in their roles as educators, perhaps? A feminist critic might also speculate on how this story might have been differently written with an aged female protagonist who had never married. Would she also have suffered from increasing isolation like Professor Revenant, or would she have sought out a cadre of other old women for activities or the sharing of thoughts and feelings? I want to say that the latter is more likely, but I may risk stereotyping older women by doing so. Yet examining gender's effects on aging through such feminist literary questions would be useful to gerontologists and general readers alike as we understand more about the different problems faced by men and women in old age and promote more humane interactions with and among elders. Reader-response critics might also look at gender in this story or in the differing reactions of male versus female readers, but they would be more likely to emphasize how our expectations about the nature of the reunion are overturned, propelling us into a fuller reception of the underlying message: that because the professor has died, his regrets come too late for true rectification (unless we believe in an afterlife). Thus, all readers are prompted to live more fully engaged while there is still time.

Finally, an important humanizing feature of this story is that readers see from inside the mind of the character (a limited omniscient narrative perspective) his own life review, that mental totaling up of life events and relationships that measures what has been accomplished and what remains to be done. The regrets of Professor Revenant humanize him and may enable readers to feel curiosity about and sympathy for the inner lives of many elderly people encountered in daily life.

In another story that also takes readers inside the protagonist's mind, Fisher offers readers a humanized depiction of dementia. This story, "A Question Answered," is narrated from within the consciousness of the elderly Mrs. Eileen Oliver Mack. Mrs. Mack worries that others are increasingly forgetting her name. She is confident that she knows who she is; however, she fails to recognize that she cannot recall others' names and identities. Readers might wonder if Mrs. Mack is projecting her identity confusion onto other people. Her confusion about her identity and her own existence, which she is able to acknowledge to herself sometimes ("I begin to wonder *if* I am"; p. 189), is conveyed through the switching of her names with other characters' names throughout the story, so that readers can experience a similar confusion. Trying to sort out their confusion with the help of literary critics, general readers will see the increasing presence of the rats in the narrative as manifestations of Mrs. Mack's own deteriorating self-image, her decline to the animalistic. Mrs. Mack's rat fantasies suggest a dis-ease within her that her "reputation" as a person is being challenged by those who (she thinks) forget her name or misname her, or by family who dismiss her as old and forgetful.

The only beings that consistently remember her name and recognize who she is are the rats in her home, with whom she begins to have vivid conversations. The elaborate dialogues and scenarios she creates involving the rat leader and his cohort are the tip-off to readers about her mental instability. Ironically, only the rat leader can soothe her agitation because he assures her that he knows her name, when no humans seem to. Hence, Fisher's literary representation of Mrs. Mack's mental meandering reveals some positive consequences of her rich inner life: its calming effect, entertainment value, and companionship. She now has what she identifies as a clearer night vision, "bright new eyes" (p. 188); this a literary critic might take more than literally: it could be a metaphor for an imagination that quickens during the dark of night when she is alone and her surroundings are quiet. Literary critics and readers familiar with the psychologist Carl Jung may recall Jung's observation that the Self is often imaged as an animal, "representing our instinctive nature and its connectedness with one's surroundings" (Jung, 1964, p. 207); if the rat is a symbolic representation in these night fantasies of Mrs. Mack's Self, it suggests to me that she is *well connected* to her surroundings at night and that she is more in touch with her instinctive nature as she fantasizes having conversations with the rat. Readers, privy to her imaginings about what is happening to her at night, can thus grasp the good as well as the disorienting aspects of dementia.

Even when, toward the end of the story, Mrs. Mack is bitten (she believes, by the rat), reader-response critics, pointing out the element of surprise to readers, may then link the surprise to an interpretation of the bite as symbolically more than a negative wound. Critics might turn again to Jung, who has written that being bitten in a dream could symbolize that the dreamer is receiving the impetus for "creative change . . . [where] we have to expose ourselves to the animal impulses of the unconscious" (Jung, 1974, pp. 219–20). Mrs. Oliver through her night visions may be more in touch with her inner Self and her basic instincts than most people would suspect in a woman who has dementia. Is she readying herself to undergo the final creative change, detachment from one's roles in life? (I'll return to this question later.) Reader-response critics might see this outcome of Mrs. Mack's story as an unsettling of the implied reader's horizon of expectations concerning someone who has dementia. Adding the feminist perspective, the literary critic contemplating Mrs. Mack's night fantasies might conjecture on whether old women in literature are more able to dwell productively within their night reveries than old men, and if so, why. To find out, I might compare Mrs. Mack to other literary female elders, such as Granny Weatherall in Katherine Anne Porter's 1930 story "The Jilting of Granny Weatherall" (Porter, 1979, pp. 80–89), the affectionate grieving widower Sam Peek in Terry Kay's *To Dance with the White Dog* (1990), and the hypochondriacal insomniac Wilkie Walker in Alison Lurie's *The Last Resort* (1998). The feminist reader-response critic, in comparing these texts of aging and in showing how readers develop sympathy for characters like Mrs. Mack, aims—like the authors of the texts—to humanize elders dealing with loneliness, sad regrets, and sometimes hallucinations in the night.

Reviewing my personal reading experience of the story (which feminist and reader-response critics often do), I recall that as I interacted with the thoughts of Mrs. Mack, I began to interrogate my own prejudices and fears about dementia: I began to feel less threatened by her confusion as I started to see more clearly the coherent structure of her thoughts about the rats, and I became more able to enter into her imagined dialogue with the rat leader as I backed off from our culture's tendencies to be dismissive, derisive, or pitying of her condition. When literary critics examine portrayals of the darker sides of aging, they have the training and the experience to show less-practiced readers how humanizing is the access they have been given to the interior landscapes and inner conversations of elders who are in the throes of declining health and deteriorating mental powers.

Readers of all stripes are persuaded through Fisher's narrator to respect Mrs. Mack's brave meditations on what is happening to her mind. When her children are visiting, she knows that she is relatively connected to reality, including her sense of self, and she says she "lost her obviously neurotic puzzlement about why people seemed to be forgetting her name" (p. 178). But when she is again left alone, the dementia intensifies, while her awareness that this is happening is also reported by the narrator, from inside her mind: "Perhaps, she thought oftener each time she got into bed, I am finally losing my mind. Before long, I shall forget who I am, the way everyone else is doing" (p. 182). She begins "to sleep patchily," fading in and out of reality, tracking the pathways of the rats and trying to engage with them when she is awake; her mental state worsened by sleep deprivation, she is in a kind of twilight zone, her inner life a "peculiar muddle" (p. 184).

One deep insight that access to the inner mental life of Mrs. Mack offers the implied reader—especially the gerontologist already attuned to issues concerning elderly people and their adult children—is the increasingly forgetful elder's feeling of growing distance from family, which may seem to the elder like abandonment by loved ones. Mrs. Mack describes her confusion about "what was happening to people she loved, and why she was not permitted to be near them, and why and how she knew that she could not be near anyway . . . Yes, things were getting worse" (p. 184). A close reading detects the tone of sadness and the sense of loss felt by Mrs. Mack in this diminished intimacy with loved ones. External projections of rats from Mrs. Mack's interior landscape can even be interpreted in this context as symbols of the "vermin" in her life: her adult children and their stress-producing interventions in her sickroom may seem ratlike and predatory to her.

Gradually, readers are also led to see Mrs. Mack intermittently through others' perspectives, although the narrative is still generally filtered through Mrs. Mack's consciousness. Especially telling is a visit to Dr. Milwright after what she tells him is a rat bite (in his office she also tells him about her friendship with one of the rats). She knows he is humoring her and treating her like a confused child, even as she recounts her "real life" with her rat friends: "His voice was too kind, too gentle. His scribble [on the chart pad] had been too discreet . . . it was plain to see that he had not noted any medical facts" (p. 186). At the end of this scene she records her own confusion over the doctor's name ("Dr. Milhouse . . . or was it Dr. Milstrom, or . . . ?" p. 187), and then she faints when (she imagines that) he calls her "Mrs. Murgatroyd" instead of Mrs. Mack (p. 187); most likely, this is once again a projection of her own identity confusion. The condescension of the mentally well to the person with dementia is not to be missed in this passage.

The story of Mrs. Mack also reveals insights about changes in elders' identities through the course of later life and how elders look on the evolution of their own identities over a lifetime. We know that most elders follow the impulse to perform a life review. Like Professor Revenant, Mrs. Mack performs some of this introspection, even while she is also experiencing some disorientation. We are told early in the story by

Fisher's narrator that she has always liked her name and her roles as single girl and then married wife and mother (p. 176). She is until near the end of the story clear about her "social label" and comfortable with her roles of "mother, friend, grandmother" (p. 184). However, as alluded to earlier, Mrs. Mack may now be in for the final role change of her life. Feminist reader-response critics, linking all these references to her life roles, might posit that when at the end of the story Mrs. Mack questions whether she had actually performed these woman's roles, it is a sign of her impending death, her way of shedding these earthly roles: "I wonder whether I have ever been the young girl and then all those other people I thought I was for so long" (p. 189).

As the rat, at Mrs. Mack's deathbed, explains the reason for her confusion and loss of memory, as she understands "everything" finally, and as he coughs the little cough associated with Mrs. Mack herself, readers put together these three clues and realize that rat and elderly woman character have now merged into one; the rat has been an emanation of Mrs. Mack's thoughts and identity and therefore stops existing when she dies. Dr. Milwright and his nurse are at her bedside too, witnessing her passing, he in apparently unsentimental recognition of her dementia refusing to agree with the nurse's words about her death, "Ah, the poor soul!" (p. 189). Readers might in themselves feel a blend of the reactions of doctor and nurse: sympathy for Mrs. Mack and for the end of a full, generous life, but no condescending pity for the forgetful woman, having seen the richness of her inner life, the range of emotions and flashes of insight she had till the end.

In her Afterword, Fisher the narrator reflects on her own old-age personality (remember that she is in her seventies writing the Afterword). There she suggests a compensation for the slowing down of physical powers and for her aches and pains in later life: "I am more openly amused and incautious and less careful socially, and . . . all this makes for increasingly pleasant contacts with the world" (p. 235). Losing social inhibitions as we age can open us to richer interactions with others, she intimates here. Yet she is realistic about the physical negatives of later life. She suggests that we should prepare for age's physical symptoms of decline, in part through help from mentors; furthermore, she desires to disrupt the American pattern of aging that ends with withdrawal "from the fray" (p. 236) in old age, such as the withdrawal that Mrs. Mack and Professor Revenant endured. Her message might be: Accept the physical deterioration and limitations, but match these with engagement in life. Fisher says, finally, that old age offers us "full use of everything that has ever happened in all the long wonderful-ghastly years to free a person's mind from his body . . . use [of] the experience . . . so that physical annoyances are surmountable in an alert and even mirthful appreciation of life itself" (p. 237). If we are able to watch elders make these trade-offs in real life and in literary depictions, we will, she argues, be more prepared to do so in our old age. Fisher the visionary thus argues against age segregation and for the generations to live together under one roof as she concludes her book. Although some readers will resist this message, most will agree that the author is effectively mentoring her readers about later life through her sympathetic character portraits of elders and through her autobiographical reflections in *Sister Age*.

A Woman of Color Ages:
Reading Maya Angelou's "Living Well. Living Good."

Maya Angelou publishes *Wouldn't Take Nothing for My Journey Now* in 1993, more than a decade after the last pieces of *Sister Age* have appeared, but ageism still is prevalent in our society at this time. Hence, Angelou has a mentoring purpose similar to Fisher's in her portrayal of 79-year-old Aunt Tee, in the chapter titled "Living Well. Living Good." The difference is that Angelou injects race into the discourse for a readership that is more comfortable with overt racial comparisons than in the decades of the 1960s, 1970s, and early 1980s, during which the chapters of *Sister Age* appeared. In Angelou's chapter, the African-American character ages well, and the whites live a dull and colorless old age in spite of their monetary wealth. No unappealing frail crone is Aunt Tee: Angelou comments on her sinewy strength and "old gold skin" (Angelou, 1993, p. 61); her skin is also likened to "old lemons" (p. 61). These are both positive images to describe an older woman of color. Black has indeed become beautiful in American society, and Angelou relies on contemporary readers' associations of blackness with "hipness" in her characterization of Aunt Tee. Aunt Tee's journey in later life is contrasted with that of the white couple that employed her as their housekeeper for thirty years. While they dry up literally and metaphorically and become mere spectators of life (especially of Aunt Tee's life), Aunt Tee lives more fully, commands her own life, "like an Indian chief" (p. 61). Readers are compelled to resist the dry old age of her employers as they "grow older and leaner" (p. 62) and to model that of the attractive and irrepressible Aunt Tee.

Reminiscent of Fisher's Frenchman Pepe, Aunt Tee enthusiastically participates in life. She begins a love affair with the chauffeur, and we see her party with him and another couple. She is a "social maven" (p. 63), drawing others to her for dinners, card games, joking, music, and dancing. Her employers have no social life or joy, so they watch hers avidly. She and her friends are examples of what might be in store for elders if we remain receptive to new relationships and venture deeper into emotional connections. Fisher would probably see Angelou's aunt as a mentor for the art of aging. The narrator affirms that "living well is an art which can be developed" (p. 65). She aims to help readers develop this art through her positive portrayal of Aunt Tee and through the contrast to the white couple. Aunt Tee teaches readers the love of life, the notion of life as a "pure adventure" into the unknown, and the "ability to take great pleasure from small offerings" (p. 65). While the narrator may sound a little like a preacher to some readers and create a bit of resistance in those who do not care to be preached to, the sparkling character and zestful attitude of Aunt Tee are sure to win over most intended readers.

The narrator also reminds us that people are born creative and can continue to "invent new scenarios as frequently as they are needed" (p. 66). Encouraging flexibility in all of us, she notes that elders can use their creative imaginations to try out new life roles, travel to new places literally and metaphorically, and thus live more intensely in the present. Reader-response critics might point out that by engaging with these imaginative literary elders, readers kindle their own imaginations and begin to consider new ways to live in later life.

Other older authors have also written of later life and its opportunities for creative living. Alison Lurie, for example, in *The Last Resort* has one of her characters say at the end of the book, "as you grow older and the future shrinks, you have only two choices: you can live in the fading past, or like children do, in the bright full present" (Lurie, 1998, p. 320). Aunt Tee lives in the bright full present. A similar philosophical outlook enables May Sarton, after having a stroke and dealing with several other serious illnesses, to declare, "I do not want to relive the past . . . I want to live in the instant, the very center of the moment" (Sarton, 1988, p. 48). Her resilience and joie de vivre are evident in these lines and are inspirational for many of her readers, as are the words of Fisher and Angelou.

Feminist Reader-Response Critics and Writers Work for Change

The feminist reader-response literary critic reading for age issues thus selects and examines deeply works by authors such as Fisher and Angelou because they are irrepressible soldiers in the war against ageism. Literary critics demonstrate for less-experienced readers how authors appeal to them and persuade them to rethink later life: portraits of attractive elderly characters who treat old age daringly when they try new ways of living and the development of new "plot elements" for later life open up new vistas for general readers. Critics track how interactions with such texts enable readers to imagine new scenarios in later life—and in real life.

Feminist reader-response critics and authors thus join together to change readers' minds. As reader-response critic Louise Rosenblatt says, "The reader's attention to the text activates certain elements in his past experience—external reference, internal response—that have become linked with the verbal symbols . . . The text may also lead him to be critical of those prior assumptions and associations" (Rosenblatt, 1994, p. 11). Readers may bring to their reading of Fisher or Angelou past memories (good and bad) of the ways their own grandparents conducted themselves in old age, or they may bring prejudices about elderly people and fears about dementia and a lonely old age based on experiences with American TV programs and films, comedians' routines, and commercials for age-related drugs. Literary critics help readers to see how their literary transactions with the texts break down these negative assumptions about old age and elderly people; critics show general readers, for example, how characters like Aunt Tee and Pepe compel them to reject the assumption that dementia in old age is inevitable.

Even when dementia is represented in literary characters, literary critics using reader-response criticism will apprehend that, because general readers are invited to navigate from within a disoriented character and follow her movements between confusion and lucidity, they may feel less threatened by the forgetful elder's mental turmoil. Literary critics model ways of reading and also point out the impact on readers of literary techniques, especially interior monologue and the perspective of the limited omniscient narrator who reports the goings-on inside the minds of both elders and their caregivers. These literary methods simulate for readers the experience of Mrs. Mack's mixed-up flood of perceptions and the deep processes of her introspection. Critics reveal how these texts invite readers to switch back and forth from elders' internal conversation to external events, to a host of distorted perceptions of other people. Narrative mimicking of elders' daily mental confusions and challenges, demented thoughts merging into more "normal" internal musings, may just confuse an inexperienced reader, but will instead prompt the reader-response critic to see the purpose behind the pattern of textual confusion: for readers to learn, cognitively and affectively, about dementia. Adding gender to the critical perspective, feminist reader-response critics will probe the inner workings of a character like Mrs. Mack and see the peculiar forms of identity confusion associated with loss of the roles of mother and wife that an old woman might have, as distinct from those of an old man like Professor Revenant, who has lost the framework of a career that defined him more than his personal relationships did.

Experienced literary critics, moreover, show general readers or implied readers (those ideal readers to whom the author implicitly addresses his or her text) how to tease out the ambiguities of texts, such as those created by the magical realism in the story of Professor Revenant. We observe recurring allusions to his present state (dead) and to his past life. We observe a pattern of passages in which he is looking back at the fruitless time devoted to his work as professor and acknowledging how it prevented him from learning about the delightful goods of a bakery to use in entertaining guests or from cultivating a relationship with a woman that never went anywhere; we hear as part of this pattern his private confessions of regret about the dissipation of friendships. We also look for recurring physical descriptions that give us cues as to his already-dead state—and to the probability that he was already emotionally dead while still alive. We "connect the dots" of these recurrences and see a life pattern that becomes a cautionary tale for those readers not yet dead, a warning against procrastination and against not living life fully.

Veteran literary critics are also aware of and can point out to less-practiced readers how comparisons between characters—characters acting as "foils" to other characters —manipulate readers for a specific end: often for the purpose of encouraging us to rethink old age. By comparing Aunt Tee to her white employers, Angelou's narrator makes us revisit the old saw that money can't buy happiness and makes us question our assumptions about a colorless old age or an old age of stasis. In a collection such as *Sister Age,* the portraits of Ursula von Ott, Pepe, Professor Revenant, and Eileen Mack complement each other, shaping readers' sensibilities about the diversity among old people and their varied ways of living out their old ages.

Feminist reader-response critics are, finally, acutely aware of the cultural and political contexts of literary texts and how writers play to, resist, and try to revise these contexts. As literary critic Steven Mailloux sums it up, "reading is historically contingent, politically situated" (1998, p. 77). This precept enables literary critics to name and emphasize the context for their reading of Angelou's character Aunt Tee: in the hip black decade of the 1990s, they understand and demonstrate how implied readers would likely turn from the dry, white "WASP" oldster stereotype to embrace the sexier figure and model of "fun aging" represented by Aunt Tee. Aunt Tee is like a black version of the women on *The Golden Girls,* American TV's hit show about older women that ran on the NBC network from 1985 to 1992. Mailloux's critical stance is my own here: "reading any text, literary or nonliterary, relates to a larger cultural politics that goes well beyond some hypothetical private interaction between an autonomous reader and an independent text" (pp. 77–78). Feminist reader-response critics, then, can uncover the cultural politics—the negative stereotypes and silencing of elders' voices, for example—as they examine texts, and they can intervene in an unhealthy cultural trend by resisting the texts that perpetuate forms of oppression, including ageism.

Feminist reader-response critics are also trained to observe how cultural politics operate in narrators who tell stories in the first person, such as in Fisher's "The Oldest Man." This story features confessions of the narrator about her own stereotyping of elderly people, derived from the mid-twentieth-century (fairly conservative) culture in which she grew up. The narrator observes her own dawning awareness and gradual dismissal of some negative associations with the very old through acquaintance with Pepe. Literary critics may point out ways in which the tale encourages general or implied readers to reassess some of their own negative stereotypes, in part by noticing stereotypical literary and media incarnations of elders in a new light. Literary critic Harold Bloom reminds us all that to be good readers we have to be creative readers:

"*One must be an inventor to read well*" (Bloom, 2000, p. 25). Feminist reader-response critics strive to be inventive or imaginative in order to enter into a text's offerings of a new place, another time, another person's psyche; we also show less-experienced readers how to be inventive and receptive to texts. We all can become more inventive if we are exposed to imaginative writers like Fisher and Angelou. Bloom reminds us that our purpose in reading is often "in quest of a mind more original than our own" (p. 25). Literary critics are practiced at discovering and demonstrating the power of these vastly original authors and texts. Imaginative authors and inventive feminist reader-response critics with gerontological interests help general readers to connect with elders and to reinvent models for elderly identity, in our cultural moment and for the future.

Texts of aging and literary critics who interpret them also do the cultural work of exposing the frequent isolation of the old from societal networks or social activities. Feminist reader-response critics recognize the importance of pointing out to less-experienced readers this isolation of elderly men and women because they are aware of the cultural context in which readers usually dwell: they are removed from and ignorant of the lives of elders who live apart. Authors and literary critics together resist the age segregation common to our society by depicting and discussing portrayals of the damaging effects of isolation on the old, such as in characters like Mrs. Mack. Literary critics may also be familiar with theories of art such as Theodor Adorno's, which argue that art by its very nature interrogates or resists society; Adorno says, "art becomes social by its opposition to society . . . By crystallizing in itself as something unique to itself, rather than complying with existing social norms and qualifying as 'socially useful,' it criticizes society by merely existing . . . Art keeps itself alive by its social force of resistance" (1997, pp. 225–26). Whether the artist consciously or unconsciously acts as a social critic while creating art, the artist must still distance himself or herself from a specific "social reality" in order to create (p. 226). A literary critic aligned to word artists is primed to observe how characters, events, and setting in a text act in opposition to a social reality, the marginalization and invisibility of elderly people, for example, by bringing an old character into the center of the text and compelling readers to interact with the character.

Conclusion

I have been examining and arguing for the powerful effects on general readers of texts peopled by elders, when these readers are guided by feminist reader-response critics attuned to the methods by which texts portray gender issues and societal oppression. The specific purposes I see in the powerful texts I have analyzed in this chapter are to defuse our culture's ageism and to lessen the marginalization of old people by increased interactions with them. Texts on later life and elders and our more informed negotiations with these texts increase "knowability" of the old and give all who read more understanding of how our culture's ageism affects all who are aging (i.e., all of us). Feminist reader-response critics expand the consciousness of less-practiced readers regarding their own feelings about aging and demonstrate how gender interacts with age in texts of later life. Literary critics who are literary gerontologists find powerful texts about senescence and help readers to read them more deeply and closely, increasing the power and reach of the texts' impact.

Feminist reader-response literary critics will be acutely aware of authors' and readers' cultural situatedness and how (or whether) American society's attitudes toward elders have changed. I have in this chapter looked at the years between the 1980s, when the last of Fisher's pieces for *Sister Age* were written and published, and the early 1990s, when Angelou's *Wouldn't Take Nothing for My Journey Now* appeared in print. I'm not so sure that attitudes toward age have changed much, although we seem more able to accept with enthusiasm the idea of sexual activity and pleasure among old people (maybe the notion of the "dirty old man" has become outmoded?). I do think that even if ageism is still rampant in our society, issues of aging are much more in the forefront in our literature and popular culture since the late 1990s, which is prerequisite to change of any kind.

The complexities and possible solutions to the issues and challenges facing elders will only increase in public consciousness as my generation of baby boomers enters "young old age," their sixties. Texts on aging and literary critics who probe them even join with films and film critics to talk about aging in new ways. Films based on literature, such as *Iris* (2001), directed by Richard Eyre, from John Bayley's memoir *Elegy for Iris* (1999) about the mental decline of his wife Iris Murdoch, and *Away from Her,* the 2007 film adaptation of Alice Munro's story "The Bear Went Over the Mountain," directed by Sarah Polley and starring Julie Christie, about a wife's descent into Alzheimer's disease and her voluntary move to an assisted-living facility, do the cultural work—together with their critics—of encouraging readers and viewers to grapple with these issues and be sensitive to the problems elders face. No longer will elders be invisible members of society, or old age seem the place that May Sarton in 1973 characterized as a "foreign country with an unknown language to the young, and even to the middle-aged" (Sarton, 1973, p. 123). Literary critics will work with readers and viewers of all generations to explore more deeply how texts evoke the issues of aging for women and men, how they move people to change their thinking, and how they help all to visit the foreign country of the old and rehearse the emotional and physical aspects of aging.

REFERENCES

Adorno, T. W. 1997. *Aesthetic Theory.* Ed. Robert Hullot-Kentor, Gretel Adorno, and Rolf Tiedemann. Trans. Robert Hullot-Kentor. Minneapolis: University of Minneapolis Press.

Angelou, M. 1993. *Wouldn't Take Nothing for My Journey Now.* New York: Random House.

Bloom, H. 2000. *How to Read and Why.* New York: Simon & Schuster.

Ephron, N. 2006. *I Feel Bad about My Neck and Other Thoughts on Being a Woman.* New York: Alfred A. Knopf.

Fetterley, J. 1978. *The Resisting Reader: A feminist approach to American fiction.* Bloomington: Indiana University Press.

Fisher, M. F. K. 1984. *Sister Age.* New York: Vintage Random House.

Jay, G. 1998. Women writers and resisting readers. *Legacy: A Journal of American Women Writers* 15 (1):104–10. Reprinted online at www.uwm.edu/gjay/women.html.

Jehlen, M. 1983. Archimedes and the paradox of feminist criticism. In *The "Signs" Reader: Women, gender, and scholarship,* ed. E. Abel and E. K. Abel, 69–96. Chicago, London: University of Chicago Press.

Jung, C. G. 1964. *Man and His Symbols.* Garden City: Doubleday & Co.

———. 1974. *Dreams.* Trans. R. F. C. Hull. Princeton: Princeton University Press.

Kay, T. 1990. *To Dance with the White Dog.* New York: Washington Square Press.

Lurie, A. 1998. *The Last Resort.* New York: Holt.

Lynn, S. 2008. *Texts and Contexts: Writing about literature with critical theory.* 5th ed. New York: Pearson Longman.

Mailloux, S. 1998. *Reception Histories: Rhetoric, pragmatism, and American cultural politics.* Ithaca: Cornell University Press.

Porter, K. 1979. The jilting of Granny Weatherall. In *The Collected Stories of Katherine Anne Porter.* 1st Harvest ed. New York: Harcourt, Brace, Jovanovich.

Rosenblatt, L. 1983. *Literature as Exploration.* 4th ed. New York: Modern Language Association of America.

———. 1994. *The Reader, the Text, the Poem: The transactional theory of the literary work.* Carbondale: Southern Illinois University Press.

Sarton, M. 1973. *As We Are Now.* New York: W. W. Norton.

———. 1988. *After the Stroke: A journal.* New York: W. W. Norton.

Selden, R. 1989. *A Reader's Guide to Contemporary Literary Theory.* 2nd ed. Lexington: University Press of Kentucky.

Woodward, K. 1991. *Aging and Its Discontents: Freud and other fictions.* Bloomington: Indiana University Press.

CHAPTER FOUR

Philosophy of Aging, Time, and Finitude

JAN BAARS, PH.D.

Human aging has not drawn much philosophical attention in the past. This is true not only of philosophy but also of other ways of reflecting human life. When the famous theologian Karl Rahner (1980) was in his late seventies, he wondered what theology said about aging. He could conclude only that it dealt with the subject neither explicitly nor in any great detail. The question arises why so much thought has been given to death in philosophy and so little to aging, as can be seen in any handbook or encyclopedia of philosophy. The reason for this may be that when only a few people in a society reach "old age" and death is a threat at all ages, death will attract more attention than aging. In the work of the eminent philosophers of the past we find references to aging only in the margins of their work. Plato, for instance, introduces the old Cephalus in his *Republic* (trans. 1941) but grants him only a short presence, as if to demonstrate that an advanced age is hardly relevant in discussing what "justice" might be. For Plato and in Greek philosophy as a whole, such matters are decided only by argument—or so they thought—and age has no role to play. When older people are considered wise in Greek philosophy, this is because they have devoted a long life to study and thought, not because of their age. It's hard to find a more negative account of "The Character of the Old" than in Aristotle's *Rhetoric* (trans. 1991), although he may occasionally make a more positive remark about aging. More interesting—but still scarce—interpretations of aging are found outside Greek philosophy, for instance, in tragedies such as Sophocles' *Oedipus at Colonus* (Cole, 1988). Because Roman philosophy is more practically oriented, we can find more relevant work here: Cicero's *Cato Maior De Senectute* (*On Old Age*, trans. 1988) is a well-known example, but still an exception. Essays such as Seneca's *De Brevitate Vitae* (*On the Shortness of Life*, trans. 2007) can be applied to aging but are meant as a more general reflection about the "Art of Life" (Hadot, 1995).

The sixteenth-century philosopher Montaigne (1993) wrote "On the length of life" in his *Essays*: "Dying of old age is a rare death, unique and out of the normal order and therefore, less natural than the others . . . we should consider whatever age we have reached as an age reached by few." Contemporary studies in historical demography show that until the earlier decades of the twentieth century there was a much greater spread of mortality over the various age categories than is currently the case in the rich countries (Imhoff, 1986). Therefore, in many respects death was much closer to people of all ages. Although the part of life that is nowadays studied and organized as "aging" can be much longer than "normal" adulthood, reflection about the possible meanings of aging has lagged behind. In trying to find answers, there has also been a renewed interest in what, however fragmented, important thinkers of the past had to say about aging (McKee, 1982; Manheimer, 2000).

In this chapter I will present another approach, as the traditions of philosophical thought have even more to offer when there is no explicit discussion of aging, but rather of themes or concepts that are crucial for our understanding of it. In this way, I have built on a long tradition of philosophical discussion of concepts of time to develop a critical approach to theories of aging (Baars, 1997a, 2007a, 2007b). In Part I of this chapter, I will argue that contemporary approaches to aging, predominant in scientific research, bureaucratic policy, planning, and even everyday discourse, pre-suppose a limited understanding of time: *chronological time*. The application of this concept of time may have some practical advantages but runs into serious problems in understanding aging processes. This diagnosis leads in Part II to another understanding of aging as living in time, where other concepts of time that have been articulated in the philosophical tradition are used to advance the understanding of aging. The first is a concept of time that aims at the *interconnectedness* of the present, the past, and the future. The second is the concept of the "right time," or *kairos*. The third is the concept of human time as articulated in *narratives*. In Part III the discussion of aging as living in time is continued in a reinterpretation of *finitude*. One of the main problems in relation to aging is the tendency to identify finitude with death or mortality. This tendency can be understood in the light of the opening paragraph, but it restricts the understanding of aging as a process of living through situations that are all finite. In this context, aging is understood as irreversibly living through unique situations with unique people, testifying at once to the vulnerability and the preciousness of living in time.

Aging as a Dialectic of Loss and Gain

Aging is part of life, and therefore interpretations of aging are as old as thinking about human life. Since the beginning of Greek thought, for instance, in seventh-century BC lyric poetry, we find that experiences of aging lead to reflections and interpretations in which we can recognize contemporary concerns. A major theme is the decline and loss of all human qualities, lamented, for example, by Mimnermus of Smyrna in his image of an old man: "sunlight gives him joy no more. He is abhorred by boys, by women scorned: so hard a thing God made old age to be" (in West, 1993, p. 28). This theme is counterpointed by an equally important theme in Greek writing: the acquisition of a more profound understanding of "reality" through aging. Mimnermus was criticized for his restricted view of aging by Solon of Athens, who emphasized the possibilities for a continuing development through the subsequent seven-year seasons of life (Lewis, 2006).

These themes of human loss and gain can still be recognized in the interpretations philosophers have given of aging in the margins of their work. In his contribution to an earlier edition of this book, Manheimer (2000) presented an overview of the basic answers of philosophers to the processes of aging as progressive changes in the bodily, personal, and social dimensions of human life. He distinguished (1) Plato's view of a "transformed outlook and unique contributive role" from (2) the Aristotelian view of withdrawal from society and resignation and (3) Cicero's plea for active involvement while striving against decrements and losses associated with aging. Manheimer added the contemporary perspective (4) of postmodern deconstruction asserting that attitudes about aging would be nothing more than "culturally imposed narratives"—"a master plot of decline" (Gullette, 1997).

To this list we can add (5) recent technocratic "antiaging" programs (De Grey, 2004; More, 2005; De Grey and Rae, 2007) that present themselves as the spearhead of fundamental scientific research but may, besides pursuing more mundane goals, also be seen as contemporary representatives of old magical traditions (Olshansky, Hayflick, and Carnes, 2002; Hall, 2003; Kass, 2003; Mehlmann et al., 2004; Post and Binstock, 2004). These programs are an interesting illustration of the thesis developed by Adorno and Horkheimer in their *Dialectic of Enlightenment* (1972). According to them, the relation to nature has been dominated by a desire to control nature from early on in history, as early as the period of magic and myth. This desire is caused by the fear of being submerged in nature and being swallowed by it. Although this fundamental historical trauma may not dominate rational or scientific efforts per se, megalomaniacal rationalistic ideas—such as "ending aging"—have often surfaced and are, according to Adorno and Horkheimer, the driving force behind the development of an ever more technically advanced control of nature. One of the fundamental paradoxes of this relationship to nature, however, is that the rational subject who wants to control nature completely remains nevertheless a part of this same nature and consequently gets confused and caught in his own actions. This results in the "Dialectic of Enlightenment," a regression from the "most advanced" forms of rationalistic Enlightenment to the "most primitive" forms of magic and myth: a fountain of youth.

As long as the aging process remains uncontrollable, the striving for complete technological control is continually confronted with mankind's shortcomings, which explains why those who are reminders of this tragic failure tend to be excluded. It comes as no surprise that a society focused on being young, dynamic, and "in control" is at a loss where aging is concerned. Here we can notice two extremes: on the one hand, the perfectly insured life of the happy pensioner, with its appealing images of staying young and being a carefree consumer (Gilleard and Higgs, 2000)—an almost magical image to ward off the uncertainties of life; on the other hand, the haunting prospect of dementia, presented by the media as a terrifying generalization of aging, in which the rational subject is lost without redemption (Robertson, 1991). These two extremes are the culmination of fears caused by the insecurities of future life in which an uncertain future of aging is not looked in the eye, but subjected to positive and negative stylization. The different dimensions of human aging are not seen as *interrelated* but are divided into an abstract positive and negative image of aging. The likely outcome is that negative aspects of aging will be denied the dignity and careful attention they deserve, even though these aspects are inherent in human lives (Overall, 2003). This fundamental dialectic of decline and growth, noticed since Solon in Greek thought but with even longer roots in Egyptian, Jewish, and Babylonian traditions of wisdom (Assmann, 1991, 1994), has profound implications for our understanding of aging (Burrow, 1986; Sears, 1986; Cole, 1988, 1992). I will return to this dialectic in my discussion of finitude in Part III.

Part I. A Philosophical Questioning of Basic Categories of Age and Aging

One of the main paradoxes we are confronted with is that all human beings are constantly aging, but at a certain moment in life one is labeled *aged* or *older* (older than whom?) and life *beyond that point* is labeled *aging*. The expressions *aged* and *aging* are without any justification understood as references to a special and abnormal group, although these expressions indicate a universal and continuous process of living in time. Individuals are transformed into an "aging," "aged," or "older" body at a particular chronological age without any evidence that important changes are taking place at that age, apart from this sudden cultural relocation. This relocation into the category of the "aged" or "older" may take place at the age of 40 years when the stigma of the "older worker" begins to hit, especially for one who has become unemployed (Hardy, 2006). In the same fashion, gerontological studies usually begin by defining their population in terms of chronological age and present their results in diagrams where the interrelation of the two axes is supposed to show that changes in certain characteristics are a function of "age." Such visualizations presuppose that "aging" processes can be clearly and unequivocally related to chronological age, although what are presented are mostly unexplained data and possible connections.

Mistaken Associations: Time Working as a Regular Cause

Generalizations about people with a certain calendar age presuppose a *causal* concept of time: because time has worked for a certain duration in aging people, certain inevitable effects should be reckoned with. Moreover, the effects are assumed to develop steadily and universally according to the rhythm of the clock. However, such a causal concept of time can never generate knowledge that might explain something of the obvious *differences* that exist between human beings of the *same* age. While it is true that all causal relations are *also* temporal relations, or relations working "in time," it would be wrong to identify causality with time or to reduce the process of aging to the "causal effects" of time.

But the grand ambition of gerontology still seems to be to establish how this chronological or calendar age of individuals determines the characteristics of aging people or even of all humans. This would eventually reduce gerontology to a straight-forward set of simple formulas in which scientific precision and practical use would be united. In the early days of gerontology this option was stated with much self-assurance: "Chronological age is one of the most useful single items of information about an individual if not the *most* useful. From this knowledge alone an amazingly large number of general statements or predictions can be made about his anatomy, physiology, psychology and social behavior" (Birren, 1959, p. 8). And yet, the author of this statement has later dealt with time extensively and has expressed serious reservations about such claims: "By itself, the collection of large amounts of data showing relationships with chronological age does not help, because chronological age is not the cause of anything. Chronological age is only an index, and unrelated sets of data show correlations with chronological age that have no intrinsic or causal relationship with each other" (Birren, 1999, p. 460). Nevertheless, explicit analysis of concepts of time that are inevitably used in the study of aging has been scarce, although there have been some notable exceptions (see Baars and Visser, 2007). Interestingly, the most recent edition of the *Handbook of Aging and the Social Sciences* (Binstock and George, 2006) opens with a section devoted to "Aging and Time," but already in the title of the second article, "Modeling the Effects of Time" (Alwin, Hofer, and McCammon, 2006), we can see how causality and time are still unjustifiably connected and distort the analysis of aging and time.

A more intrinsic measure of aging, at least from a biological perspective, would re-quire establishing clear indicators of "normal" functioning. If we follow biological reli-ability theory (Gavrilov and Gavrilova, 2006) and define aging as an increasing risk of failure with the passage of time, the question remains in what way the statistical notion of increasing risk might contribute to an understanding of aging processes. Even if we would have reliable biomarkers of *age* (such as the aspartate racimization in the teeth used in forensics), this would not allow us to explain *aging*, nor would it even be helpful in predicting an increasing risk of death or any other type of biological failure.

If aging would develop in synchrony with chronological time, the differently marked *ages* would have to be included in a continuum, as subsequent *phases* that demonstrate a structured development away from a state of adult "health" or "normality." It is doubtful whether all biological processes can be adequately seen as *continuous* functional deterioration; some may suddenly deteriorate or collapse. Moreover, human aging appears to imply many distinct but interrelated processes that are relatively independent but still interact with other processes in the same body (Kirkwood et al., 2006). The many different processes of aging may have their specific dynamic properties, but these are usually affected by the environments inside and outside the human body (e.g., ecological or social contexts and personal lifestyles). This explains their intrinsic malleability (Kirkwood, 2005; Westendorp and Kirkwood, 2007), which is seen in the large differences in life expectancy and health that we can observe when we compare several historical and contemporary countries or regions with each other.

How important such contexts are can be gathered from the enormous change in life expectancies that has taken place in the rich countries during the last 150 years (Oeppen and Vaupel, 2002), which still awaits explanation. A major shift or mutation in the evolutionary substrate of human life seems not very likely. Seen from this perspective, our bodies basically have not changed since the ancient Greeks, let alone since the nineteenth century. All this defies the possibility that chronological age could by itself give any explanation of aging processes.

The Age-Period-Cohort Problem as Epistemological Riddle

We cannot study the processes of aging as we would study other processes, because we cannot isolate "aging" in an experimental group and compare the results with a control group that does not age. Moreover, all aging takes place in specific contexts that co-constitute its outcomes. This fundamental human condition haunts even the most sophisticated research strategies (see Baars, 2007a; Schaie, 2007). The notorious age-period-cohort problem confronts us with the question of what we have established when we have found, for instance, that a high percentage of a group of 70-year-olds has obesity. Is this because of their age? Is it part of their specific "cohort identity"? Is it because they lived for a certain period of years in a culture of fast junk food? Is it "a little bit of all that"? Human aging cannot be studied in a *pure* form: even a scientifically controlled life in a laboratory would be a life in a specific context that would co-constitute the processes that would take place.

The search for general aging characteristics based on chronological age has produced much counterevidence, testifying to the many differences in aging processes. This counterevidence hardly comes as a surprise when we try to imagine people with the same chronological age but living in very different circumstances. Think, for instance, of "60-year-olds": one would expect major differences in many important respects among, say, a contemporary poor Russian farmer, a wealthy Japanese person, and a homeless American of that age—not to mention 60-year-olds in ancient Egypt, in classical China, or among nineteenth-century factory workers.

Approaches to aging in terms of chronological age are likely to result in establishing many *differences* in aging processes among people with the same age. Therefore, they should not (implicitly) be used to *explain* aging processes without a further gerontological clarification. Problems resulting from an unreflective overemphasis on chronological age are likely to occur, as the concept of chronological time has been institutionalized to measure and coordinate processes and actions in modern societies. This leads also to the idea that societal processes can be optimally organized on the basis of the ages of the people concerned. In turn, this can easily lead to self-fulfilling prophecies: if in a given society the dominant agents in the labor market are under the impression that productivity is declining after the age of 50, this will most likely become true, not because this is inherent in their aging process, but as an artifact of the "chronological regimes" that define these people as "older workers."

Confronted with the enormous quantity of empirical data gathered in the last decade that demonstrate the differences among "the aged," Settersten (2005, 2006) has given an overview of what gerontologists say makes "old people" different from other adults: losses in physical and cognitive capacities; increased likelihood of failing health and a centrality of health concerns in self-definitions; shorter time horizon and a more pressing need to come to terms with one's mortality; personal loss, bereavement, and more restricted social networks; being perceived and treated by others in ageist ways; and a greater acceptance of things that cannot be controlled *in* life, coupled with a greater fear of losing control *over* one's life.

These important issues for adult aging show how limited the concept of chronological age is. It is always possible to establish averages, but losses in physical and cognitive capacities, failing health, and bereavement are not evenly distributed according to chronological age but are in an essentially *uncertain* way part of finite human lives. There may be different forms of "increased likelihood," for instance, according to the socioeconomic contexts of the people concerned, but these demonstrate once more that chronological age cannot give an explanation of the processes involved. Moreover, we can see in the problem of ageism (Gullette, 2004) how problematic generalizations about people above a certain age can be. Finally, themes such as "a shorter time horizon" and "mortality" presuppose a more personal involvement in temporal living than can be understood from chronological time.

Part II. Aging and Experiences of Living in Time

Statistical overviews and average estimates on the basis of chronological time may be needed for planning purposes, but they cannot satisfy the need to understand the passage of time in one's personal life. From philosophy we can derive three approaches to (living in) time that allow for more elaboration of personal experiences. A first has been initially developed by the fifth-century theologian Augustine and had a major influence on such contemporary philosophers as Husserl, Heidegger, and Merleau-Ponty (see Ricoeur, 1988; Baars, 2007b). This approach offers opportunities to understand that we experience a *present*, in which we read a text, speak with somebody, or listen to music. Such an experience of the present gets completely lost in the blur of rapidly rolling digital numbers; moreover, although the duration of each event or experience could be measured, such measurements are completely irrelevant for the intensity of the experience or the way it may be unforgettable and life changing.

One's experience of the present is inherently connected with a remembrance of the past and an anticipation of the future. Hence, something that happened "a long time ago" (from a chronological perspective) can be vividly experienced in the present and remembered as if it happened yesterday, whereas something (for instance, a personal relationship) that was important a year ago can be experienced as taking place in the distant past. Experiences of the past, present, and future do not follow the orderly arrangements of chronological time even though we have, a posteriori, the possibility to locate or date the situations and experiences in chronological time.

Memory as presence of the past does not just comprise what or how we *want* to remember. We only evoke a part of our memories consciously; a much greater part evokes us or keeps troubling us just when we would like to forget. In this context, Hannah Arendt (1958) referred not only to memory but also to forgiveness as a typically interhuman characteristic. Resentment or bitterness can be a destructive form of what Augustine called the presence of the past in which painful events remain as vivid as if they took place only recently and no time seems to have passed since. Ultimately, nonforgiving obstructs one's openness to the present and to the future so that the past cannot be a source of inspiration for the future.

We may be able to understand our life backward, but we must, as Kierkegaard (1987) remarked, live life forward and are inevitably confronted with uncertainty about the future—an uncertainty that opens, however, the opportunity to live one's life. That there are nowadays no generally accepted structures of meaning in aging can be seen as a loss, but the obligation to follow fixed patterns or phases of life might weigh heavily and frustrate creativity. The awareness that our confrontations with the contingencies of life are not based on unquestioned structures of meaning makes life more insecure but also potentially richer. We may not know how to live with fundamental uncertainty, but we cannot live well without it either.

A second temporal concept is even older than Augustine's pathbreaking work and can already be found in Hesiod (2006). The idea of *kairos*—that the present offers or denies a particular opportunity—plays an important role in early Greek Pythagorean philosophy and in Stoic thought: this idea has clearly pragmatic origins in experiences of sailing, fishing, and agriculture. For the Stoics it was important to live according to what opportunities were given (ευκαιρια) or denied (ακαιρια) by the gods or the course of nature. This concept of time is still presupposed when we are thinking about when the "time is ripe" to do or say something and when not. We know this from everyday expressions such as "If you want to do it, do it now"; "It's now or never"; or "Now is not the right time." This has in the past often been interpreted in relation to life's phases or seasons, but it can also be applied to important situations in life. In all these cases, *kairos*, the eminent moment, is not regulated by chronological time.

A third temporal concept is that of narrative, the arrangement of chronologically separated events in time into a coherent story. One of the remarkable aspects of narrative is its ability to integrate in a loose but potentially meaningful way the most diverse events, actions, and their evaluations. According to Ricoeur, a central role in composing loosely integrative configurations is played by the *act* of *emplotment*. In creating a *plot*, unrelated incidents are integrated into a meaningful whole, making them part of a story that contains a beginning, middle, and end.

Through the plot, *events and story* are connected reciprocally so that the story changes when other events or interpretations are introduced and vice versa. This implies that the "same" events can be integrated into different stories, where the elements are arranged differently, with other emphases or from other points of view. Such differences are not due to a lack of precision, as it may appear from the point of view of methodically controlled intersubjectivity. Different stories may express other experiences, other evaluations, or different points of view precisely. Another important achievement of emplotment is the integration of the *configurational* dimension of the narrative (where the emphasis falls on the meaningful pattern) with its *chronological* dimension (where the emphasis falls on the timing and succession of events). In this context a reference should be made to Paul Ricoeur's *Time and Narrative*, in which the hermeneutical circle is fruitfully applied to an unfolding understanding of lived time in *prefiguration, configuration,* and *refiguration* of time (Ricoeur, 1988).

Part III. Aging and the Reinterpretation of Finitude

As said earlier, much thought has been given to death in different traditions, whereas aging has been relatively neglected. Now that mortality has been substantially reduced in childhood, adolescence, and much of adulthood, death occurs much more commonly in older individuals. In a culture that tends to be dominated by idols of dynamic life, success, and invulnerability, this has led to a continued neglect of aging and a tendency to approach it as an unimportant residue of life. The growing numbers of "aged" people and the sheer quantity of years that can be spent in "aging" already make it understandable that such an exclusion from the most central domains of society, merely because of the attainment of a certain age, will provoke massive resistance. Not only gerontological programs of "successful aging" but also a more informal culture of "staying young" have been among the one-sided answers to this one-sided vision of aging. The finitude of human life contradicts such superficial answers, but it also deserves to be reinterpreted with regard to aging (see Baars, 1997b).

First of all, finitude in the sense of an awareness of one's mortality does not have to lead to a vision of aging as a residue of life that is of little importance. On the contrary, the awareness of finitude relativizes cultural idols and poses the question of what our life (as a "whole") is really about. This fundamental questioning has been part of our cultural traditions but has been radically elaborated by philosophers such as Martin Heidegger (1996). Especially in his early work *Being and Time,* he presents a fascinating attempt to break away from the modern Cartesian emphasis on the rational subject who is confronted with the world outside of him as his object. Heidegger does break with the rationalism of this tradition by emphasizing the fundamental meaning of the human temporal existence (*Da-sein*), which can be found in open confrontation with one's inevitable death. But he also continues the monological orientation of modern rationalism and its individualistic bias.

The importance of an awareness of finitude in the sense of mortality cannot be denied, yet I am not convinced that Heidegger's isolated heroism in the confrontation with one's inevitable personal death offers the most important perspective in life, as he maintains. The *Angst* of death is supposed to "disclose Da-sein as *being-possible,*" but this would also "individualize and thus disclose Da-sein as '*solus ipse*'" (a "solipsistic self") (Heidegger, 1996, pp. 176, 188). Other people enter this solipsist universe only as temptations to deviate from this authentic *Da-sein*. Although this is presented as being-in-the-world, this world is narrowed down to "*individualized, pure, thrown potentiality for being*" (p. 176, Heidegger's italics). Heidegger's view leaves us with two unresolved problems.

First, facing death includes the lives of others who tend to be regarded by Heidegger as anonymous representatives of inauthenticity (*They*), a criticism that has been articulated by thinkers such as Levinas (1969, 1987; see Baars, 2007b). Finitude should not, as has traditionally been the case, be seen as an aspect of the human condition, but as a quality of the *inter*human condition (see Baars, 2002).

Second, the tendency to identify finitude with mortality indicates that the finitude *throughout* human life, its finitude *as such* is not sufficiently acknowledged. Finitude also applies to the particular qualities and limitations of individuals, to relationships with others, to specific situations in life and their irrevocably transitory uniqueness. The wish to ignore this fundamental quality leads to an abstract image of a world that revolves around success, perfection, infinite youth, and innovation, in which, so it seems, failing, decay, and vulnerability do not occur. Not only does such a culture exclude the "aged," the disabled, or mentally disabled young people, as well as the sick and the weak, but also it creates stressful and superficial environments for young healthy people who must try to keep up with these idols.

Finitude and the Constitution of Meaning

An early text of Homer arouses again our attention. In her book *The Fragility of Goodness,* Martha Nussbaum (1986) refers to Odysseus's passionate embrace of finite, mortal life at the very moment that he is offered not only a pleasant life but also immortality by the goddess Calypso. In Homer's *Odyssey,* Odysseus is faced with a far-reaching choice: either he will share his life with the wonderful goddess Calypso and will not die, or he will have to leave her island and may have to fight for his life in order to return home to Ithaca. Odysseus, however, informs Calypso that he chooses mortal life, although he does not look forward to all the dangers he may have to face. However, so he emphasizes, he wants to return home, to his wife Penelope, although she is mortal and not as perfect as Calypso, who has "immortality and unfading youth." Odysseus trusts his "heart that is inured to suffering" (Homer, 1991, p. 76), which helped him endure the hardships of the past. And so he trusts that he will endure what is to come. He does not aspire to live forever, even when he has the choice in this magical narrative, but wants to live with other human mortals.

This episode presents an interesting contrast with the many stories about paradises where eternal life was lost in punishment of sinful behavior. Homer lets Odysseus make a positive choice for a finite and vulnerable life, a profound choice with far-reaching implications. If everything could always be postponed, nothing would matter. Simone de Beauvoir articulated a similar vision in her novel *All Men Are Mortal* (1992), in which the person who became immortal loses all meaningful understanding of finite living in human worlds. Only in a finite life can something be at stake.

Facing Limit Situations

One way to approach the finitude of human life in a broader sense is through the example of "limit situations" (*Grenzsituationen*) (Jaspers, 1971; Blattner, 1994) such as, indeed, death, but also depression, sorrow, disease, and suffering, and not only one's own but also of beloved others. These situations are not connected with chronological age but with human life as such: even a young child may become seriously ill or lose a parent or a friend. Loss, suffering, and death are inherent to human life; we can try to avoid or postpone them, but we cannot eradicate them from our lives. In this sense we cannot change these limit situations, but they will change *us*. As Jaspers emphasizes, the way we should confront them is not through planning and calculation, but through becoming ourselves in surrendering acceptance. However, as in Heidegger's resolute confrontation with death, there is an almost heroic tendency, a melancholic counterpart to "successful aging"—to idealize suffering as if this would be the only way to live authentically. When one could become oneself in confrontation with the limit situations, as Jaspers maintains, the question arises whether the person who becomes "oneself" did not have a self before that. It appears to be important to acknowledge the *dignity* of suffering, but also to say that if we are not suffering that much, this does not mean that we fail to lead a fully human life.

There are, however, still good reasons to heed the finitude of the interhuman condition as the highly cultivated ability of the Western world to cure disease, create safer environments, and postpone dying has created the illusion that people suffer or die *because* the efforts to help them have failed. This may be occasionally true, but eventually there are limitations inherent to human life. The highly specialized and often effective technology tends to occlude the fundamental character of the interhuman condition and create the illusion that people are dying because medical technology has not yet found the means to cure the diseases they are dying from (see Hayflick and Moody, 2002).

Aging as a Radicalization of Human Vulnerability

"Aging" people have no monopoly on human vulnerability, and their lives should not be considered as the opposite of the "invulnerable" lives of "normal" adults, which could be put under great stress without any negative effects. Still, as we saw earlier, a persistent theme through the ages has been the decline and loss of all human qualities: failing organs, brittle bones, and stiffening muscles, but also an increasing risk that beloved others may die. In other words, the vulnerability inherent in human life radicalizes as people get older.

The other important theme has been that inherent to human aging is a deeper meaning that will present itself or that has to be discovered during its process (Cole, 1992; Randall, 1997; Randall and Kenyon, 2000). Not only are healthy aging people capable of a continuing growth in experience and competence in the specific activities and fields they are interested in, especially when they find that their competences are acknowledged, but also they develop—even when they are chronically ill or disabled— important skills when dealing daily with problems and restrictions facing them. But on another, more existential level, a growing depth in experience and vision of aging people may be intimately connected with an increasing vulnerability, although this will not be the automatic result of "a higher age," "the passing of time," or the "seasons of life." By itself, a confrontation with limit situations does not give a deepening of understanding. This presupposes attention to and "working through" the crucial moments of life in which its hidden meaning may be discovered (Kierkegaard, 1987; Birren and Deutchman, 1991; Birren and Cochran, 2001). The meaning of human aging may be found in a radicalization of the vulnerability of unique human life, which is not the monopoly of "aged" people, but inherent to the interhuman condition.

REFERENCES

Adorno, T. W., and M. Horkheimer. 1972. *Dialectic of Enlightenment.* New York: Herder & Herder.

Alwin, D. F., S. M. Hofer, and R. J. McCammon. 2006. Modeling the effects of time: Integrating demographic and developmental perspectives. In *Handbook of Aging and the Social Sciences,* ed. R. H. Binstock and L. K. George. Boston: Academic Press.

Arendt, H. 1958. *The Human Condition.* Chicago: University of Chicago Press.

Aristotle. 1991. *On Rhetoric: A theory of civic discourse.* New York: Oxford University Press.

Assmann, A., ed. 1991. *Weisheit: Archäologie der literarischen Kommunikation III.* Munich: Wilhelm Fink Verlag.

———. 1994. Wholesome knowledge: Concepts of wisdom in historical and cross-cultural perspective. In *Life-Span Development and Behavior,* ed. D. L. Featherman, R. M. Lerner, and M. Perlmutter. Hillsdale: Erlbaum.

Baars, J. 1997a. Concepts of time and narrative temporality in the study of aging. *Journal of Aging Studies* 11:283–96.

———. 1997b. A reinterpretation of finitude: An introduction to three articles on philosophy of aging. *Journal of Aging Studies* 11:259–62.

———. 2002. *Ouder worden en de Fragiliteit van de Intermenselijke Conditie.* Utrecht: Universiteit voor Humanistiek.

———. 2006. Beyond neo-modernism, anti-modernism and post-modernism: Basic categories for contemporary critical gerontology. In *Aging, Globalization and Inequality: The new critical gerontology,* ed. J. Baars, D. Dannefer, C. Phillipson, and A. Walker. Amityville: Baywood.

———. 2007a. Introduction. Chronological time and chronological age: Problems of temporal diversity. In *Aging and Time: Multidisciplinary perspectives,* ed. J. Baars and H. Visser. Amityville: Baywood.

——. 2007b. A triple temporality of aging: Chronological measurement, personal experience and narrative articulation. In *Aging and Time: Multidisciplinary perspectives*, ed. J. Baars and H. Visser. Amityville: Baywood.

Baars, J., and H. Visser, eds. 2007. *Aging and Time: Multidisciplinary perspectives*. Amityville: Baywood.

Binstock, R. H., and L. K. George, eds. 2006. *Handbook of Aging and the Social Sciences*. Boston: Academic Press.

Birren, J. 1959. Principles of research on aging. In *Handbook of Aging and the Individual: Psychological and biological aspects*, ed. J. Birren. Chicago: University of Chicago Press.

——. 1999. Theories of aging: A personal perspective. In *Handbook of Theories of Aging*, ed. V. L. Bengston and K. W. Schaie. New York: Springer.

Birren, J., and K. N. Cochran. 2001. *Telling the Stories of Life through Guided Autobiography Groups*. Baltimore: Johns Hopkins University Press.

Birren, J., and D. E. Deutchman. 1991. *Guiding Autobiography Groups for Older Adults: Exploring the fabric of life*. Baltimore: Johns Hopkins University Press.

Blattner, W. D. 1994. Heidegger's debt to Jaspers's concept of the limit-situation. In *Heidegger and Jaspers*, ed. A. M. Olson. Philadelphia: Temple University Press.

Burrow, J. A. 1986. The Ages of Man. A study in medieval writing and thought. Oxford: Clarendon Press.

Cicero, M. T. 1988. *Cato Maior De Senectute*. Ed. J. G. F. Powell. Cambridge: Cambridge University Press.

Cole, T. R. 1988. Aging, history and health: Progress and paradox. In *Health and Aging: Perspectives and prospects*, ed. J. J. F. Schroots, J. Birren, and A. Svandborg. New York: Springer.

——. 1992. *The Journey of Life: A cultural history of aging in America*. Cambridge: Cambridge University Press.

de Beauvoir, S. 1992. *All Men Are Mortal (Tous les Hommes sont mortels)*. New York: Norton.

De Grey, A., ed. 2004. *Strategies for Engineered Negligible Senescence: Why genuine control of aging may be foreseeable*. New York: Academy of Sciences.

De Grey, A., and M. Rae. 2007. *Ending Aging: The rejuvenation breakthroughs that could reverse human aging in our lifetime*. New York: St. Martin's Press.

Gavrilov, L. A., and N. S. Gavrilova. 2006. Reliability theory of aging and longevity. In *Handbook of the Biology of Aging*, ed. E. J. Masoro and S. N. Austed. San Diego: Academic Press.

Gilleard, C., and P. Higgs. 2000. *Cultures of Aging: Self, citizen and the body*. Harlow: Prentice Hall.

Gullette, M. M. 1997. *Declining to Decline*. Charlottesville: University Press of Virginia.

——. 2004. *Aged by Culture*. Chicago: University of Chicago Press.

Hadot, P. 1995. *Philosophy as a Way of Life: Spiritual exercises from Socrates to Foucault*. Oxford: Blackwell.

Hall, S. S. 2003. *Merchants of Immortality: Chasing the dream of human life extension*. Boston: Houghton Mifflin.

Hardy, M. 2006. Older workers. In *Handbook of Aging and the Social Sciences*, ed. R. H. Binstock and L. K. George. Boston: Academic Press.

Hayflick, L., and H. Moody. 2002. *Has Anyone Ever Died of Old Age?* New York: International Longevity Center.

Heidegger, M. 1996. *Being and Time.* New York: SUNY Press.

Hesiod. 2006. *Theogony, Works and Days, Testimonia.* Ed. G. W. Most. Cambridge: Harvard University Press.

Homer. 1991. *The Odyssey.* New York: Penguin.

Imhoff, A. E. 1986. Life course patterns of women and their husbands: 16th to 20th century. In *Human Development and the Life Course: Multi-disciplinary perspectives,* ed. A. Sørensen, F. E. Weinert, and L. R. Sherrod. London: Lawrence Erlbaum.

Jaspers, K. 1971. *Philosophy.* Chicago: University of Chicago Press. Original edition, 1932.

Kass, L. 2003. Ageless bodies, happy souls: Biotechnology and the pursuit of perfection. *The New Atlantis* (spring):9–28.

Kierkegaard, S. 1987. *Either-Or.* Princeton: Princeton University Press.

Kirkwood, T. B. L. 2005. Understanding the odd science of ageing. *Cell* 120:437–47.

Kirkwood, T. B. L., R. J. Boys, C. S. Gillespie, C. J. Procter, D. P. Shanley, and D. J. Wilkenson. 2006. Computer modeling in the study of aging. In *Handbook of the Biology of Aging,* ed. E. J. Masoro and S. N. Austed. San Diego: Academic Press.

Levinas, E. 1969. *Totality and Infinity: An essay on exteriority.* Pittsburgh: Duquesne University Press.

———. 1987. *Time and the Other.* Pittsburgh: Duquesne University Press.

Lewis, J. D. 2006. *Solon the Thinker: Political thought in archaic Athens.* London: Duckworth.

Manheimer, R. 2000. Aging in the mirror of philosophy. In *Handbook of the Humanities and Aging,* ed. T. R. Cole, R. Kastenbaum, and R. E. Ray. New York: Springer.

McKee, P. L. 1982. *Philosophical Foundations of Gerontology.* New York: Human Sciences Press.

Mehlmann, M. J., et al. 2004. Anti-aging medicine: Can consumers be better protected? *Gerontologist* 44:304–10.

Montaigne, M. de. 1993. *The Complete Essays.* New York: Penguin.

More, M. 2005. *Superlongevity without Overpopulation,* February 6, 2005, www.longevitymeme .org/articles/viewarticle.cfm?article_id=24.

Nussbaum, M. 1986. *The Fragility of Goodness.* Cambridge: Cambridge University Press.

Oeppen, J., and J. Vaupel. 2002. Broken limits to life expectancy. *Science* 296:1029–31.

Olshansky, S. J., L. Hayflick, and B. A. Carnes. 2002. No truth to the fountain of youth. *Scientific American* 286:92–95.

Overall, C. 2003. *Aging, Death and Human Longevity: A philosophical inquiry.* Los Angeles: University of California Press.

Plato. 1941. *The Republic.* Cambridge: Harvard University Press.

Post, S. G., and R. H. Binstock, eds. 2004. *The Fountain of Youth: Cultural, scientific and ethical perspectives on a biomedical goal.* New York: Oxford University Press.

Rahner, K. 1980. Zum theologischen und anthropologischen Grundverständnis des Alters. In *Schriften zur Theologie XV: Wissenschaft und Christlicher Glaube.* Zurich: Benziger Verlag.

Randall, W. L. 1997. *The Stories We Are: An essay on self-creation.* Toronto: University of Toronto Press.

Randall, W. L., and G. M. Kenyon. 2000. *Ordinary Wisdom: Biographical aging and the journey of life.* Westport: Praeger.

Ricoeur, P. 1988. *Time and Narrative.* 3 vols. Chicago: University of Chicago Press.

Robertson, A. 1991. The politics of Alzheimer's disease: A case study in apocalyptic demography. In *Critical Perspectives on Aging: The moral and political economy of growing old,* ed. M. Minkler and C. E. Estes. New York: Baywood.

Schaie, K. W. 2007. The concept of event time in the study of adult development. In *Aging and Time: Multidisciplinary perspectives,* ed. J. Baars and H. Visser. Amityville: Baywood.

Sears, E. 1986. *The Ages of Man. Medieval interpretations of the life cycle.* Princeton: Princeton University Press.

Seneca, L. A. 2007. *Dialogues and Essays.* New York: Oxford University Press.

Settersten, R. A. 2005. Linking the two ends of life: What gerontology can learn from childhood studies. *Journal of Gerontology Series B: Psychological Sciences and Social Sciences* 60: S173–80.

———. 2006. Aging and the life course. In *Handbook of Aging and the Social Sciences,* ed. R. H. Binstock and L. K. George. Boston: Academic Press.

West, M. L., ed. 1993. *Greek Lyric Poetry.* Oxford: Oxford University Press.

Westendorp, R. G. J., and T. B. L. Kirkwood. 2007. The biology of aging. In *Ageing in Society: European perspectives on gerontology,* ed. J. Bond, S. Peace, F. Dittmann-Kohli, and G. Westerhof. London: Sage.

CHAPTER FIVE

Aging in World Religions

An Overview

STEPHEN SAPP, PH.D.

Definitions and Limitations

After devoting an early chapter of *The Varieties of Religious Experience* to "Circumscription of the Topic," that is, to considering the definition of "religion," William James begins the next chapter by affirming that "in the broadest and most general terms possible . . . it consists of the belief that there is an unseen order, and that our supreme good lies in harmoniously adjusting ourselves thereto" (1958, p. 58). That harmonious adjustment has been a goal of humankind since our beginning, perhaps especially as a person's earthly life draws ever nearer to its end. It is not surprising therefore that many ways have been and are advocated for achieving it. This chapter will consider only five such ways that are generally acknowledged to be among the major "world religions," four chosen for their size and the other because of its wideranging influence: Hinduism, Buddhism, Christianity, Islam, and Judaism. No disrespect is meant by their exclusion to any of the many other religions practiced today (worldwide, as of mid-2008 "all distinct organized religions" were estimated to total 11,300, with approximately 150 having 1 million or more followers), but together these five claim approximately 5 billion adherents, or roughly three-quarters of the world's population (Barrett, Johnson, and Crossing, 2008, p. 30).

More specifically, Hinduism, the predominant religious tradition of the Indian subcontinent and of many emigrants to other places, has almost 900 million adherents. Buddhism, also originating in India but now widely disseminated throughout Asia and beyond through the efforts of one of its two major branches, Mahayana ("the Big Raft"), numbers about 400 million (Barrett, Johnson, and Crossing, 2008, p. 30). Of the remaining 5.5 billion people estimated to live on earth, a little over 2

An earlier version of this chapter appeared as "Mortality and respect: Aging in the Abrahamic traditions," *Generations* 32 (2), Summer 2008. Copyright © 2008. American Society on Aging, San Francisco, California. www.asaging.org. Used with permission.

billion are Christians, somewhere between 1.25 and 1.5 billion are Muslims, and about 12 to 14 million are Jews.

Thus, almost one-half of humans alive today are followers of these three religions that together are known as "the Abrahamic religions," named for the man they all claim as their ancestor. As Feiler (2002, p. 9) puts it, "The great patriarch of the Hebrew Bible is also the spiritual forefather of the New Testament and the grand holy architect of the [Qur'an]." Feiler's statement suggests the reason that a religion of fewer than 15 million is included with four others that number in the multiples of billions: the influence of Judaism goes far beyond its current size. It is unquestionably the spiritual forebear of the world's two largest religions, Christianity and Islam, but Judaism is also the source of the formative worldview, beliefs, and values of what has been called "Western civilization" and that give it its distinctive character, even now when many people no longer accept the theological claims on which those beliefs and values rest.

An important caveat should already have been entered, and it is necessary for what follows: it is easy to speak of "religions" or a specific "religion" as if such entities exist independently of their varied practitioners or as monolithic institutions in which the beliefs and practices of all adherents throughout the millennia have been the same. However, within Christianity alone, as an example, 39,000 denominations are estimated to exist around the world (Barrett, Johnson, and Crossing, 2008, p. 30), and it is perhaps better to speak of a tradition as old as Hinduism as "Hinduisms" because of the vast diversity it contains.[1] Furthermore, some scholars assert that one should always say, "Muslims affirm . . . ," or, even better, "*Some* Muslims affirm . . . ," rather than "Islam teaches . . . ," because "Islam" in the sense implied by the last statement simply does not exist; in fact, the same can be said of all the religions to be considered. Nonetheless, acknowledging this limitation, some generalizations can and must be drawn to make possible a consideration of their views of aging.

But what constitutes a "humanistic" study of aging in world religions, the task of this chapter? Thomas Cole, one of the editors of this volume, provides a helpful response when he writes in the introduction to the first edition of the *Handbook of the Humanities and Aging*, "Defined by its subject matter, the humanities reflect on the fundamental question 'What does it mean to be human?' " (1992, p. xiii). Taking direction from this question, we can now ask what these five major religious traditions say about what it means to be human with regard to arguably the *most* human of all experiences, one that is shared by *every* human being who ever lives, namely, aging.[2] This question will be considered under two major headings, the transience of life and respect for elders.

The Transience of Life

Writing from the Tibetan Buddhist perspective, Maitland asserts that the "path of knowledge is not a quest for identity or an attempt to find ourselves . . . The path of knowledge is a journey of awakening to our true nature and the highest reality" (2004, p. 103). All of the religions considered in this chapter agree, although they differ radically on what "our true nature and the highest reality" are. To grasp their teachings about that nature, however, one must acknowledge that aging is inevitable and is in fact taking place with every breath—an admission that is also the first requirement for dealing successfully with growing older. Furthermore, only one, unavoidable outcome of aging awaits all human beings. Thus, truly to recognize one's own (and others') aging is of necessity to acknowledge the transient nature of human existence, that is, to accept one's own *mortality*, which in a fundamental sense is also the *cause* of aging.

Although it is dangerous to claim that "all religions" share any particular belief or teaching,[3] if such a concept exists, it may well be this one: All of the religions under consideration here have at their core an affirmation of human mortality, which seems always to have been at odds with what human beings have wanted and is especially so today (see the "antiaging" movement). Indeed, as Tilak aptly observes, "The quest for longevity and youthfulness predates all organized religions and cultures and is as universal as people's consciousness of the inevitability of their own death and the roots of that quest stretch back to the dawn of time" (1989, p. 137).

Each of the religions considered in this chapter can be said in its own way to place this question at the center of what it characterizes as *the* human problem that must be overcome if human beings are to find fulfillment, as differently as that concept (and goal) may be understood by each of them. Thus, any consideration of aging in the religions of the world must begin by acknowledging that in their views *death* is the real issue insofar as it is the only result of growing old and in fact is simply another term for mortality.

The Indian Religions

Hinduism and Buddhism agree that "no human life can be filled with a sense of meaning and efficacious action unless it is lived in full acceptance of the fact of death . . . To meet death, not only as an event at the end of life but as an ever-present ingredient in the life-process itself, is the final goal to be sought in both Hinduism and Buddhism" (Long, 1975, p. 65). To understand why this is so, it is necessary to understand how the perspectives of each tradition arose.

The earliest stage of the development of the religion called Hinduism likely began roughly 1500 BCE with the merging of the religion practiced by inhabitants of the

Indus Valley and that of a group of people known as Aryans who migrated into the subcontinent from the northwest. The Aryans brought with them a priestly religion that produced the foundational Hindu scriptures known as the *Vedas* (or "knowledge"). These hymns offer a picture of a universe that is basically ordered as it should be by gods whose favor can be gained through proper performance of sacrifices and other rituals. The later notion of an endless cycle of rebirths (*samsara*) governed by the results of actions in previous incarnations (*karma*), in which humans are implicated by their ignorance of the nature of true reality, is only inchoate if present at all (Long, 1975). Overall the Vedic peoples appear to have been most interested in living this one life as well as possible. Therefore, during most of this period death itself was not viewed as something unexpected that evoked terrible dread; rather, it was premature or untimely death that caused anxiety and that Vedic people sought to avoid. Thus, instead of fearing or resenting growing old, precisely because they recognized and accepted the transient and fleeting nature of life on earth, they desired to extend it as long as possible; in short, one knows what one has here, but the future is not so clear! Hence, aging and its result, old age, were valued and to be sought.

Although the Vedic understanding of the world has long ago been superseded by views to be considered shortly, the association of old age with a good life—or more properly that untimely or premature death is still viewed in a negative light—lingers in popular Indian culture. This persistence is demonstrated by records from a *muktibhavan* ("place people go to die") in the holy city of Kashi that indicate that almost no one dies there below the age of 60 (even if it requires exaggeration of the dying person's age by the person or accompanying family members). Why? The basic rule is that death in a *muktibhavan* requires one to die a good death (*acchi maut*), and death before 60 is by definition *akal mrityu* or "untimely death," understood to be a result of "bad *karma*—of past sins. It is a morally bad death because it is caused by morally bad behavior" (Justice, 1997, p. 192).[4] Thus, it follows that the older one is at the time of death, the higher the assessment of the person's morality. In addition, dying "young" prevents one both from reaching the stage of life in which enlightenment is most likely to be reached and from satisfying the accumulated debt of karma, which will then carry over into subsequent incarnations, causing them to be worse than they might have been otherwise.

Returning to the survey of the historical development of Hindu thought, the worldview associated with philosophical Hinduism arose from a series of reflections on the Vedas that began to appear in the eighth to seventh century BCE, often in the form of master-pupil dialogues and thus known as *Upanishads* (from the Sanskrit "to sit under," i.e., at the feet of a learned master). Unlike the Vedic worldview, Upanishads are radically monistic, leading to the appellation for this approach of Advaita Vedanta, the "non-dualist end [or core] of knowledge." *Brahman* (often called the

"World Soul [or Self]," the "Absolute," or something similar) is Utter Reality and is in fact *all* that is real; furthermore, Brahman is eternal and unchanging. This view is clearly expressed, for example, in the Maitri Upanishad (6:17): "In the beginning all was Brahman, ONE and infinite . . . In the consciousness of Brahman the universe is, and into him it returns . . . He who is in the sun, and in the fire and in the heart of man is ONE. He who knows this is one with the ONE" (Mascaró, 1965, p. 101).

Because Brahman is one, inseparable, and the only Reality, each human self must in some way also be that reality, much as every raindrop—despite all its apparent separateness from other drops—is actually the ocean, of which all water on earth can be said to be part. The task for each human being, then, is for this "inner self" or *Atman* to recognize its essential unity—indeed, *identity*—with Brahman, that which Atman has in truth always been. The problem, however, is that humans live in a world of *maya* or "illusion" that appeals so strongly to the senses that it seems to be what is real, making realization of the essential unity of Atman and Brahman difficult to perceive.[5] This almost universal misperception of the true nature of reality leads to many mistaken notions, such as the belief that human existence as separate individuals is real and indeed that *any*thing other than Brahman exists.

When a breakthrough to illumination or liberation (*moksha*) from normally mistaken perceptions of reality takes place, however, the physical body, which is subject to the ravages of aging and death, can be left behind as the Atman—perhaps here appropriately called "individual consciousness"—returns to the "cosmic consciousness."[6] As the Chandogya Upanishad (8.7) affirms, "There is a Spirit which is pure and which is beyond old age and death . . . and sorrow. This is Atman, the Spirit in Man" (Mascaró, 1965, p. 121). The Hindu philosophers have long advocated this realization as the only solution to the human problem of aging, death, and rebirth, that seemingly endless samsaric cycle that leads to going through it all again and again and . . . .

Thus, the Upanishadic view of human life—as different as it from the Vedic—nonetheless also recognizes and accepts the inevitability of growing old and dying, in part as an incentive to seek liberation from them by recognizing one's true unchanging nature. The Brhadaranyaka Upanishad (3.36) makes the point using the familiar image of the fate of fruit when it becomes ripe:

> When this [body] becomes thin—is emaciated through old age or disease—then, as a mango, or a fig, or a fruit of the peepul tree is detached from its stalk, so does this infinite being, completely detaching himself from the parts of the body, again go, in the same way that he came, to particular bodies, for the unfoldment of his vital force. (Rambachan, 1997, pp. 74–75)

In fact, probably under Buddhist influence, the view of aging as a natural and inevitable aspect of human existence of the Vedic period continued to evolve until, by the end of the first millennium CE, the important Hindu metaphysical commentary *Yogavasistha* asserts that "old age, which preys on the flesh of the human body, takes as much delight in devouring its youthful blossom as a cat does in feeding upon a mouse" (quoted in Tilak, 1989, p. 79).

Not surprisingly, because the Upanishad's highly philosophical path to escape from the seemingly endless samsaric cycle of growing old, dying, and being reborn was hardly accessible to ordinary folk, the final "stage" in the historical development of the tradition today called Hinduism was its "popularization" through the rise of devotional movements (or sectarian Hinduism), which allowed people to move toward *moksha* by becoming followers of various deities who assist in the quest. This path to liberation (*bhakti yoga*, the way of devotion) has become the form of Hinduism adopted and practiced by the vast majority of contemporary Hindus and the most widely known manifestation of the tradition. Its approach is best illustrated in the great epic poem *Mahabharata*, the most famous portion of which is the *Bhagavad Gita* (*Lord's Song*). In this widely known story the god Vishnu appears on earth as his avatar Krishna and instructs the young warrior Arjuna on the eve of battle in the importance of fulfilling his *dharma* or duty[7] regardless of how unpleasant or difficult it may appear.

This notion of *dharma* is relevant to a discussion of Hinduism's view of aging because it looms large in a widely noted and striking feature of traditional Indian culture, the division of the life span into four distinct stages (*ashrama*). Laid out in a codification of the Hindu view of the proper ordering of society known as the *Laws of Manu* (Desai, 1989), these stages of about 25 years each spell out the *dharma* appropriate to each. The first is the *student* stage, a time of celibate study with a spiritual master to learn as much as possible to lay the foundation for the rest of life. Next comes the *householder* phase, where one's energy and attention are directed toward creating and providing for a family and serving one's community. As early as the birth of the first grandchild, one can begin to leave behind these worldly attachments and enter the *hermit* or *forest-dweller* stage (sometimes referred to as *retirement*, but our very different understanding of this term makes such usage here misleading), in which through meditation and study of the scriptures a person embarks on "his true adult education, to discover who he is and what life is about" (Smith, 1958, p. 66). Finally, if desired, a person can become a *sannyasin* or renunciant, leaving behind all traces of former identity and setting out as a wandering mendicant who is, as the *Bhagavad Gita* puts it, "one who neither hates nor loves anything" (quoted in Smith, 1958, p. 67).

Through this mechanism Hinduism has in a sense institutionalized its recognition of the transient quality of human life, recognizing different duties, responsibilities, and abilities at different times in the life course. Hindus traditionally have seen the last two stages as precisely that period of life in which one can finally devote total energy and concentration to attaining spiritual enlightenment. In this role, older people function as models for younger members of society, and their personal needs are to be met so that they can pursue their quest without distraction.

Anyone familiar with contemporary gerontology will hear echoes of several recent theories of aging in this staged approach to life, especially the last two stages, and it should be noted that the relinquishing of personal identity and relationships in the fourth stage can be interpreted to some extent as "practice" for the ultimate loss of all earthly possessions that awaits every human at death. Indeed, much recent writing in the area of "spirituality and aging" advocates turning one's attention inward as old age approaches to discover the meaning one's life holds and to prepare for the end of it.

As much as Hinduism affirms the transience of earthly existence (as humans mistakenly understand it), its offshoot Buddhism goes even farther. Buddhism—and certainly its perspective on aging—cannot be understood without knowing that Siddhartha Gautama (fifth century BCE), the "historic Buddha" who provided the tradition its fundamental teachings, was driven to embark on his journey to enlightenment when, after a childhood and youth spent in luxury as the son of a wealthy minor ruler in northern India, he saw "Four Sights" from which his father had managed until then to shield him: a sick person, an old person, a corpse, and a wandering monk. From this experience he learned that human existence is not at all as he had lived it up to that point but instead consists of becoming ill, growing old, and dying; seeing the monk, however, suggested to him that at least some people believed that a way of release from such a life of suffering exists.

After a lengthy and arduous quest, Gautama became the "Enlightened [or Awakened] One" (the literal meaning of *Buddha*), and he gave to the world the Four Noble Truths, the core of what he had discovered from which all of his other teachings derive: (1) to live is to suffer (*dukkha*, even translated by some scholars as "transient"; Mascaró, 1973, p. 22); (2) the cause of life's suffering is selfish craving (*tanha*), leading to "attachment" to the things we crave, which causes us to continue to be reborn and thus to suffer; (3) a way exists to end our desire and thereby eliminate our suffering; and (4) that way is via the Noble Eightfold Path (*Dhamma*), a way of training for life that remakes the entire person. Thus, it can be said that Buddhism came into existence because of human mortality and the impossibility of finding in embodied, material existence spiritual fulfillment and escape from life's inherent and unavoidable suffering. The Buddha is reported to have said, "Life is subject to age and death. Where is the realm of life in which there is neither age nor death?" Given the obvious answer, he saw no choice but to look elsewhere, beyond the physical realm.

So far, little difference from Hinduism may be apparent, not surprising given Gautama's early life and the fact that he spent the first phase of his quest for enlightenment learning all he could from two Hindu gurus. A major difference between

Hinduism and Buddhism, however, lies in their understandings of the fundamental nature of reality (and especially of the "self"), with obvious implications for their assessments of what it means to grow old.

Indeed, in contrast to Upanishadic Hinduism's notion of Brahman/Atman as the eternal, unchanging Self that is all that is real, the Buddha's teaching about the nature of selfhood represents a radical departure. Commonly called the doctrine of nonself (*anatman*), his view stems from his observation that the phenomenal world humans inhabit consists solely of impermanence (*anitya*) and constant change. Rejecting *maya* as an adequate explanation—although acknowledging from his own experience that humans are woefully ignorant of how things really are—the Buddha asked how there can be an unchanging Reality like Hinduism's Brahman/Atman. Instead, what a person speaks of as "I" is merely a conglomeration of constantly changing, transient, and therefore impermanent thoughts, feelings, sensory experiences, and physical matter.

This concept is well illustrated by the answer given to me recently by the Venerable Geshe Sopa, Professor Emeritus at the University of Wisconsin and one of the Dalai Lama's examiners, when I asked him how he felt about his own aging: "Why should I even think about that? All is impermanent and constantly changing. So where is this *self* you are asking me about that is growing old?" Much the same view is expressed by the contemporary Japanese Zen master Roshi Yasatuni: "If we do not change, we are lifeless. We grow and age because we are alive . . . We die because we are alive. Living means birth and death. Creation and destruction signify life" (Kapleau, 1971, p. 8). This view is graphically demonstrated by the fact that Buddhists seeking to become monks are often sent to a graveyard and told to sit in meditation on the reality of human existence displayed there. This first step toward their enlightenment entails visualizing their bodies as the corpses or ashes strewn about until they realize that such is the fate that awaits all living beings, indeed, all *existent* entities.

With this understanding of the nature of reality in general and human existence in particular, Buddhism counsels its followers to discipline their minds to accept that nothing endures, however much it might be valued, such as youth, beauty, wealth, power, indeed, embodied existence itself. Recognizing this (no simple task, of course), the seeker can let attachment to all these things begin to recede in importance and move toward final release from life after life after life of *dukkha*. The implications for attitudes toward one's aging are apparent (see Geshe Sopa's remark above).

The Abrahamic Religions

Many fundamental differences exist between the religions of Indian origin just considered and Judaism, Christianity, and Islam. One of the most relevant here is the

Abrahamic tradition's markedly different view of reality, influencing its attitudes toward a number of issues pertinent to aging. All three of these religions unequivocally affirm the existence of both the material world and individual human beings within it, each of whom is seen in some way to continue to exist after this life ends.[8] Because the God of these religions chose to create the world and its inhabitants, the physical order possesses not only a reality but also a value not possible in a worldview that considers that realm at best *maya* and at worst the arena within which humans must suffer constantly until they can end their "attachment" to it by eliminating their desire to continue as embodied beings. Despite this basically positive evaluation of the created world and human life, however, Judaism, Christianity, and Islam agree with Hinduism and Buddhism that human life is transitory and that recognizing one's mortality is a necessary step to achieving life's goal, in their case following God's way as laid out in their respective scriptures.

The Hebrew Bible is the oldest of the Abrahamic religions' sacred books and thus provides the foundation for the worldview of all three, and from the outset it makes clear that human beings' existence on earth is limited. The second of the two creation stories that open the Bible (Genesis 2–3) states the point graphically: "then the Lord God formed man from the dust of the ground, and breathed into his nostrils the breath of life; and the man became a living being" (2:7; all quotations from the Bible are from Meeks, 1993). Life thus belongs intrinsically only to God, who freely bestows it on humankind, made of dirt like all other creatures, as a gift. To erase any possible misunderstanding, after the first couple disobey God's command to leave one tree alone, God levies several punishments, concluding with a vivid reminder of the constant suffering and labor that will thenceforth mark human life "until you return to the ground, for out of it you were taken; you are dust, and to dust you shall return" (Gen. 3:19). Note also that God expels them from Eden explicitly because God fears that "the man . . . might reach out his hand and take also from the tree of life, and eat, and live forever" (Gen. 3:22). It is hard to imagine a blunter way for the storyteller to convey his key point: only God is eternal, God is the source of the life humans have, and life is *not* forever. This recognition of human mortality continues to be stated throughout the Hebrew Scriptures (e.g., Josh. 23:14; Job 9:10; Pss. 39:4–6; 90:3–6, 9–10, 12; and Eccles. 3:1–2; 12:7, among many others).

The Hebrew Bible is also forthright about the losses resulting from the aging that mortality makes inevitable. For example, in Numbers 4, a maximum age of 50 is set for Levite priests' service in the tent of meeting, implying that their ability to perform their duties was thought to decline with age. Elsewhere, other losses such as blindness, inability to conceive (women) and sexual impotence (men), obesity, foot problems, and general waning of sensual acuity and the attendant pleasures of life appear. A particularly candid example is the lengthy allegory of Ecclesiastes 12:1–8 that describes the negative effects of aging on the human body, which opens by calling old age "the days of trouble . . . when you will say, 'I have no pleasure in them' " (v. 1).

Although this brief look at the Hebrew Bible's affirmation of human mortality, its acknowledgment of the inevitability of aging, and its blunt statements of the losses of growing older might seem to paint a uniformly gloomy picture, the prophet Isaiah expresses another important element in ancient Israel's outlook: whatever aging may entail for humans, no one will face it alone because God, speaking through the prophet, promises that "even to your old age I am he, even when you turn gray I will carry you" (46:4). Furthermore, age offers compensations, both in the respect and solicitude of those who are younger (see next section) and in the acquisition of wisdom. The clearest statement of this more positive note occurs in Deuteronomy 32:7, and it is corroborated throughout the Hebrew Bible and later Jewish tradition: "Remember the days of old, consider the years long past; ask your father, and he will inform you; your elders, and they will tell you." Those who had the qualifications to be leaders thus came to be called "elders"; although this designation may not always have referred to age, it surely originated there, or why else was this particular term chosen? Indeed, Feldman observes that Judaism considers the soul in part to contain one's memories, feelings, and experiences, in which case "the older the person the greater the capacity of the soul" (1986, p. 98).

As one would expect, the Christian Scriptures continue these central themes of their spiritual predecessor, with vivid reminders of human mortality and the transience of life serving as the context for the central message of the New Testament. This includes the teachings of Jesus insofar as unavoidable death and what lies beyond provide the setting for many of them (e.g., Matt. 6:27; 19:16–26; Luke 12:20; John 5:24; 11:25–26). The emphasis on human mortality is most explicitly expressed, however, in the writings of the Apostle Paul, who provided the new faith much of the shape it still has today. The inevitable decay and death that characterize the post-Fall world (Rom. 8) are a constant theme in Paul's theology (e.g., Rom. 5:12–14), and his first letter to the Christians in Corinth contains his most direct and lengthy treatment of the topic. He claims that Christ's resurrection proves that his followers also will be raised and concludes, "For as all die in Adam, so all will be made alive in Christ" (v. 22); he then asserts that when Christ destroys "every ruler and every authority and power" of evil, "the last enemy to be destroyed is death" (vv. 24–25). Interestingly, in an extended description of the "resurrection body," Paul contrasts the earthly body that must perish (i.e., mortal and subject to decay) with the spiritual body that does not perish: "The first man was from the earth, a man of dust; the second man is from heaven . . . For this perishable body must put on imperishability, and this mortal body must put on immortality" (vv. 47, 53).

The Qur'an, the holy scripture of Islam, continues this emphasis, only enhanced by constant reference to the Day of Doom and its impending judgment, which serve as regular reminders that humans' time on earth is limited. Islam thus takes a typically straightforward stance on this question: Only Allah is God, which means that "all that is seen and unseen is God's creation, and all that is created shall perish. Death (*mawt*) is not a punishment but a natural termination of life" (Kassis, 1997, p. 49). Using the imagery of the Genesis creation story, the Qur'an often refers to the human life span as beginning from a lump of clay or dust (22:5), through strength, and back to weakness, concluding, "Then after that you shall surely die, then on the Day of Resurrection you shall surely be raised up" (23:15; all quotations from the Qur'an are from Arberry, 1982). As do the Hebrew Scriptures, the Qur'an accepts the realities of growing old, calling old age "the vilest state of life, that after knowing somewhat, they may know nothing" (16:70, repeated in 22:5). The aptly titled sura "Afternoon" affirms this understanding: "Verily, by the Afternoon, Man is in the way of loss" (103). And Sura 30 asserts, "God is He that created you out of weakness, then he appointed after weakness strength, then after strength He appointed weakness and grey hairs" (30:50). Furthermore, "to whomsoever we give long life, we turn back in the process of creation" (36:68), that is, when old a person becomes like a child once again, both dependent physically and deficient mentally.

Still, old age is understood to be an important time because, as at the outset of life one cannot avoid acknowledging dependence on others, so at the end one is reminded of the fundamental human condition, utter dependence on Allah and God's endless mercy (see 22:5–7). This recognition is in fact the very meaning of Islam (derived from the Arabic *salaam*; cf. Hebrew *shalom*): that perfect peace that one finds only from acknowledging one's dependence on Allah and submitting one's will completely to God. Thus, in addition to frank recognition of the losses of aging, Islam also offers it as a reminder (*zidhkar*) of the most fundamental lesson a person can learn in order to please Allah.

The basic lesson, then, from the Abrahamic religions' teachings about aging is the same as that of the two religions of Indian origin already considered (although of course the details differ markedly): growing old *will* happen because human beings are mortal, created by God from the dust and destined to return to it. This message is critical today because the first step in addressing any issue is acknowledging that it exists, and as long as humans deny their mortality and aging (as is increasingly the case today), they cannot deal with it in a healthy, positive way. Perhaps our culture can take a lesson from these ancient traditions rather than pretend that the losses do not occur or can be avoided, delayed, or at least covered up, thus eliminating the possibility of finding any compensation for such losses. The unified voice of the Abrahamic religions on this point—supported by the same message from two very different religions—offers a vivid reminder to everyone who stands in those traditions that growing old is not something to be denied or overcome but instead something to be accepted either as simply the way things are or as part of their one God's plan for humankind, and thus it is to be accepted and dealt with on those terms. Given this ineluctable reality, all these religions provide guidance about how to live the allotted "threescore and ten" years (or many more today!) in ways that offer humans the greatest fulfillment possible and, in the case of three of them, ways that also please God. One crucial component of this guidance with regard to growing older and those who are doing so merits brief attention.

Respect for Elders

If the world's major religions present acceptance of human mortality as the starting point for learning to deal successfully with *one's own* aging, they share a second cardinal principle that informs their teachings on how to treat *others* who are older. Some hints of this have appeared already, but a few explicit aspects need to be considered.

The Indian Religions

As already suggested, in Hinduism the division of life into four stages provides a natural structure within which age can be respected and valued. By making explicit that the third and fourth stages represent not only a legitimate but also an expected time of separation from the productivity and the values of youth that contemporary American society values so highly and pursues so frantically—and for the express purpose of seeking spiritual fulfillment and liberation, the highest goal in Hinduism —Hindu culture assigns great inherent value to old age, contrary to its devaluation in our culture. Furthermore, because such enlightenment is usually the result of many years of seeking, those who are recognized as the greatest spiritual masters and guides tend to be old. Because the value of this period of life is thus recognized, not only is respect accorded those embarked on it, but their material needs are also supposed to be met by younger people so their quest can continue unhampered by daily concerns.

Buddhism's emphasis on the necessity of overcoming attachment to this world through eliminating one's craving for embodied existence suggests a similar basis for respect for the old because it is that last period of life—although not formally structured as in Hinduism—in which such a pursuit is most likely to be able to be undertaken. In addition, regarding appropriate behavior for Buddhist laypeople, the *Sangala Sutta,* a discourse of the Buddha delivered to Sangala, stresses relationships and duties among family members, one of which is that children should care for their elderly parents. Indeed, the Buddha refers to the parents as *Brahma,* "a word which denotes the highest and the most sacred in Indian thought" (Chit, 1988, p. 42). After parents, reverence is prescribed for teachers and elders, whether related or not. If one lacks parents, other elderly people should be sought because the good life requires that every person is to have others to revere and respect because the "tradition of paying respects to elders is a source of spiritual strength" (p. 43).

Beyond respect, the elderly Buddhist should be able to expect all the blessings of old age, "such as honor, love, obedience and troops of friends." In accord with the law of karma, good deeds are important to influence one's future rebirths in a positive direction, and showing respect to parents and other elders is "one of the best deeds of merit" (Chit, 1988, p. 44). In fact, the Buddha himself said, "He who wishes to serve and attend on the Buddha, Such a one should serve and attend on the sick and the aged" (p. 58).

It should be noted, however, that the Buddha taught that age alone is not adequate to make a person worthy to be called "elder," as is made clear in the *Dhammapada* (19.260–61), a collection of early Buddhist poems from the third to second century BCE:

> A man is not old and venerable because grey hairs are upon his head. If a man is old only in years then he is indeed old in vain.
>
> But a man is a venerable "elder" if he is in truth free from sin, and if in him there is truth and righteousness, non-violence, moderation, and self-control. (Mascaró, 1973, p. 73)

In short, one must earn the fruits of old age by one's own good conduct and practice, perceived to be increasingly important as death draws near.

The Abrahamic Religions

Judaism, Christianity, and Islam all command their followers to practice respect for their elders.[9] As expected, the content of that respect is similar for all three, stemming as it does from a key text in the Hebrew Bible: the Fifth Commandment of the Decalogue (Exod. 20:12), the Abrahamic tradition's basic statement of proper relationship with God and one's fellows.

The axial position of this commandment between those referring to the relationship with God and those ordering interactions with other humans suggests the weight Torah gives to proper generational relationships in making a human community pleasing to God. Although popularly understood to refer to obedience of young children to their parents, most scholars agree that the commandment intends to guarantee that adult offspring will take care of their parents in their old age (see, e.g., Knierim, 1981, p. 29); this interpretation finds support in the use of the word "honor" (instead of "obey," for example), which in Hebrew includes the idea of "personal service" and thus demands genuine caring for elderly parents. Further, this commandment is the only one that contains a promise ("so that your days may be long in the land that the Lord your God is giving you"), again implying that its fulfillment confers particular blessing from God. Finally, although formally extending the obligation of the commandment beyond one's own parents may go too far, nonetheless "society's protection of the elderly begins with protection by the family, basically expressed in the fifth commandment" (Knierim, 1981, p. 28).

This last point suggests another important verse, Leviticus 19:32, which states, "You shall rise before the aged, and defer to the old; and you shall fear your God. I am the Lord." Beyond explicitly enjoining respect for all old people, not parents alone, the depiction of honor toward elders in strikingly similar language to fear of God significantly heightens its importance and mandatory nature. Also, the verse's location immediately before verses 33–34 (forbidding marginalizing and oppressing resident aliens) and verses 35–37 (commanding honesty in weights and measures) has prompted both rabbinic commentators and more recent interpreters to reach the same conclusion as presented earlier about the Fifth Commandment, that is, that the honor due the old includes not only respect for their innate worth but also concern for their material welfare. In fact, Feldman asserts that respect for age in Judaism is commanded partly because of the greater wisdom it is presumed to confer "but even more so because of greater infirmities" (1986, p. 98).

As for Christianity, two incidents in the life of Jesus of Nazareth offer clear examples of the importance he gave to his tradition's injunctions on this issue. In Mark 7:1–23 Jesus engages in his first major confrontation with Jewish leaders, this one concerning the practice of *Corban* (declaring one's possessions "an offering to God"), which some people seemed to be using to justify their failure to provide for their parents' needs. Jesus appeals to the Fifth Commandment to highlight the prior demand of Torah itself to support parents, thus reasserting that mandatory obligation. And as Jesus hangs dying on the cross in John 19:26–27, he commands his "beloved disciple" to assume the son's role of caring for his mother in her old age: "And from that hour the disciple took her into his own home." In both of these stories, Jesus unequivocally demonstrates support for his tradition's respect for parents and its commitment to care for them, and the religion that arose from his life and teaching continued in the path of its Lord (see, e.g., 1 Tim. 5:3–16; Acts 6:1).

Islam offers much the same perspective, in part because it holds "a profound respect for knowledge and experience. As these qualities are normally associated with age, respect for one's elders is deeply ingrained" (Roberts, 1981, p. 124). But Sura 17 of Islam's holy book, the Qur'an, provides a much more compelling reason:"Thy Lord has decreed . . . to be good to parents, whether one or both of them attains old age with thee; say not to them 'Fie,' neither chide them, but speak unto them words respectful, and lower to them the wing of humbleness out of mercy." The passage concludes, "My Lord, have mercy upon them, as they raised me up when I was little" (17:23–24; see also 46:15). As with Leviticus 19:32, the structure of this passage heightens the substance considerably because it begins, "Set not up with God another god, or thou wilt sit condemned and forsaken. Thy Lord has decreed you shall not serve any but Him, and to be good to parents." The Qur'an's central message is the uniqueness of Allah (*tawhid*), and placing the command to honor elderly parents in this relationship with the command to serve God alone gives much greater significance to that obligation. Muslims obviously cannot refuse to respect elderly parents any more than they can engage in idolatry (*shirk*). Based on this and other passages, Moody (1990) asserts that "respect for parents in their old age is of utmost importance. Except perhaps for Confucianism, no religion is as insistent as Islam on the importance of filial respect" (p. 15). Said (1989) goes so far as to claim, "There is no exaggeration in the fact that it is the Qur'an which has most vividly laid stress on the rights of the old and disabled in human society" (p. 29).

The centrality of belief in the oneness of the God who creates all that exists leads Muslims to emphasize also the commonality of human experience, including aging, thereby precluding differentiation among people based on mere external changes. Said (1989) thus can affirm, "In an Islamic society an old person has as much right to safety of life and property as a young man has" (p. 28), leading him to conclude that although parents remain most important, "in an Islamic society, every old and disabled person deserves the same respect, compassion, and solicitude that the parents do because Islam stands guarantor to the security of life" (p. 31).

The divine emphasis on respect for parents, extended to all older people, greatly influenced the treatment of elders in the early communities of the three Abrahamic faiths, as well as in those that followed for many centuries. Recently, however, this core teaching has come to be neglected more and more in the constantly increasing rise of individuality and the consequent quest for *self*-fulfillment. At the same time, acceptance of the even more basic assertion of human mortality and the transience of life, essential to acknowledging the inevitability of aging and thus dealing with it positively, has also diminished drastically. The same can be said of the two religions of Indian origin considered in this chapter as the phenomenon known as "globalization" leads to "emerging global techno-economic and sociocultural networks . . . [that] transcend national boundaries and . . . challenge previous forms of authority and identity" (Esposito, Fasching, and Lewis, 2008, p. 3). Still, the foundation exists for adherents of these religions who want to return to the core teachings of their traditions, a foundation from which to reassert a healthier, more constructive attitude toward both their own aging and that of others.

Conclusion

Although this consideration of "aging in world religions" has been necessarily selective and superficial relative to the vastness of its topic, it provides a starting point for further examination of an issue that will only become increasingly important for all those who are themselves aging and who interact with elders (in short, for *every* human being). In keeping with a major theme of the chapter, the words of the Swedish diplomat, second Secretary General of the United Nations, and Christian mystic Dag Hammarskjöld serve as both an appropriate conclusion in light of what we have learned about the teachings of these religions and an admonition that all of these traditions would likely affirm: "No choice is uninfluenced by the way in which the personality regards its destiny, and the body its death. In the last analysis, it is our conception of death which decides our answers to all the questions that life puts to us. That is why it requires its proper place and time—if need be, with right of precedence. Hence, too, the necessity of preparing for it" (1966, p. 136).

NOTES

1. As Gene R. Thursby aptly says, "No single founder, savior, or scripture is acknowledged by all who are given or who actively accept the label 'Hindu' " (1992, p. 181). In fact, because the name "Hinduism" was introduced during British colonial rule to facilitate census taking, some people today prefer the term *Sanatana Dharma* ("eternal [or ageless] religion [or order]"; Fisher, 2008, p. 72).

2. In common parlance today, "aging" of course has come to mean "growing old" and to be associated with issues addressed by various disciplines within the broad field of gerontology, but it should be noted that aging begins to occur the moment a person is born (and some would claim at least nine months before that!). Thus, one can argue that it is the only one of the several characteristics by which human beings categorize and therefore evaluate and separate themselves that is common to *all.*

3. A story related by the eminent historian of religion Huston Smith is instructive: A colleague of Smith spent his professional life trying to discover what all the religions of the world have in common, ultimately concluding that they share two things: " 'Belief in God—if there is a God,' and 'Life is worth living—sometimes' " (1958, p. 319). Nonetheless, despite this valuable warning not to overgeneralize among religions, it can be asserted that all agree that embodied life in this material world is not the point and that the true goal and fulfillment of human existence lie in some other realm; furthermore, they all emphasize in their various ways that recognizing and accepting that fact are central—indeed, *essential*—to finding the point of it all.

4. That 60 is widely accepted in India today as the beginning of "old age"—and that that stage of life is seen as fraught with difficulty—is illustrated by the use of the term "sixtyishness" (*sathiyana*), defined in the 1987 *Sanskrit Hindi Sabdsagar* dictionary this way: "1. To be sixty years old. 2. To be old . . . Due to old age, to have a diminished intellect." The Hindi word

literally means "to go sixtyish," a euphemism for showing signs of cognitive decline (Cohen, 1998, p. 156).

5. The best contemporary explanation of this universal human condition (and of the solution to it) may be found in the trilogy of *Matrix* films, in which dwellers in the Matrix refuse to believe that the illusory world in which they live is not reality until shown the truth by a guru such as Morpheus, who reveals to them their real nature and situation and leads them out of the Matrix into the world of True Reality.

6. It is important to note that, contrary to some misinterpretations, the *water* in the raindrop (which is what is real in the earlier analogy) does not cease to exist. What ceases to exist is the drop's perception of itself and by others as a *separate* entity, which was illusory all along! Indeed, it can be claimed that the consciousness of the *individual* is infinitely enhanced when it recognizes that it is in fact the consciousness of the *cosmos*.

7. "Duty," although probably the best English translation of this word, does not fully capture the concept. It is important to keep in mind that one's particular *dharma* is dependent on one's *karma*, the accumulation of actions in all of the person's past lives, and is thus unique to each individual. To state that a person has a duty as, say, a warrior means far more than to affirm that "a warrior has a duty to do this or that." Although that statement is true, e*ach* person has his or her own particular *dharma* to fulfill as well (see Sharma, 1993, pp. 25–26, for further amplification).

8. This claim is not so clear-cut among contemporary Jews as it is for the other two religions, but historically it has been a tenet of Jewish belief and remains so for many Jews today (see Solomon, 2005, pp. 294–97, for a brief but complete treatment of this matter; see also Feldman, 1986, pp. 100–102).

9. For more detailed information about Judaism and Christianity, see Knierim (1981), Stagg (1981), Sapp (1987), Daniels (1988), and Harris (2007). Islam has not received nearly as much treatment on this topic as have the other two, and the best sources for concise presentations of Islamic views remain Said (1989) and Moody (1990).

REFERENCES

Arberry, A. J., trans. 1982. *The Koran: Interpreted.* New York: Oxford University Press.

Barrett, D. B., T. M. Johnson, and P. F. Crossing. 2008. Missiometrics 2008: Reality checks for Christian world communions. *International Bulletin of Missionary Research* 32 (1):27–30.

Chit, D. K. M. 1988. Add life to years the Buddhist way. In *Religion, Aging and Health: A global perspective,* ed. W. M. Clements. Binghamton: Haworth Press.

Cohen, L. 1998. *No Aging in India: Alzheimer's, the bad family, and other modern things.* Berkeley: University of California Press.

Cole, T. R. 1992. The humanities and aging: An overview. In *Handbook of the Humanities and Aging,* ed. T. R. Cole, D. Van Tassel, and R. Kastenbaum. New York: Springer.

Daniels, N. 1988. *Am I My Parents' Keeper? An essay on justice between the young and the old.* New York: Oxford University Press.

Desai, P. N. 1989. *Health and Medicine in the Hindu Tradition: Continuity and cohesion.* New York: Crossroad.

Esposito, J. L., D. J. Fasching, and T. Lewis. 2008. *Religion and Globalization: World religions in historical perspective.* New York: Oxford University Press.

Feiler, B. 2002. *Abraham: A journey to the heart of three faiths.* New York: William Morrow.

Feldman, D. M. 1986. *Health and Medicine in the Jewish Tradition: L'Hayyim—to life.* New York: Crossroad.

Fisher, M. P. 2008. *Living Religions.* 7th ed. Upper Saddle River: Pearson Prentice Hall.

Hammarskjöld, D. 1966. *Markings.* Trans. L. Sjöberg and W. H. Auden. London: Faber and Faber.

Harris, J. G. 2007. *Biblical Perspectives on Aging: God and the elderly.* 2nd ed. Binghamton: Haworth Pastoral Press.

James, W. 1958. *The Varieties of Religious Experiences.* New York: Mentor Books.

Justice, C. 1997. *Dying the Good Death: The pilgrimage to die in India's holy city.* Albany: SUNY Press.

Kapleau, P., ed. 1971. *The Wheel of Death: A collection of writings from Zen Buddhist and other sources on death, rebirth, dying.* New York: Harper & Row.

Kassis, H. 1997. Islam. In *Life after Death in World Religions,* ed. H. Coward. Maryknoll: Orbis Books.

Knierim, R. 1981. Age and aging in the Old Testament. In *Ministry with the Aging: Designs, challenges, foundations,* ed. W. M. Clements. New York: Harper & Row.

Long, J. B. 1975. The death that ends death in Hinduism and Buddhism. In *Death: The final stage of growth,* ed. E. Kübler-Ross. Englewood Cliffs: Prentice Hall.

Maitland, A. 2004. *Living without Regret: Human experience in light of Tibetan Buddhism.* Cazadero: Dharma Publishing.

Mascaró, J., trans. 1965. *The Upanishads.* New York: Penguin Classics.

———, trans. 1973. *The Dhammapada.* New York: Penguin Classics.

Meeks, W. A., ed. 1993. *The HarperCollins Study Bible: New revised standard version.* New York: HarperCollins.

Moody, H. R. 1990. The Islamic vision of aging and death. *Generations* 14 (4):15–18.

Rambachan, A. 1997. Hinduism. In *Life after Death in World Religions,* ed. H. Coward. Maryknoll: Orbis Books.

Roberts, D. S. 1981. *Islam: A concise introduction.* San Francisco: Harper & Row.

Said, E. 1989. Islam and the health of the elderly. In *Religion, Aging and Health: A global perspective,* ed. W. M. Clements. New York: Haworth Press.

Sapp, S. 1987. *Full of Years: Aging and the elderly in the Bible and today.* Nashville: Abingdon Press.

Sharma, A. 1993. *Our Religions.* New York: HarperSanFrancisco.

Smith, H. 1958. *The Religions of Man.* New York: Mentor Books.

Solomon, N. 2005. Life after death from a Jewish perspective. In *Abraham's Children: Jews, Christians and Muslims in conversation,* ed. N. Solomon, R. Harris, and T. Winter. New York: T & T Clark.

Stagg, F. 1981. *The Bible Speaks on Aging.* Nashville: Broadman Press.

Thursby, G. R. 1992. Islamic, Hindu, and Buddhist conceptions of aging. In *Handbook of the Humanities and Aging,* ed. T. R. Cole, D. Van Tassel, and R. Kastenbaum. New York: Springer.

Tilak, S. 1989. *Religion and Aging in the Indian Tradition.* Albany: SUNY Press.

PART II

INTERDISCIPLINARY PERSPECTIVES

CHAPTER SIX

The Value and Meaning of Friendship in Later Life

BRIAN DE VRIES, PH.D.

Friendship is the Rodney Dangerfield of social relations: it gets no respect, to quote one of his most famous lines (Dangerfield, 2004). Although it is frequently referenced in academic texts, friends are most often noted in some wide-ranging sentiment, such as "friends and social networks," as if friends count only in the aggregate. Such references mark the generalities of friends and friendship and not the particulars.

Moreover, friends appear to be of greatest relevance to the lives of children and adolescents. The central relational theories (e.g., Selman and Schultz, 1990) and foundational studies (e.g., Serafica and Blyth, 1985) of friendship focus on such age ranges. This is similarly the case in more popular venues in which writings about friendship appear; for example, an internet search on "friendship" conducted on popular search engines is likely to generate a disproportionate number of "hits" for children's friendship. A surprising second in the "hit frequency" are those relating to sexual exchanges and sexual encounters—"find a hot friend for tonight"—previewing the many and varied meanings of the term "friend" in our lives.

An alignment of demography and geography, among other factors, has led to renewed interest in the meaning and function of friendship in later life. That is, life expectancies have made impressive gains in the past century, resulting in unprecedented numbers of old and very old adults; many of these people have survived other family members and potential caregivers (Johnson and Barer, 1997), and many of these families find themselves increasingly dispersed across cities, countries, and even continents. Moreover, the related, contested, and evolving conceptions of "family" provide a unique contemporary platform for the recognition of the meaning, value, and experience of non-kin relationships and especially friendship. Friends have entered the public and professional discourse as holding promise in addressing some of the social issues revealed in the wake of these life-course and societal shifts; for example, a friend is a role that can continue even as other family and social roles (e.g., spouse, parent, worker) change, potentially increasing the value of friendship in later life (Blieszner, 2001).

This discourse, however, particularly in the social sciences, reveals a position that might best be described as ambivalent. On the one hand, recent research proclaims the salutatory benefits of friendship for individual well-being (e.g., Blieszner, 1995) and even longevity itself (Michael et al., 2002). On the other hand, it is kinship that occupies the position of prominence with its favoring social, cultural (Johnson, 1983), and legal (Montgomery, 1999) sanctions. A thorough reading of the friendship literature reveals the many family references that implicitly organize the field and cast friendship in secondary roles. Friendship is diminished by this framework; it is misunderstood in the process.

An incremental accounting of the friendship literature is a goal of this chapter, attempting to build the following case along both empirical and conceptual lines: current understanding of friendship has been both informed and limited by researchers' quantitative assessments and their focus on friendship in a family-dominant context; gerontologists can gain a deeper and finer understanding of the *experience* of friendship through consideration of its transactional roles and relational meanings in the lives of older adults, particularly those living beyond heteronormative roles and the traditional family context. My argument rests in large part on the evolution of my own research and understanding of friendship in later life, as references to several of my studies, in chronological order, will reveal. In tracing how my own understanding of friendship has deepened over time through both quantitative and qualitative research, I hope to encourage readers to generate richer studies that explore the full potential of friendship across the life course and in later life.

Counting Our Friends
Friendship Number

North American society has somewhat of a fixation on the number and/or size of things, as witnessed in the number or size of one's automobile(s), the square footage of one's dwelling, the amount of money one earns, and other metrics used in colloquial discussions. Friendship is not immune to this societal influence, in which it is often assumed, although sometimes implicitly, that more is better. That is, a bigger social sphere suggests, and with some accuracy and empirical support (e.g., Antonucci and Akiyama, 1987), a greater range of and potential for support. Researchers have often turned to number of friends as a measure of one's social support, social capital, or social worth.

Large social surveys often include a question about friendship number; in an early investigation into this area and with a sample of more than 11,200 women and men ranging in age from 18 to over 85 representing the Canadian adult population (de Vries, 1991), I explored the responses to the following question: "Apart from family, how many friends do you have, that is, people you can confide in and feel close to?" The responses to this question ranged in number from "0" to "over 99" and averaged about 6, with provocative age and gender differences.

The pattern of friendship number across age groups is best represented by a modified sine-shaped curve: those adults in earlier stages of adulthood identified on average 9 friends; those in the middle stages of adult development identified the fewest number of friends, averaging about 5; those in the preretirement and early retirement years averaged about 7 friends; and those in the late years averaged about 6. This is a sensible and predictable pattern: the consequences of the friendship network-building efforts in adolescence and early adulthood are often challenged by the tasks of early and middle adulthood, including the raising of children, for example, which may take a toll on nonfamily factors, of which friendship is included. (It is worth noting, however, that even those with no children demonstrated a pattern similar to this and so family factors do not account for the complete picture.) The later middle years, as neatly described by Huyck (1989) and others, may be characterized by a reaching outward from family resources and the formation of new friendships or renewing of old relationships; this trend is once again compromised by the losses of later life and a retreat from broader social ties (Carstensen, 1995).

The gender comparison was more surprising: men reported a greater number of friends than women at almost all junctures of the family life course, excepting the stage of widowhood. On average, men identified 7 friends and women identified 5. With amazing consistency, upon learning of these results, individuals will often say, "Well, that's because women and men mean something different when they talk about friendship."

I agree—mostly. Arriving at an individual definition of "friend" sufficient to address the question posed above is a complex task and is made even more complex by the fact that friends are not like numbers of cars, or square footage, or dollars earned— all categories that all have some reliable and fixed metric. The work of definition, inferred by the number offered, remains the hidden and essential feature. An effort to further uncover this complexity and to provide some foundation for the inference of meaning by the presentation of number may be found in inquiries into spheres of support and social networks, suggesting levels of connection and relationships and implicating meaning in a special way.

Friendship Number in Context

An interesting and distinguished literature has emerged describing convoys of social support within which appears a more contextualized consideration of friendship. The term *convoy* has been used to describe the protective layer of family and friends who surround the individual and help in the negotiation of life challenges (Antonucci and Akiyama, 1987). The convoy is an evocative metaphor constructing for individuals the image of a group of ships traveling life's sometimes turbulent waters, supporting, guiding, and aiding each other.

A notable feature of the convoy model, as articulated by Kahn and Antonucci (1980), is its dynamic nature and life-span emphasis; it is an attempt to characterize social support in the context of social networks over time and circumstance—a contrast to the static or "snapshot" view of social networks typically found in social relations and gerontological literatures. That is, this model proposes that individuals pass through the life course surrounded by and embedded in a convoy of others—a set of people to whom the individual is connected through the giving and/or receiving of social support. The specific people who make up an individual's convoy may change over time as a function of the interacting properties of the person (such as age, sex, and health; e.g., Carstensen, 1995) and situational forces (such as finances, residential mobility, role changes, and role losses; e.g., Tesch, Nehrke, and Whitbourne, 1989). The understanding and conceptualization of social support in the context of the social network convoy provide a lens through which both may be viewed and interpreted.

Convoys are typically accessed by way of modified network mapping procedures in which participants are provided a series of three concentric circles that are said to represent the psychological-emotional space in which they, their family, friends, and the other significant people of their lives are enclosed. Participants are asked to consider themselves as the center of their network circles, and then to graphically distribute the significant people around them, with no specific guidelines offered in terms of how these individuals were to be drawn in terms of number, size, placement, or orientation. In our assessments of the convoys of women and men across the adult life course, we found that individuals included friends and family in roughly equal proportions (de Vries and Watt, 1996, 1998). That is, just over one-half of the social space within which individuals embed themselves is populated by friends. For the most part, this pattern applied equally to men and women of all ages, even those over the age of 80, as did the more preliminary results reported below.

The distribution of friends and family over the three circles differed; there was a linear decrease in the number of family members from circle 1 to 3 (i.e., from the "inner" circle to the "outer" circle), whereas the number of friends was curvilinearly related to circle, with the greatest proportion of friends congregating in circle 2, followed closely by circle 3. Circle 1 contained, on average, 3 friends and 5 family members; circle 2 contained 5 friends and 2 family members; circle 3 contained 3 friends and 1 family member. Participants were asked to rate those nominated in their convoy on a range of measures, including satisfaction with the relationship, levels of reciprocity, and emotional closeness. Importantly, the ratings for individuals, within circles, did not differ, even as ratings on these measures decreased from circle 1 to circle 3. Just as the gender difference reported above typically draws comments on definitions, there is often some initial surprise at hearing this finding. This frequently assumes the form of follow-up questions about the presence of these friends in this family space with ready-made responses that often implicate fictive kin or other honorary kin titles (e.g., Johnson, 1999), as if the only expression of deep intimacy with friends has to be in the language of family.

Notwithstanding North America's "family-centrism" (de Vries and Hoctel, 2007) or "family-first" psychology, discussed below, participants of all ages included friends (and not all family ties) in the most intimate psychosocial emotional space of their social worlds (the inner circle). Furthermore, those within this space did not differ on important measures of intimacy (i.e., friends in circle 1 were rated just as highly as were family members). That is, located in the psychosocial emotional space nearest the self are those intimate others nominated by adults of all ages to be their companions on their shared voyage through life's waters. Perhaps the broad labels that are commonly applied to social relationships (i.e., friends, family, acquaintance), along with all that such labels entail and entitle, count for less when the focus is on the nature of the tie rather than its form.

Counting On Our Friends

Implied in the approach to and results of the research reported above, there is mounting research evidence describing the many benefits of friendship for individuals of all ages (Sherman, de Vries, and Lansford, 2000), along with some cautionary acknowledgment of friendship's imperfections (e.g., Yager, 2002). Such benefits are noted in both members of the friend relationship, although research has disproportionately highlighted what individuals receive from their "collection of friends" (de Vries, 2005) in more of a commodity perspective. For example, individuals with a greater number of friends, and greater contact with them, describe themselves as happier (Blieszner, 1995), more satisfied with life (Siebert, Mutran, and Reitzes, 1999), and more likely to be engaged in their civic setting (McPherson, Smith-Lovin, and Brashears, 2006). A variety of studies have reported a general tendency of increased positive and decreased negative effect in close relationships as individuals age (Akiyama et al., 2003).

Physical benefits have also been noted with studies revealing, for example, that women with breast cancer fared better (e.g., higher vitality, better physical functioning) when they were also more socially integrated (e.g., Michael et al., 2002). Recent Australian research has revealed that having a network of good friends may even be more important than contact with children and other family members in increasing longevity and improving survival rates (Giles et al., 2005): in a 10-year study of approximately 1500 people over 70 years of age, those with the most friends tended to live longer, whereas contact with children and other family members had little impact on survival.

A few studies have explored more directly the tangible support offered by friends. In a variety of surveys, estimates are that up to 10 percent (and perhaps more) of caregivers are non-kin. Although the particular ties between these non-kin individuals are rarely further elaborated, the vast majority are likely to be friends. And, there is strong reason to suspect that these numbers greatly underestimate the proportions of friends providing care. For example, Barker (2002) found great reticence on the part of her community non-kin respondents to identify themselves as caregivers. Instead, these women and men describe their behavior as neighborly and just doing what good friends do for each other.

Non-kin caregiving often included the provision of personal, even intimate, care, with some relationships between physically dependent older adults and non-kin caregivers persisting over five or more years (Barker and Mittness, 1990). Importantly, Barker (2002) reported that in many cases the caregiving efforts of friends were largely indistinguishable from those of family members (what emerges as an "inner circle phenomenon"). Barker (2002) reports that friend caregivers may refuse to engage in some tasks so that their actions are not perceived as inappropriate, greedy, or self-serving. Frequently, it is not that these caregivers are unwilling to perform these tasks; it is that they fear societal reprisal for their performance. Poignantly, Barker commented that some friend caregivers have even had to go to probate court to continue their care provision; they usually have been brought there by suspicious health professionals who question the integrity of the relationships or feel that their relationship to the patient does not have the moral obligation to carry them through when demands become higher. The friend caregivers report the opposite and resent having to go to court to continue caring for a person they love.

Friends, as supporters and caregivers, play an important role in allowing older adults to remain in community settings in a lifestyle of their choice (sometimes being the sole providers of support; sometimes supplementing or complementing the efforts of family); as such they support "current public policy goals of delaying or preventing institutionalization of dependent older adults" (Piercy, 2001, p. 43). Perhaps the true significance of friends emerges from what they are not—they are not (conventionally) family (i.e., they are chosen, not ascribed) and hence they are free of many of the more formal role prescriptions that govern family relations (de Vries, 1996)—a double-edged sword, as noted below.

The Search for a Definition

In all of the research cited so far, researchers have expended considerable effort to infer the meaning and benefits of friendship to these women and men of all ages. Surprisingly absent in much of the literature are more direct efforts at exploring what friendship means to those whose experiences are under scrutiny. Most researchers in the area of friendship either allow study participants to use the word "friend" in widely varying ways, thereby ignoring complexity and variability, or provide a limited definition of friend for the purposes of the study, thereby risking relevance for the respondent. Alternatively, researchers dodge the definitional issue entirely, resigning themselves to statements such as, "What is true of friendship is true of jazz: 'If you need a definition for it, you'll never understand it' " (Donelson and Gullahorn, 1977, p. 156).

Some attempts have been made, however, at exploring the personal working definitions of friendship (e.g., Roberto and Kimboko, 1989; Patterson, Bettini, and Nussbaum, 1993) and their consequences. Matthews (1983), for example, in guided conversations with women and men aged 60 or older, found that individuals adopted two distinct orientations toward friendship: one, *friend as individual*, focuses on a specific person who alone could qualify for such a term; another, *friend as relationship*, focuses on the nature of the association between people rather than the people involved so that the number of people who might qualify was greater. Matthews (1983) suggested that the use of individual definitions may be associated with precarious social support networks given that as friends leave the networks (through relocation, death, immobility, etc.), they are unlikely to be replaced as other individuals cannot substitute, potentially leaving the respondents feeling isolated and lonely.

We (Adams, Blieszner, and de Vries, 2000), too, have waded into these definitional waters, examining the verbatim interview transcripts of 120 women and men ranging in age from 55 to 87, drawn from two independent studies in Canada and the United States. As part of these studies, participants responded to a short series of questions, including the following: "What is your definition of friend? What makes someone a friend and someone else not?" The responses were reliably coded according to a framework we developed (e.g., Parker and de Vries, 1993; Adams and Blieszner, 1994), which identified a series of processes: *behavioral processes* were articulated by the dimensions of self-disclosure, sociability (i.e., "being" with your friend), assistance, and shared activities (i.e., the things we do with our friends); *cognitive processes* included the dimensions of loyalty/commitment, trust, shared interests and values, empathy, and appreciation or respect (the ways in which we think about our friends); and *affective processes* were articulated in terms of compatibility (e.g., liking each other's company) and care. Also included were structural characteristics, such as solidarity (or lack of social distance) and homogeneity (frequently identified as belonging to the same group, religion, or occupation), as well as proxy measures of process, including frequency of contact, length of acquaintance, and duration of contact.

There were surprisingly few age or gender differences; the most provocative and significant differences uncovered in these analyses were attributable to the study location effects. Specifically, the Canadian sample named more affective and cognitive processes than did the U.S. sample, which, in turn, named more behavioral, proxy, and structural characteristics. These significant effects involving study location point to the importance of considering the influence of culture (broadly defined) and national identity on friendship. Examining contextual effects is complicated, however, because it is difficult to determine where they operate. For example, at what level(s) are definitions of friendship socially constructed—individual, dyadic, network, immediate social environment, community, or societal (see Adams and Blieszner, 1993)? To some extent, the answer is probably "at all levels" (Adams, Blieszner, and de Vries, 2000).

This position has often been treated as the frustrating and dangling, albeit provocative, ending point of analyses and inquiries into the friendship domain; researchers have typically resigned at this juncture, offering some comment on the contested and valuable notion of friendship. It is precisely this incompleteness and ambiguity that could spur researchers on to consider more deeply the complexity of friendship in its many manifestations, looking beyond the traditional fields and outside of standard protocols.

Searching outside of Convention

The dominant, quantitative approaches more typical of research in the field of friendship have obscured and/or been unable to consider the lived experiences of friends—the deeper meanings and appreciation of the person, the relationship, and the experience of the "inner circle" and beyond. Moreover, just as this quantitative logic eclipses the lived experiences, so too does the heteronormative and traditional conceptualization of friend (particularly vis-à-vis family) hide the malleability and diversity of this important social tie. Less conventional approaches to understanding friendship and recent explorations of friendship in the lives of those outside of heteronormativity ideals have yielded provocative insights into this important social relationship and its potential in the lives of older adults.

Friendship Grief

Poignant and moving examples of the meaning and full potential of friendship in adult lives are to be found in the neglected area of the death of a friend, the most frequent loss of later life (de Vries and Blando, 2002). Each year, an estimated one in three people over the age of 65 (Ministry of National Health and Welfare, 1993) and almost one in two people over the age of 85 (Johnson and Troll, 1994) lose a close friend through death. A literature search reveals only a handful of empirical studies into this sadly common loss.

We (de Vries and Johnson, 2002) conducted one such study in which we explored the representation and meaning of the death of a friend in the life narratives of 145 women and men aged 70 and older. This sample of San Francisco Bay Area residents were members of a longitudinal study of daily life experiences among community-dwelling older adults. The data considered in this study stem from responses to the question about the death of friends within the 12 months preceding the interview and derive from focused interviews lasting 2 to 3 hours typically held in respondents' homes. Verbatim notes were taken and later transcribed.

A number of broad themes were distilled from the focused reading and coding of these transcripts, as reported in de Vries and Johnson (2002). Contained in these themes are the central meanings and features of friendship, as illuminated through loss. For example, these older adults spoke of the large number of friends they had lost through death, including poignant accounts (in approximately one-third of the interviews) of having lost all of one's friends. These individuals identified themselves as the sole survivors of a cohort, a circle of friends. Examples include the following:

— "All those people who are close to me are dying or dead."
— "All of them, gone. I am the sole survivor. I am the only one left of the old gang."
— "All my friends passed away. I'm the only one left of my friends. Isn't that awful when you get to live that long and all your friends are gone?"

The fact that numbers dominate considerations of friendship discourse (i.e., the number of friends identified by respondents, as reported above, and the number of friends lost through death) reveals an interesting parallel. The latter example suggests a deeper meaning than has been attributed to the former, rightly or wrongly.

Many of these older adults made reference to the quality of the relationship and what was now lost to them with the death of their friend. These comments ranged from the emotional closeness of the relationship, to an explicit reference of the length of the relationship, to events and activities now lost to them attributed to the death of the friend, to pointed accounts of the ties embedded in such relationships. Respective examples of these comments follow:

— "My best friend died; I have no best friend anymore."
— "Two weeks ago a schoolmate friend died—a friend for 60 years."
— "I miss not having anyone to share memories with. I miss not being necessary to anyone."

— "You feel lonely in that no one that you really have roots tied to—you're left alone by yourself."

The last example in particular reveals an undervalued point in the friendship ties of individuals: these are individuals with whom we are connected to other places, times, and people (including ourselves), and such connections are severed through death. Older adults spoke of the emotional toll that these deaths had taken, using a language not unlike that reserved for the death of a family member. Again, this parallel is noteworthy: as with the sharing of the "inner circle" of the convoy intimated above, the distinction between friends and kin may be more apparent than real—more form than function.

Articulating this emotional toll assumed several forms, as reported below. Description of the loss experience ultimately reveals further the central, meaningful, and personal role that friends assume in the lives of individuals. For example, several participants spoke of how the death of their friend was a turning point, causing them to reflect on their own longevity or life-course position:

— "It was a turning point when all the people who depended on me passed away. My husband's gone, my daughter's gone, my friends are gone. I'm the only one left. I'm lonely."
— "I just noticed that I'm at the stage in my life where in one page of obituaries, among the decedents, one half are below my age and one half are above. Up to now, they were always older than me. Now, I've found as many who are younger."
— "I figure I passed my years—that I should have gone long ago. I've lived too long."

Together, these suggest how the self is experienced and reflected in the lives of friends. Perhaps not surprisingly, many respondents adopted a philosophical tone of personal reflection when discussing the death of a friend:

— "I ask, 'why not me?' I've been thinking about it. I see in the paper that this one died. It makes you stop and think."
— "I've lost a lot of friends. I'm just losing interest in life. Being a survivor is tough. You don't make friends like you do in your youth. It's another feeling that surviving is not easy. Your peers die and you're still living. I consider surviving the worst part of life. You hear of people your age who have died and you wish it could be you. You're existing, not really living."
— "You become conscious of your age when your friends die."

Uncovered by these themes and quotes are core statements about the ways in which friendship is considered in the lives of older adults (de Vries, 2001). A stronger sense emerges of the bridge that friendship provides to other times, places, and experiences. This connection is emotional, tangible, and meaningful. It is biographical and self-revelatory. The self is further considered by way of friends, as noted in the reflections of the bereft. This association raises awareness of the dyadic nature of the friendship—a consideration of the influences and perspectives of the self and the other in social relations (e.g., Parker and de Vries, 1993). Not only do individuals have friends, but also they are friends, as Davis and Todd (1985) suggested. It is not only what friends can do for us but also what we can do for our friends. The self-other/having-being dimension reflecting this ongoing negotiation provides a more holistic and gestalt image of the relationship (de Vries and Blando, 2002). Friends inhabit many domains of our lives.

These themes further develop the conceptions and complexity of friendship as suggested by previous research. That there is grief following the death of a friend comparable to that which follows the death of a family member signals common experiential ground. Unlike many family relationships, however, there are no terms to describe the loss of a friend: in contrast to the widow role or orphan role accompanying the loss of a spouse or parents, there are no titles that signal the identity and role losses that accompany the death of a good friend (Deck and Folta, 1989). A similar observation has already been offered: there is a paucity of language by which to characterize friendship.

"Friend-grievers" (Deck and Folta, 1989) or "survivor-friends" (Sklar and Hartley, 1990) are a hidden population experiencing "the social and emotional transformation of bereavement, while they are forced to suffer the lack of institutional outlets that act as support" (Sklar and Hartley, 1990, p. 105). Friends are left to find their own way in the world of grief; health care facilities often exclude friends during the dying process, and family rights predominate (de Vries and Johnson, 2002). Admission personnel in institutional settings rarely consider the fact that an individual may prefer that non-kin be notified "in case of emergency." In studies of bereavement, friends are most often identified as support givers, not receivers; they are not perceived as legitimate grievers according to society. In fact, "society often considers interest in the deceased by non-kin as an infringement upon family rights and prerogatives, and any say in funeral or burial arrangements is considered an intrusion on the sanctity of the family" (Deck and Folta, 1989, p. 82).

Such conditions exist, in part, because of a family-centered society in which virtually no rights are granted to surviving friends, disenfranchising them from the grief systems of North America (Doka, 1989). Sklar (1991–92) commented that grief "is an emotional role whose rights, privileges, restrictions, obligations, and entry requirements tend to be confined to family members" (p. 110). There exists a "cultural lag between the social definition of rights and responsibilities of family members, and the reality of social relationships . . . The legal rights of kin appear to outweigh the intimate personal concerns" of individuals (Deck and Folta, 1989, p. 81).

In pilot research on friendship grief (de Vries, 2005), one man offered the following in his description of the circumstances following the death of his friend for whom he had provided care:

> His family didn't seem to care much about him in his life. After his accident, they all came out to the coast, formed a sort of human shield around him denying us access to him or even knowledge about his condition. They swept through the house taking his belongings and left us with nothing—not even a chance to speak at the funeral. (p. 27)

Pogrebin (1987) also quoted an individual's experience of the death of his friend:

> When Josh was dying, his wife and children monopolized every last minute for themselves; they couldn't share him. Someone from the family was always around the hospital bed. I wanted to ask them to leave us alone for a minute, but they seemed to resent that I was there at all. I wasn't able to tie up the loose ends before he died. People should realize that friends too need to say good-bye. (p. 107)

These practices, policies, and legal barriers are problematic in themselves and representative of a society in which friendship is misunderstood, taken for granted, and neglected. Perhaps nowhere is this more apparent than in the clumsy vocabulary of North America, where we use the term to refer to objects (i.e., diamonds), animals (e.g., dogs), and humans alike (de Vries, 2005). When used to describe other people, this single term (sometimes awkwardly modified to suggest varying levels—e.g., close friends, best friend, good friend, only friends) is intended to refer to many relationships of varying degrees of intimacy, a sharp contrast to the language of family in which there exist very particular, clearly delineated, and legally sanctioned labels. We have had to "borrow" kinship terms (e.g., fictive kin labels) to legitimize and bolster the nature of our connections with our friends. These linguistic practices speak volumes about North American friendship, and perhaps nowhere is the contrasting language and the prominence of family more notably apparent than in the experiences of lesbians and gay men.

Gay Men, Lesbians, and Friendship

Older gay men and lesbians are said to have lived "uncharted lives" (Siegel and Lowe, 1995), coming of age in the absence of historical experience and/or explicit cultural guides (Beeler et al., 1999). In a poignant and frequently quoted statement by Kochman (1997), these men and women bring to their later years a lifetime of having been "labeled as sick by doctors, immoral by clergy, unfit by the military, and a menace by the police" (p. 2). This harassment from multiple directions led to few protected places, even (or especially) in known gay establishments; for example, de Vries and Herdt (forthcoming) provide the example of one 78-year-old gay man in San Francisco who reported the following:

> We would go to this bar in North Beach; the lights were dim and men would dance with drinks in hand. When someone unknown to the door man would approach the club, he would turn the lights brighter and everyone adopted a neutral standing position, as if engaged in conversation. When the approaching person either was cleared for or dissuaded from entry, the lights would again dim and festivities would continue. (p. 10)

Biological families infrequently provided the safe base to ward against the attacks gay men and lesbians routinely endured; friends were frequently the ones to whom individuals turned in these turbulent times—those who were known to be "like them." As such, several authors have posited that the positive contributions of friends to the well-being of individuals should be even more dramatic in the lives and experiences of lesbians and gay men (Grossman, D'Augelli, and Hershberger, 2000; Barker, Herdt, and de Vries, 2006). Nardi (1982), for example, wrote that gay and lesbian friendships develop

> out of a need to find role models and identity in an oppressive society. The friendship group for heterosexuals may be close and important, but it occurs as an option in the context of a heterosexually dominant society. However, the gay person must create, out of necessity, a meaningful friendship group to cope with threats to identity and self-esteem in a world of heterosexual work situations, traditional family systems, and stereotyped media images. (p. 86)

Along these lines, Adelman et al. (2006) reported that more than 20 percent of gay men and just under 10 percent of lesbians (in their life-span sample of more than 1300) would turn exclusively to their friends in times of need, with an additional 25 percent of gay men and more than 40 percent of lesbians including friends in combination with others. This pronounced outreach to and connection with friends gained prominence, visibility, and even acclaim during the crisis years of AIDS; gay men and lesbians cared for each other when other individuals, families, and governments turned away from those who were ill, frightened, and in greatest need. Several authors have described these intense communities as families of choice, or what Maupin (2007) describes as "logical" families, in contrast to biological procreative families.

There are several examples of this framework in popular gay and lesbian media.

Manasse and Swallow (1995), for example, in photographs and essays characterizing 24 gay families, report that friendships exist at the core:

> The way a lot of gay men and lesbians come out in the world is very alienating. For many of us, building families of linkage and connection is very healing. It's important for us to feel that love and connection because it's the antithesis of the alienation of homophobia. It's important for us to say, 'This is the innermost circle.' (p. 153)

The use of the "inner" circle is especially provocative, given the discussion above.

The presence of such families has been noted in empirical accounts as well. Beeler et al. (1999), for example, report that two-thirds of their sample of middle-aged and older gay men and lesbians held that they had a family of choice. The MetLife survey of 1000 gay, lesbian, and bisexual baby boomers (MetLife Mature Market Institute, 2006) revealed that over three-quarters of the sample report that their friends are like their family or like their second family. Weinstock (2000) makes reference to this complexity in the patterns she identified in her sample of midlife lesbians: friends as substitute family members, friends as a challenge to the core structure of the family, and friends as in-laws. Not surprisingly, the concept of "friends as family" is contested; Weston (1991) reports that critics have challenged the use of the phrase "chosen family," opposing the underlying attempts to achieve heterosexual ideals, while others view the phrase as a political challenge to the traditional family in which biological ties are privileged.

De Vries and Hoctel (2007) explored the role and appraisal of friends, in the context of chosen families, in open-ended and in-depth discussions with 20 lesbians and gay men ranging in age from 55 to 81. Verbatim responses were transcribed, as were the extemporaneous comments offered by participants. In general, the role of choice was particularly emphasized by respondents; for example, one woman said:

> — "A family is a circle of friends who love you. You can't choose your family, but you can choose your friends and make a family. Creating a family of friends is really a joy. The rewards are immense."

Although respondents often searched for ways to describe these relationships, often engaging terms such as "alternate," "extended," or even "different" (echoing both the language issues raised above and the contested nature of the concept), many of the gay men and lesbians of this sample elaborated on these friendships in a manner that replicates what one might expect from family ties:

> — "I think we know that we can depend on each other for the kinds of things that families do."
> — "If I were impaired in any way, they are the ones who would take care of me, and I them."

A noteworthy minority of respondents believed that friends could offer more than biological kin and could therefore be there for each other in ways less constrained. Examples include the following:

— "With a friend, there isn't an obligation to rescue, whereas with a family member there is."
— "To my family of choice, I am a whole person."
— "They [friends] provide the sustenance that you ordinarily would want a family to provide."

In both contrast and extension, however, significant numbers of the respondents also spoke of their chosen families as having arisen through alienation from biological kin, some through having been disowned, others disowning, and some from death and distance. For example:

— "I see my friends as my family, because I don't have any connections with my birth family."
— "A lot of times, people's families aren't around—that's just the way society is."
— "They're all I have left."

About half of the respondents believed that friendships were more important to gay men and lesbians than they were to heterosexuals—a view often formed on a sense of mutual dependence. For example, one man said:

— "Gay people have to make their friends their family. If my brother and sister-in-law's friends fell away, they'd still have their family. If my friends fell away, I would have nothing."

For those for whom friendships are not seen as more important, respondents adopted either a historical or normative perspective, as revealed in the following quotes:

— "Although friendships were probably more important to gays and lesbians in the past, when you had to have that certain thing with people to be protected, this was no longer the case because it was so easy to be out."
— "We're all social beings regardless of our sexual orientation; friendships are important to everyone."

This relatively recent charting of the lives and experiences of gay men and lesbians in the later years offers much needed insight into an understudied and growing group of older adults (de Vries, Croghan, and Worman, 2006); although notoriously difficult to estimate, the size of this population is expected to be 4 million by the year 2030 (Cahill, South, and Spade, 2000).

Friends are often seen in relation or contrast to family by gay men and lesbians, but not as the "poor second cousins," as might be expected in a family-dominant frame-work. Friendship groups were sought or created as the "logical" connections in times of need and in search of a safe haven (de Vries and Megathlin, 2009). The absence of an agreed-upon term for their reference is at once limiting and freeing: while there is little language and little consensus on the constituents of chosen family, there is freedom to construct new relationships and new meanings.

The pioneering experiences of living open lives as lesbians and gay men have been as a result of, and have resulted in, pervasive social movement. This includes many public declarations of pride and group membership well known in North American communities, including redefining terms and reshaping concepts. Studying the lives of these older men and women requires a sensitivity to evolving norms and social experiences.

The study of LGBT older adults is a timely addition to theoretical, empirical, and practical literatures in gerontology; it has much to contribute to our understanding of aging in minority communities and under stigmatized conditions (de Vries, 2006). It also offers much to an analysis of aging more generally (de Vries and Blando, 2004), fostering a more holistic and inclusive view of the experiences of older adults.

Reviewing Friendship

Work from outside the quantitative paradigms and beyond traditional norms reveals much about the meaning of friendship and its potential in the lives of older adults. Those left to their own devices to include, characterize, and consider their friends (e.g., several of the groups as summarized above) have unearthed a path for us to follow in better exploring the meaning and value of friendship in the lives of adults of all ages. In the absence of a neatly defined and articulated system of friendship (that might parallel kinship, for example), friendships have been developed and enacted in ways that best suit the participants and function in ways that best fit the needs and desires of those who have chosen to be each other's friends. The shifted paradigm from one of hierarchy, in which friends are placed somewhere beneath kin in terms of societal importance and esteem, to one of cholarchy, in which friends and other intimates are placed alongside one another, offers a new vantage point from which to reconsider this relationship.

In the spirit of Bronfenbrenner (1977, 1979) and others (e.g., Belsky, 1980), several layers of the construct of friendship may be gleaned from the accounts described above: personal and developmental features, interpersonal dynamics, social and community influences, and cultural, institutional, and political factors. For example, the pivotal role of choice in the selection and development of friendships is ultimately an expression of the self: who becomes a friend and why? This most interesting question has rarely been considered in the friendship literature yet probably lies at the core of the experience of this relationship. In the symbolic presence of a friend, an individual understands him- or herself in unique ways; in the symbolic presence of a friend, an individual may become or enact the self to which he or she aspires.

Similarly, much has been made, in childhood and beyond, about how one is judged by the "company one keeps," ostensibly a statement of personal and interpersonal values. What effects do friends have on us and what effect do we have on our friends? What do we create in our friendships? Grieving friends speak of their friends as lifelines and connections to other places and other selves—extending ourselves over time and being recognized for who we want to be or who we once were. Often as age-congruent peers, friends may serve as support for each other through the crises and challenges of life, including old age, in ways and with knowledge unique to their relationship.

It is in the community of our friends and others that we learn the "ropes," rules and rituals of nonfamily life and to be in the company of those "like us," much like widows who, for example, frequently report this experience as they evolve into their new public and relational status among their "society of widows" (e.g., Lopata, 1973). Communities also reflect the convoys we identify and the "chosen families" we create. These individuals are the implicit response to questions such as, on whom do we rely in times of need?

Friends are identified in this context often in spite of rather than guided by social structure. Just as this chapter was introduced and notwithstanding the demonstrated centrality of friendship in the lives of women and men of all adult ages, friends are trivialized by society ("you can always make another friend"), dismissed by social institutions ("next of kin only"), and ignored by policy makers who focus instead and exclusively on family roles and responsibilities ("family care leaves" or "family bereavement policies").

Just as social science research has tentatively and inadequately explored the depths of this relationship, popular culture has represented friendship in complex and many ways; the humanities stand poised to carry this forward. After all, a humanities approach to friendship has a deep history. Cicero, for example, wrote on friendship and old age; Aristotle, similarly, wrote about the bases and types of friendship.

More recently and popularly, there are dozens of songs, perhaps many more, that speak to the ways in which individuals turn to their friends for support and comfort (e.g., "You've Got a Friend," by James Taylor) or experience with and through their friends' memories and connections over time ("In My Life," by John Lennon and Paul McCartney). There are many songs that address the long-term commitments that friends make to each other ("I Will Be Your Friend," by Amy Grant), their role in personal growth ("That's What Friends Are For," by Dionne Warwick and friends), and the grief experienced following the death of a friend (e.g., "Good-bye My Friend," by Linda Ronstadt). The songs of our times have similarly addressed explicitly the meaning of friend, something social sciences have particularly avoided (e.g., "Whenever I Call You Friend," by Kenny Loggins).

Television and film have similarly treaded into this territory in ways that suggest their value, relevance, and significance for many. Some of the most popular television series have focused on friend relations (e.g., *Golden Girls*, which also broke ground by dealing with healthy, active, sexual older women; *Friends*, focusing on the lives and friendships of six Generation Xers; and *Will and Grace*, addressing the friendship between a gay man and his female best friend). Friendships often figure prominently in the relationships of many other prime-time television characters. A cursory review of feature films similarly yields a wide array of examples dealing with friendship centrally. Examples include films dealing with the development and flow of friendships over a lifetime (e.g., *Beaches*, featuring Bette Midler and Barbara Hershey, and *Whales of August*, with Lillian Gish and Bette Davis), the navigation of the unclear and uncertain paths that friendships follow (e.g., *When Harry Met Sally*, featuring Meg Ryan and Billy Crystal), and the bonds that are formed through crises and challenging circumstances, including the later years (e.g., *Driving Miss Daisy*, with Jessica Tandy and Morgan Freeman).

An analysis of popular music, films, and other media for its representation of friendship could yield a great deal, both for what it reveals about friendship per se and for what it reveals about a culture and its values. What are the friendship themes and central issues presented in different media and over time? Similarly exciting are the possibilities of exploring the role of friend and friendship in the life stories of women and men across the adult life course, a rare point of intersection of the humanities and social sciences. Narrative gerontology (Ruth and Kenyon, 1996), encompassing reminiscence, life review, and autobiography, is an emergent and appealing field designed to explore the variety of "ways in which stories function in our lives, as well as how we ourselves function as stories" (Kenyon and Randall, 2001, pp. 3–4).

Life stories embrace the narrative terms of plots, events and scripts of life, the characters, heroes and villains, and the themes and settings in which events and interactions take place. Analyses of the terms and features included in life stories have recently been undertaken, and of particular relevance here are those reports detailing the social nature of these stories. For example, in a reanalysis of data, I (de Vries, 2002) found that 43 percent of the events identified in the life reviews of the adult sample I studied concerned other people explicitly, many of which (just under 10% of all events) were specific to friends and friendship. (This is a slippery coding dilemma; when is an event about the self with friends playing roles, and when are events about friends with the self playing a role?) The more particular "friend" events tended to describe beginnings of significant friendships, the deepening or changing of a friendship, and/or the death of a friend.

On the one hand, the presence of others is not surprising; many theorists speak of the interpersonal worlds into which we are born and in which we live and grow. On the other hand, these are stories that are told by individuals about themselves and their lives, often initiated by comments such as "tell me a little about yourself." To understand these individuals, you have to understand the others in their lives. Friends are presented in ways that suggest deep connections with or even manifestations of the self, much like the narrative accounts of the friend grievers and of gay men and lesbians; parts of the self are lost with the death of a friend just as parts of the self are only expressed through the presence of a friend. This is a provocative point and has significant potential for a more complete understanding of selves and relationships, and friendships in particular, across the life course.

These data prime questions on the particular roles and functions of friends for women and men of different ages and at different life stages; these data suggest how the path of life is illuminated, at least in part, by the friends with whom we travel. Even at this broader level, these statements speak to the implicit value and meaning of friends to individuals and the respect they deserve.

REFERENCES

Adams, R. G., and R. Blieszner. 1993. Resources for friendship intervention. *Journal of Sociology and Social Welfare* 20 (4):159–75.

———. 1994. An integrative conceptual framework for friendship research. *Journal of Social and Personal Relationships* 11:163–84.

Adams, R. G., R. Blieszner, and B. de Vries. 2000. Definitions of friendship in the third age: Age, gender, and study location effects. *Journal of Aging Studies* 14:117–33.

Adelman, M., J. Gurevitch, B. de Vries, and J. Blando. 2006. Openhouse: Community building and research in the LGBT aging population. In *Lesbian, Gay, Bisexual, and Transgender Aging: Research and clinical perspectives*, ed. D. Kimmel, T. Rose, and S. David. New York: Columbia University Press.

Akiyama, H., T. Antonucci, K. Takahashi, and E. S. Langfahl. 2003. Negative interactions in close relationships across life span. *Journal of Gerontology Series B: Psychological Sciences and Social Sciences* 58:P70–79.

Antonucci, T., and H. Akiyama. 1987. Social networks in adult life and a preliminary examination of the convoy model. *Gerontologist* 42:519–27.

Barker, J. C. 2002. Neighbors, friends and other non-kin caregivers of community-living dependent elders. *Journal of Gerontology Series B: Psychological Sciences and Social Sciences* 57:S158–67.

Barker, J. C., G. Herdt, and B. de Vries. 2006. Social support in the lives of lesbians and gay men at midlife and beyond. *Sexuality Research and Social Policy* 3 (2):1–23.

Barker, J. C., and L. S. Mitteness. 1990. Invisible caregivers in the spotlight: Non-kin caregivers of frail older adults. In *The Home Care Experience: Ethnography and policy*, ed. J. F. Gubrium and A. Sankar. Newbury Park: Sage.

Beeler, J. A., T. D. Rawls, G. Herdt, and B. J. Cohler. 1999. The needs of older lesbians and gay men in Chicago. *Journal of Gay and Lesbian Social Services* 9 (1):31–49.

Belsky, J. 1980. Child maltreatment: An ecological integration. *American Psychologist* 35:320–35.

Blieszner, R. 1995. Friendship processes and well-being in the later years of life: Implications for interventions. *Journal of Geriatric Psychiatry* 28 (2):165–82.

———. 2001. "She'll be on my heart": Intimacy among friends. *Generations* 25 (2):48–54.

Bronfenbrenner, U. 1977. Toward an experimental ecology of human development. *American Psychologist* 32:513–31.

———. 1979. *The Ecology of Human Development*. Cambridge: Harvard University Press.

Cahill, S., K. South, and J. Spade. 2000. Outing age: Public policy issues affecting gay, lesbian, bisexual, and transgender elders. Washington, D.C.: National Gay and Lesbian Task Force Policy Institute.

Carstensen, L. L. 1995. Evidence for a life-span theory of socioemotional selectivity. *Current Directions in Psychological Science* 4:151–56.

Dangerfield, R. 2004. *It Ain't Easy Being Me: A lifetime of no respect but plenty of sex and drugs*. New York: Harper Entertainment.

Davis, K. E., and M. J. Todd. 1985. Assessing friendship: Prototypes, paradigm cases, and relationship description. In *Understanding Personal Relationships: An interdisciplinary approach*, ed. S. Duck and D. Perlman. Newbury Park: Sage.

Deck, E. S., and J. R. Folta. 1989. The friend-griever. In *Disenfranchised Grief: Recognizing hidden sorrow*, ed. J. K. Doka. Lexington, MA: Lexington Books.

de Vries, B. 1991. Friendship and kinship patterns over the life course: A family stage perspective. In *Caring Communities: Proceedings of the symposium on social supports*, ed. L. Stone. Ottawa: Industry Science and Technology.

———. 1996. The understanding of friendship: An adult life course perspective. In *Handbook of Emotion, Aging, and the Life Course*, ed. C. Magai and S. McFadden. New York: Academic Press.

———. 2001. Grief: Intimacy's reflection. *Generations* 25 (2):75–80.

———. 2002. Narrating friendship: Cultural representations of the meaning of friend. In *Annual Meeting of the Gerontological Society of America*. Boston, MA.

———. 2005. Making a case for friendship. *Healing Ministry* 12:25–28.

———. 2006. Home at the end of the rainbow: Supportive housing for the LGBT elders. *Generations* 29:64–69.

de Vries, B., and J. Blando. 2002. Friendship at the end of life. In *Annual Review of Gerontology and Geriatrics*, ed. M. P. Lawton. New York: Springer.

———. 2004. The study of gay and lesbian aging: Lessons for social gerontology. In *Gay and Lesbian Aging: Research and future directions*, ed. G. Herdt and B. de Vries. New York: Springer.

de Vries, B., C. F. Croghan, and T. Worman. 2006. "Always independent, never alone": Serving the needs of older LGBT persons. *Journal of Active Aging* 4:45–52.

de Vries, B., and G. Herdt. Forthcoming. Gay men and aging. In *Handbook of GLBTI Aging*, ed. T. M. Witten and E. Eyler. Baltimore: Johns Hopkins University Press.

de Vries, B., and P. Hoctel. 2007. The family friends of older gay men and lesbians. In *Sexual Inequalities and Social Justice*, ed. N. Teunis and G. Herdt. Berkeley: University of California Press.

de Vries, B., and C. L. Johnson. 2002. The death of friends in later life. In *Advances in Life-Course Research: New frontiers in socialization*. New York: JAI Press.

de Vries, B., and D. Megathlin. 2009. The meaning of friends for gay men and lesbians in the second half of life. *Journal of GLBT Family Studies* 5:82–98.

de Vries, B., and D. Watt. 1996. A lifetime of events: Age and gender variations in the life story. *International Journal of Aging and Human Development* 42:81–102.

———. 1998. The network locations of friends and family: Evidence of subjective appraisal. In *Self-Reported Qualities of Family Relationships*. Symposium conducted at the meeting of the Gerontological Society of America (C. L. Johnson, Chair). Philadelphia, PA.

Doka, J. K., ed. 1989. *Disenfranchised Grief: Recognizing hidden sorrow*. Lexington, MA: Lexington Books.

Donelson, E., and J. Gullahorn. 1977. *Women: A psychological perspective*. New York: Wiley.

Giles, L. C., G. F. V. Glonek, M. A. Lusszcz, and G. R. Andrews. 2005. Effect of social networks on 10 year survival in very old Australians: The Australian longitudinal study of aging. *Journal of Epidemiology and Community Health* 59:574–79.

Grossman, A. H., A. R. D'Augelli, and S. L. Hershberger. 2000. Social support networks of lesbian, gay, and bisexual adults 60 years of age and older. *Journal of Gerontology Series B: Psychological Sciences and Social Sciences* 55:P171–79.

Huyck, M. H. 1989. Models of midlife. In *Midlife Loss: Coping strategies*, ed. R. Salish. Newbury Park: Sage.

Johnson, C. L. 1983. Fairweather friends and rainy day kin: An anthropological analysis of old age friendships in the United States. *Urban Anthropology* 12:102–23.

———. 1999. Fictive kin among oldest old African Americans in the San Francisco Bay Area. *Journals of Gerontology* 54:368–75.

Johnson, C. L., and B. M. Barer. 1997. *Life beyond 85 Years: The aura of survivorship*. New York: Springer.

Johnson, C. L., and L. E. Troll. 1994. Constraints and facilitators to friendship in late late life. *Gerontologist* 34:79–87.

Kahn, R. L., and T. Antonucci. 1980. Convoys over the life course: Attachments, roles, and social supports. In *Lifespan Development and Behavior*, ed. P. Baltes and O. G. Brim. New York: Academic Press.

Kenyon, G. M., and W. L. Randall. 2001. Narrative gerontology: An overview. In *Narrative Gerontology: Theory, research and practice*, ed. G. M. Kenyon, P. Clark, and B. de Vries. New York: Springer.

Kochman, A. 1997. Gay and lesbian elderly: Historical overview and implications for social work practice. In *Social Services for Senior Gay Men and Lesbians*, ed. J. Quam. New York: Haworth Press.

Lopata, H. Z. 1973. *Widowhood in an American City*. Cambridge: Schenkman.

Manasse, G., and J. Swallow, eds. 1995. *Making Love Visible: In celebration of gay and lesbian families*. Freedom: Crossing Press.

Matthews, S. H. 1983. Definitions of friendship and their consequences in old age. *Ageing and Society* 3:141–55.

Maupin, A. 2007. *Michael Tolliver Lives*. San Francisco: HarperCollins.

McPherson, J., L. Smith-Lovin, and M. Brashears. 2006. Social isolation in America: Changes in core discussion networks over two decades. *American Sociological Review* 71 (3):353–75.

MetLife Mature Market Institute. 2006. Out and aging: The MetLife study of lesbian and gay baby boomers. Westport, CT: MetLife Mature Market Institute.

Michael, Y. L., L. F. Berkman, G. A. Colditz, M. D. Holmes, and I. Kawachi. 2002. Social networks and health-related quality of life in breast cancer survivors: A prospective study. *Journal of Psychosomatic Research* 52 (5):285–93.

Ministry of National Health and Welfare. 1993. Aging and independence: Overview of a national survey. Ottawa, Canada: Ministry of National Health and Welfare.

Montgomery, R. J. 1999. The family role in the context of long-term care. *Journal of Aging and Health* 11 (3):383–416.

Nardi, P. M. 1982. Alcohol treatment and the non-traditional "family" structures of gays and lesbians. *Journal of Alcohol and Drug Education* 27 (2):83–89.

Parker, S., and B. de Vries. 1993. Patterns of friendship for women and men in same and cross-sex relationships. *Journal of Social and Personal Relationships* 10:617–26.

Patterson, B. R., L. Bettini, and J. F. Nussbaum. 1993. The meaning of friendship across the life span: Two studies. *Communication Quarterly* 41:145–60.

Piercy, K. W. 2001. "We couldn't do without them": The value of close relationships between older adults and their nonfamily caregivers. *Generations* 25 (2):41–47.

Pogrebin, L. C. 1987. *Among Friends*. New York: McGraw Hill.

Roberto, K. A., and P. J. Kimboko. 1989. Friendship patterns in later life: Definitions and maintenance patterns. *International Journal of Aging and Human Development* 28:9–19.

Ruth, J. E., and G. M. Kenyon. 1996. Biography in adult development and aging. In *Aging and Biography: Explorations in adult development*, ed. J. Birren, G. M. Kenyon, J. E. Ruth, J. J. F. Schroots, and T. Svensson. New York: Springer.

Selman, R. L., and L. H. Schultz. 1990. *Making a Friend in Youth: Developmental theory and pair therapy*. Chicago: University of Chicago Press.

Serafica, F. C., and D. A. Blyth. 1985. Continuities and changes in the study of friendship and peer groups during early adolescence. *Journal of Early Adolescence* 5 (3):267–83.

Sherman, A. M., B. de Vries, and J. Lansford. 2000. Friendship in childhood and adulthood: Lessons across the life span. *International Journal of Aging and Human Development* 51:31–51.

Siebert, D., E. Mutran, and D. Reitzes. 1999. Friendship and social support: The importance of a role identity to aging adults. *Social Work* 44 (6):522–33.

Siegel, S., and E. Lowe. 1995. *Uncharted Lives: Understanding the life passages of gay men*. New York: Plume.

Sklar, F. 1991–92. Grief as a family affair: Property rights, grief rights, and the exclusion of close friends as survivors. *Omega: Journal of Death and Dying* 24:109–21.

Sklar, F., and S. F. Hartley. 1990. Close friends as survivors: Bereavement patterns in a "hidden" population. *Omega: Journal of Death and Dying* 21:103–12.

Tesch, N. A., M. F. Nehrke, and S. K. Whitbourne. 1989. Social relationships, psychosocial adaptation, and intrainstitutional relocation of elderly men. *Gerontologist* 29 (4):517–23.

Weinstock, J. S. 2000. Lesbian friendship at midlife: Patterns and possibilities for the 21st century. *Journal of Gay and Lesbian Social Services* 11 (2/3):1–32.

Weston, K. 1991. *Families We Choose: Lesbians, gays, kinship*. New York: Columbia University Press.

Yager, J. 2002. *When Friendship Hurts*. New York: Simon & Schuster.

CHAPTER SEVEN

Encountering the Numinous

Relationality, the Arts, and Religion in Later Life

SUSAN H. MCFADDEN, PH.D., AND JANET L. RAMSEY, PH.D.

> I will also praise you with the harp for your faithfulness, O my God;
> I will sing praises to you with the lyre, O Holy One of Israel. My
> lips will shout for joy when I sing praises to you; and my soul also,
> which you have rescued. —*Psalms 71:22–23*

> Whatever is true, whatever is honorable, whatever is just, whatever
> is pure, whatever is lovely, whatever is gracious, if there is any
> excellence, if there is anything worthy of praise, think about these
> things. —*Philippians 4:8*

What does it mean to seek God? And what does it mean to be human and aging through time, destined for death? What is an authentic community, and how can humans in all their uniqueness trust one another enough to create such community? These ancient and enduring questions reverberate through the disciplines we usually consider under the rubric of the "arts and humanities." This chapter brings one domain of the humanities—religion—into conversation with the arts to provide a fresh perspective on older people's religiousness and spirituality.

Throughout history, the arts and religion have been intimately connected both institutionally and in individuals' lives. However, in the last 200 years, the forces of secularism and pluralism tended to split apart artistic and religious institutions (Harris, 2001). In contrast to the suspicion and even hostility often found between artistic and religious institutions, several large national research studies have shown that in the United States, religious *persons* value, support, and participate in a broad variety of art forms (Harris, 2001; Wuthnow, 2003), and many artists conceive of their work as expressive of their spirituality (Wuthnow, 2001). Indeed, Arthurs called the arts and religion "two strongholds of spirituality in American life" (2001, p. 270).

This chapter uses a relational lens to explore how older adults employ the arts in their quests to locate, experience, and incorporate transcendent meaning into their lives. Such a quest is spiritual, for it is part of a meaning-seeking enterprise that transcends the world of material existence. Although not all people use art in their search for meaningful connectedness with the sacred, some participants in faith communities want more than what is traditionally supplied by formal religious beliefs, symbols, and rituals. They long for a unique, creative experience of the sacred sublime, the dimension that psychologist of religion Rudolf Otto (1958) called "the numinous." When he sought a word for the experience of the holy that would not be associated with its moral significance or the discourses of theology, Otto found that this term best described the religious emotion that grips the mind in the presence of mystery. Although he described the numinous as containing elements of awe and overpoweringness, he also stated that it could be experienced in tranquility as well as in ecstasy. Offering examples of indirect expressions of the numinous, he described "the sublime" in Gothic cathedrals, the music of Bach and Mendelssohn, and classical Chinese landscape painting. He reserved special praise for the latter because in those paintings he found exquisite representations of emptiness, silence, and darkness—effects he saw as particularly expressive of the numinous.

Experiences of light and dark, sound and silence, fullness and emptiness can orient human beings to the numinous. They remind us of the distinctive way that both the arts and religion illuminate the polarities and paradoxes of life. In old age it is precisely these tensions that we experience with particular urgency, for growing old provides numerous opportunities that challenge us to live life between poles and to tolerate paradox. The pressing dialectics of loss and gain, despair and hope, engage us daily. Actions, which we organize somewhere between productivity and play, and thoughts, which we orient to both reality and imagination, point to a "duality of human existence" (Bakan, 1966) that is inescapable. Most important, we are called on to live wisely and creatively somewhere in between individual agency and interpersonal communion.

Woven throughout this chapter is our emphasis on relationality, an emphasis that arises from our conviction that personal identity is socially constructed and develops dialogically. Slife (2004) refers to this theory of human development as "strong relationality," or "ontological relationality," agreeing with object relations theorists (e.g., Klein, Winnicott, Bowlby) that each person "is first and always a nexus of relations" (p. 159). This model of the origins of selfhood contrasts sharply with Western individualism and with the atomism of "weak relationality" that envisions self-contained, autonomous beings, interacting reciprocally and independently. Although we recognize the solitary nature of many peoples' experience of the numinous through the arts or religious practices, nevertheless we argue that this experience itself is always relational, because there is, in any artistic event, both a creator and an audience, real or imagined. Similarly, relationality is at the heart of faith in the Abrahamic traditions of Judaism, Christianity, and Islam. In these religions, people are linked to each other through spiritual community and linked to a relational God through spiritual encounters, such as prayer. Thus, experiences of creating art and experiences of participating in religious community occur within the context of relationality and facilitate encounters with the holy.

We open this chapter by offering evidence for an emerging convergence of scholarship and practice in gerontology that connects religion and spirituality to the arts. Next, we briefly present the psychological and theological assumptions that ground our thinking, namely, that a relational understanding of religion, creativity, and the arts can best equip us for scholarship in this area. After examining connections between religion and the arts in late life, we test these connections with snapshot descriptions of older adults' encounters with the arts and reflect on our own imaginative acts, placing the holy within all of these experiences. Finally, we acknowledge the vastness of religion, art, and aging as a topic for writing and research, and we reference several issues outside the range of this chapter, thus posing challenging questions for future scholars and gerontological practitioners.

Religion and the Arts in Gerontology

Tantalizing suggestions about connections between religion and the arts appear in the first and second editions of the *Handbook of the Humanities and Aging* (Cole, Van Tassel, and Kastenbaum, 1992; Cole, Kastenbaum, and Ray, 2000). For example, writing about artistic representations of aging, Mary Winkler (1992) reflected on the "almost priestly function in which the artist offers ourselves *to* ourselves" in order to convey "knowledge of the meaning of our humanity" (p. 282). In addition, in his review of studies of aging artists and their creativity across the life span, Robert Kastenbaum suggested that "creative artists may still have a sense of connection with the divine or the mysterious." (2000, p. 383). He noted, however, that this connection has received little scholarly attention.

Kastenbaum's observation is verified by reviewing the research literature on religion, spirituality, and aging. With the exception of occasional references to the role of music in worship, the arts have been nearly invisible in most social scientific and biomedical accounts of late-life religiousness and spirituality. This academic gap does not, however, reflect the actual experiences of aging persons. In places where people gather to worship—whether humble or grand—we often find paintings, sculptures, tapestries, stained glass, and artful arrangements of flowers. Admittedly, some worship settings are the architectural cousins of high school gymnasiums, but many, both large and small, have been designed to evoke reverence for the holy. We find it odd that efforts to deduce the "mechanisms" whereby religious attendance can explain some percentage of the variance in older adults' well-being have ignored the aesthetics of the worship environment and its meaning for old people, the same people who often make a valiant effort to be present there week after week. Edward Heenan (1972) once famously stated that aging was an "empirical lacuna" in the sociology of religion, and we believe that the arts are equally a lacuna in the contemporary study of religion and aging. We are encouraged, however, by the emerging attention given to the arts among gerontologists, by national surveys that show significant connections between adults' religiousness and arts involvement, and by the support of organizations such as the Henry Luce Foundation for scholarship on the arts and religion (Arthurs and Wallach, 2001; Heller, 2004). The present day appears to be a good time to begin a deeper exploration of the role of the arts in aging peoples' religious and spiritual lives.

As a discipline, gerontology continues to mature. Scholars in the second generation of gerontologists, whose work emerged in the latter part of the twentieth century, have now begun to experience firsthand the existential and spiritual aspects of human life that are thrown into stark relief as the years pass. These existential experiences by scholars who are themselves aging have coincided with interest in how the arts portray the polarities and paradoxes of later life. For example, recently a number of photographers have created exhibits portraying the psychological, social, and spiritual exigencies of old age (e.g., Kashi and Winokur, 2003). Similarly, the well-known journal *The Gerontologist* always features a photograph of at least one elder on its cover, and evidence of growing gerontological interest in the arts can be seen in publications such as those of the American Society on Aging, which devoted an issue of *Generations* to "aging and the arts" (Perlstein, 2006). A year later, the *Journal of Aging, Humanities and the Arts* was launched by the Gerontological Society of America, and its first issue contained a research report by Gene Cohen and his colleagues on health-related outcomes of participatory arts programs in three cities in the United States (Cohen et al., 2007). Other evidence of increased interest in the arts and aging has come from the proliferation of arts programs that have older people (including those with memory impairment) acting, dancing, painting, sculpting, making music, taking photographs, and writing stories and poetry. Although we are not aware of empirical studies to confirm this hunch, we suspect that one form of older adults' arts involvement remaining constant through the years is the vital music ministry in many faith communities. Although not purposefully designed to engage elders with the arts, congregational choirs and instrumental groups have long included older people, some of whom have been involved in these programs for their entire adult lives.

Why does there seem to be such hunger among older people for participating in the arts? One reason may be that acts of imagination foster relationships with the holy and with other spiritual seekers. Many of the ways older adults engage with the arts are "spiritual" precisely because they elicit a sense of meaningful connectedness with other persons and with God. People come together to tap their own wells of creativity, share their creative achievements, and experience the arts in a variety of forms. Sometimes this happens within settings explicitly "religious" or "spiritual," but, at other times, awareness of the numinous erupts unbidden into secular arts venues or into the intimacy of the home studio. God can relate to us during a church service, but also in the midst of a boisterous rock and roll concert or as we listen to a Baroque chamber orchestra, visit the Hermitage, or share a grandchild's first painting.

Most emphatically, we do not wish to paint a pallid portrait of older people being passively entertained by "pretty" or "harmonious" art. Sadly, we have found, in some arts programs for elders as well as in some "senior programming" in religious settings, the ageist assumption that older people will not tolerate "modern" art, in either secular or religious settings, and that they do not want to be disturbed by anything that might challenge their "comfort zones." In this rapidly changing world, as older people increasingly access digital media and the Internet (Shapira, Barak, and Gal, 2007), the assumption that all, or even most, elders automatically resist change and exposure to new ideas must be vigorously refuted.

This flexibility is not merely wishful thinking. It is confirmed by research, and it counters the misconception that art and religion for the old are harmless placebos, activities that, at best, distract and calm. Although it is true that psychological research has noted older adults' efforts to optimize positive affect, studies on affect complexity by Labouvie-Vief (1994, 2000) and colleagues (Labouvie-Vief et al., 2007) present a counterargument to any facile (and defensive) expectation that older people always prefer to "look on the sunny side." Recognizing that the optimization of positive affect lies at one end of a continuum, Labouvie-Vief suggests that a richer spiritual and creative life is found at the other end; it requires tolerance for the complex and sometimes disturbing tension between joy and sorrow. This implies to us that religious expressions erected on a foundation of positive emotions alone—for example, the themes found in contemporary Christian Evangelical "praise music"— are inadequate to sustain an elder through the dark valleys of loss that inevitably accompany the aging process. Neither the arts nor any religious expressions that aim to be "pretty," "nice," or "pleasant" offer insight or assistance for the profound moral and spiritual struggles of humankind, particularly during the later years of life. If the arts and religion are expected to support only positive affects, they shrivel and shrink to accommodate individual narcissistic demands and remain apart from the messy mix of emotions found in real human community. Labouvie-Vief wrote that the experience of affect complexity (which we believe can be expressed through the arts and in many forms of religious faith) represents a goal realized "by opening ourselves to all forms of human experience, whether positive or negative, whether in self or others. This goal is achieved through widening our emotional horizons to achieve fuller intersubjective partnership between individuals, and between individuals and institutions and cultures" (2000, p. 376).

"Intersubjective partnership" (or "relationality" as we are calling it here) supports the development of affective complexity and provides a zone of safety for older adults to embrace "creativity and transformation" (Labouvie-Vief, 2000, p. 376). In this zone, which is described by object relations theorists as recognizing and respectful of intersubjective space (Benjamin, 1998), people can engage in a creative dialogue between two modes of knowing: the logic and rationality of "logos" and the imagination and emotion of "mythos" (Labouvie-Vief, 1994).

Carl Jung's account of post-midlife development, which affords the opportunity to integrate the visions and insights of mythos into selfhood and to reconcile with the shadow side of the personality, provides an additional understanding of the dynamics of older adults' encounters with the numinous through the arts and religious beliefs and practices. We agree with Labouvie-Vief's (1994) assertion that Jungian psychology offers a corrective to narratives of aging based solely on the acquisition and loss of cognitive capacity and rationality. However, we find in feminist object relations theory and feminist Christian theology a stronger position regarding the relational foundation on which late-life creativity and transformation can be built. Although Jung taught us much about the collective unconscious, he conceptualized it in individual terms, whereas we locate the dynamics of the collective unconscious in the intersubjective space where people tell stories and pass their narratives along to other generations.

Psychological and Theological Perspectives on the Arts and Religion

Theologically, the most respectful and appropriate argument for an intersection of the arts, religion, and aging is based not on *doing* but on a kind of *being*, namely, on our existence as persons created for relationships by a loving, just, and relational God. Because status as God's beloved creatures does not change as people age and lose significance in a youth-centered society, belief in God's justice requires that elders be given the same opportunities to experience agency—the capacity for self-expression— as those of any other age. Belief in God's love precludes utilitarian attitudes toward human beings in planning for and evaluating the value of their artistic experiences. Thus, we do not encourage people working with older adults, or older adults themselves, to focus on the arts in later life primarily because they are enjoyable or distractive. Such motivations are insulting to the dignity of older adults. Belief in a relational God reminds us that none of us want to be treated as objects—in this case, objects of care needing to be "kept busy."

In light of the ageism that surrounds us in Western culture, and in light of the objectification and disrespect that ageism arouses, this emphasis on the relational aspects of spirituality offers a particularly helpful corrective in our discussion of the arts, religion, and aging. Relationality requires respectful subjectivity, and because creative expression has hopeful and vital power and is part of what it means to be fully alive and at peace in the world, to be creatively involved is not to be an object that is acted on. Rather, it is to be a subject, an agent who is a living, unique creation, a child of God and a cocreator with God who participates in the continual re-creation of our beautiful world. This ongoing creation, visualized as humble yet agentic partnership with God, then becomes both particular and universal, both immediate and timeless.

Relational language in theology, which reinforces this respectful vision of human beings and their creativity, is nothing new. In Judaism, for example, it is at the heart of Martin Buber's "I-Thou" vision. In traditional Christianity, a relational emphasis lay dormant for some time, overcome by a post-Enlightenment preference for Platonic, material categories. Recently, relationality has regained its place in the conversation, largely through the work of feminist scholars (e.g., Lacugna, 1993) and those influenced by them (e.g., Shults and Sandage, 2006). Similar to feminist artists such as Nancy Azara, who helped to recover maternal aspects of the divine in their art while drawing on Christian and Buddhist themes (see further Wuthnow, 2001), feminists working today in theology and philosophy wish to correct static, paternal images of the divine. These women have been particularly interested in the deep, primordial themes of human experience that trace back to our early human relationships (e.g., Johnson, 1993; Lacugna, 1993). Against modern conceptualizations of faith that viewed God as a divine *substance*, most postmodern Christian theologians envision a dynamic, social (trinitarian) God, a God who creates, restores, and renews people and thus transforms the dynamics of their lives. Such a God partners with human beings to open up radically fresh possibilities for healthy and repaired relationships with God and with one another.

The implications of belief in a social God, a "God for us" (Lacugna, 1993), are important for the intersection of art and religion, for, like any creator, God makes something new according to God's own preferences and according to God's own ideas of beauty. Thus, it should be no surprise that God also made people "in God's image," that is, as deeply social beings—so much so that from the moment of our birth when we separate from our mother's body, we are psychologically and biologically oriented toward forming and maintaining close interpersonal relationships. In other words, we are made for love, at the deepest level, whether or not we are aware of feeling this love at any particular moment of life. However, although humans are "hardwired" for relationships, we are never at a place where we get them quite right. Thus, across the life span, we move between the poles of freedom and destiny; we hurt one another, experience guilt and remorse, mourn our disappointments, and stand in need of forgiveness. When artists are able to capture these fundamental, defining experiences of human life, we sense the presence of the numinous, perhaps even more strongly than when we hear or see works that try to capture transcendence alone.

There are also psychological arguments for the relationality of artistic activity. The potential for creativity appears to be located deep within us as is obvious from its timeless, worldwide nature. Although it is risky to speculate on the origins of a phenomenon so mysterious and so hidden from human consciousness, psychodynamic theory takes that risk and goes deep into the shadow lands of human personality. These theorists ask questions about both the meanings and origins of human creativity. Early on, Freud, ever the risk taker, believed that human beings are creative because of the need to find ways out of the conflicts that arise from unconscious attempts to reconcile contradictory drives, such as love and hate, death and life forces, the desire to self-protect and the desire to explore. For Freud, art was a kind of privileged neurosis (Glover, 2005); he claimed that creative experience is best understood as an extension of the artist's troubled inner world. Writing of Freud's work on Leonardo, Glover stated:

> Freud's approach centers on the experience of the individual artist, and like a detective, he reconstructs his subject's past, discovering possible complexes, repressions, and neuroses. The artist is treated as a patient and his products are analyzed in terms of these psychological considerations. The artwork is seen as a means of giving expression to, and/or dealing with, various psychic pressures. (2005, p. 2)

Although we see the limits in Freud's mechanistic paradigms today, at least he did not visualize art as simply an object for psychoanalysis (see Freud, 2002). As his work on jokes shows, there was also room in his theory for viewing human creativity as a playful process. In this way he helped, albeit inadvertently, to pave the way for what is sometimes called the "British School" of psychoanalysis, where relationality came to trump Freud's emphases on drives and the mechanics of forces.

Although she, too, was the child of her times and believed in the power of drives and forces, the founder of object relations theory, Melanie Klein, used her own creativity to both embrace and challenge Freud's authority. She dared to go earlier into the mysteries of human psyche, using her observations of infants (including her own children) and her analytical case studies of adults to postulate that creativity, like the capacity for empathy and envy, begins very early, during the early months of life. Klein's work was extended by Winnicott, Bowlby, and others, who recognized the importance of early experiences for shaping our lifelong styles of attaching to one another and for being creatively alive in a complex world. More recently, interpreters of Klein such as Judith Edwards (2005) have gone further, suggesting that even children whose early years were highly disadvantaged psychologically and socially could begin to create when they began to trust their therapist. A safe, holding place for creative expression allowed them to cope with the disorder in their own lives even before they reached the stage of taking responsibility for others and for themselves.

Perhaps the origins of creativity can be found in all of the above, reflecting both the diversity of human personality and the enormous variety with which people express their freedom and resiliency. There are no doubt infinite numbers of ways human beings can experience and express the *spark toward new ways of thinking, doing, and being* that we call creativity. Certainly, to be creative does not require an older person to paint a picture or write a song. Rather, a creative spark may be felt by an old man sitting in his favorite chair looking through a book about Renaissance painting, or by an old woman resting on her bed in the nursing home, listening to a Saturday radio broadcast of the Metropolitan Opera. In other words, what is sometimes called the "Big-C" creative expression by eminent artists (Beghetto and Kaufman, 2007) can activate a more humble yet powerful creative spark in people of any age, as well as a connection with the numinous.

Whatever its origins or forms of expression, creativity clearly requires a place of safety. The language of intersubjective space used by object relations theorists is one way to envision this location, where agents (subjects) meet with mutual respect, encouragement, and freedom (Benjamin, 1998). This is the opposite of what feminist philosopher Kelly Oliver calls "colonized" space (2004), space that has been taken over by invasive forces of oppression. Colonized space is not an environment where new things are likely to develop and be born. In the case of older adults, interpsychic spaces can too easily be colonized by the forces of ageism, by ideas that one is "too old" to create, "too stuck" to think in new ways, "too dependent and/or disabled" to contribute or even appreciate something of beauty and meaning.

As object relations theorists teach, relationality is not merely an add-on to life experiences, not merely an optional dimension of life among others. Rather, we are, as persons, literally constituted by our human relationships. Or, using the language of narrative theory, we not only *have* a story—we *are* our stories. Thus, drive for self-expression, for creating and re-creating our very selfhood, cannot be divorced from relationality, from the circle of others who make up our lives. Contrary to an obsolete, modern vision of the isolated artist, postmodernism suggests that art, like all of reality, is "made up"—created both for and by the Other. This includes not only those others who are physically present or who will recognize and appreciate our creative expressions, but also all of the introjected others who form us as unique selves. It also includes our "audience," those whom we imagine listening to, looking at, and touching our creations, thus cocreating with us a fresh perception of reality.

One approach to art that can be highly privatized, but that also allows for shared communal experience, is expressed by Romantic theorists. Here, artistic expression becomes a mystical and transcendent encounter, leading to what Bernard Berenson called the "aesthetic moment," which is a "flitting instant, so brief as to be almost timeless, when the spectator is at one with the work of art he is looking at, or with actuality of any kind that the spectator himself sees in terms of art, as form and colour. He ceases to be his ordinary self, and the picture or building, statue, landscape or aesthetic actuality is no longer outside himself . . . In short, the aesthetic moment is a moment of mystic vision" (Berenson, 1954, quoted in Morgan, 2004, p. 32).

Friedrich Schleiermacher's theology, with its emphasis on the feeling of *absolute dependence* on God (1996), echoes this trust in the sublime possibilities of religious aesthetic experience and hints of intimate, albeit romantic, relationality. Although a friend of many in the German Romantic movement, especially its poets, Schleiermacher viewed religion and theology as originating in the human experience of contingency. He "did not succumb to the temptations of romantic fantasy and sentimentality" (Redeker, 1973, p. 63), nor did he conflate art and religion. Rather, he wished to explore how the arts could liberate the human imagination in its intimate encounter with the numinous.

The idea that the arts can draw people into closer relationship with God has also been both embraced and rejected in American religious history (Harris, 2001). However, today we find many voices in religious institutions calling for scholarship on religion and the arts. Indeed, since the late twentieth century, a number of endowed chairs for this kind of scholarship have been established at theological seminaries (Heller, 2004). In addition, ordinary people are seeking opportunities to come together to share the ways their experiences of the arts contribute to spiritual development. In the last section of this chapter we suggest several ways local religious congregations might enable such a conversation to take place among older adults, including those with dementia.

Imaginative Moments with Elders, Art, and the Numinous

Turning from theological and psychological reflections, we now present "imaginative moments" to illuminate older people's encounters with the numinous. These vignettes have three sources: the experiences of both authors with older women in faith communities, a documentary film, and a visit the first author (McFadden) made to an elderly sculptor's studio. In the first and last cases, we did not specifically ask individuals about their awareness of the holy. Rather, we use our acts of imagination to connect human stories to the abstractions presented in this chapter, thus honoring those older adults who inspired our reflections and graciously absorbed our projections.

Imaginative Moment 1: "Church ladies" gather in the basement. It is highly unlikely that Rudolf Otto would have searched for the numinous on a Tuesday morning, in a church basement. Amidst fabrics, yarns, needles, and empty coffee cups, elderly women gather to talk and sew a bright-colored banner to hang in the modest sanctuary where they have worshipped for many years. The skeptic might ask, "Is this art or craft?" Surely the skills required of craft are here, but there is more: the creation of something new, something born from the imagination and spirit. Even though these women would modestly assert that they do not see themselves as artists, there is a sense in which they are entering into a holy process. They are not alone. In faith communities of all sizes and denominations, one finds older adults working together to create, engaging the religious imagination of fellow congregants, and motivated by the possibility of selling their creations to support the local congregational budget, a community cause, or mission outreach. Creation here joins faith seamlessly (pun acknowledged); they believe that God, the creator, is present with them. And although they may not know the language of the numinous, when their work is complete they will see what they have made, feel a sense of awe for what has emerged, and likely express gratitude for the opportunity they have had to contribute to this creation.

Imaginative Moment 2: Lloyd Herrold goes to a museum. In one of the most poignant and moving moments of *Almost Home* (2005), a documentary film about culture change in long-term care, the administrator of a long-term care facility in Milwaukee takes a resident, Lloyd Herrold, to the Milwaukee Art Museum. Herrold, whom viewers of the film have come to know as a dignified and wise man struggling with Parkinson's dementia and loneliness, was once president of the board of this very museum. The administrator, John George, comments on what an honor it is to know Herrold, who has had such an exalted position. Herrold replies, "It is noticed by some." Later, George pushes Herrold in his wheelchair to view *The Two Majesties (Les Deux Majestes)*, by Jean-Leon Gerome. In this luminous painting, a lion sits on a promontory high over a valley and watches the sun set (or, perhaps, rise). George describes how he sees a lion boldly claiming, at the end of his life, that he has done what was needed and is now satisfied. Herrold softly replies that he disagrees. Instead, he says, the lion is longing for companionship and is "aware that most of us are going to be alone most of the time." Nothing is said about the holy in this scene, but viewers may catch a glimpse of the numinous in the intersubjective space in which an old man with multiple disabilities quietly teaches a younger man about strength, loss, and courage.

Imaginative Moment 3: Alfred Tibor gives a tour. On a humid summer day in Columbus, Ohio, Alfred Tibor graciously walks a middle-aged woman through his home, yard, and studio—all filled with his art. He talks about life as a gift to which he must witness every day. Now in his mid-eighties, Tibor is a sculptor whose work is displayed in several places in his adopted city, as well as in museums and private collections around the world. His life's journey to this studio has been arduous. He lost nearly all of his family to the Holocaust, was enslaved by the Germans, and spent several years as a Russian prisoner of war. Fleeing the Hungarian revolution, he made a new life in the United States in 1957, and since then, he has dedicated his life to expressing his enduring faith in God and humanity. His faith endures in spite of the terrible suffering and many losses he has experienced, and he honors the dead through bronze representations of Biblical figures, Jewish families who perished in the Holocaust, African-Americans escaping from slavery into Ohio, and even a young woman's horse commissioned to rest on her grave. Having learned to live between dramatic and dangerous polarities, Tibor's expansive love and compassionate empathy are visible in his art, along with his knowledge that although life is transient, God is eternal.

These snapshots of artistic moments represent our own acts of imagining the numinous that is present in older peoples' encounters with the arts. We find in them "a whiff of the divine," as Robert Kastenbaum (2001, p. 277) depicted in the feeling of being creatively inspired. We offer these vignettes to stimulate our readers' own imaginations, hoping that you will picture for yourself older people as they play instruments in community orchestras, or as they paint, quilt, knit, do wood carving, or participate in any of the myriad forms of artistic expression. We hope to call up images of elder poets, actors, and dancers sharing their arts with their communities in cultures around the world. We challenge you to engage in thought experiments by simply varying the age, gender, race, class, cognitive status, and culture of the elders you know who make or experience the arts. Although some of these imagined people would undoubtedly deny any numinous element to their artistic creations or their appreciation of the arts, many others would unabashedly affirm that the arts have nourished their spirituality. Wuthnow's (2001) interviews with artists confirm our imagining and attest to the many artists who invoke spirituality as central to the meaning and the beauty of their work.

Perhaps some of the people we observed also exemplify what Lars Tornstam called "gerotranscendence"—a shift in "metaperspective" from a materialistic view of the world to one that is more transcendent and may or may not include any religious referents. In his many papers (e.g., Tornstam, 1999), he described gerotranscendence as a developmental possibility for later life that consists of three dimensions: cosmic, self, and relational. According to Tornstam, older people may reorder their sense of time, experience more openness to life's mysteries, and feel a deep sense of joy that transcends their daily encounters with human limitations. He also characterizes older people who exhibit gerotranscendence as being less self-centered and as appreciating relationships with others more deeply than those who have not achieved this worldview.

Although appealing in its hopeful vision of old-age potential, gerotranscendence has not lacked its critics. Some, including Kastenbaum (1999), believe that it may imply a kind of gerontological "cheap grace"; he suggested that gerotranscendence could become "a popular quick fix for what ails us about growing old" (1999, p. 210). Others note its weak empirical support and theoretical essentialism (Jönson and Magnusson, 2001), both of which can lead to the unfortunate conclusion that elders who do not demonstrate gerotranscendence have somehow failed to age well.

Undoubtedly, some elders do undergo the kinds of metaperspectival shifts Tornstam describes, finding inspiration in the arts and their own creative output. On the other hand, however, in the arts, the polarities and paradoxes of life are not transcended so much as they are held in creative tension. Furthermore, religion offers diverse symbols, narratives, and rituals that can enable humans to encounter the numinous in the midst of precisely these tensions—between the restraints of our human destiny and our freedom to create a new future, and between our drive to differentiate and our longing for community. More specific to the theological position taken here, these symbols, narratives, and rituals reveal and nurture the capacity, at any age, for a relationship with a loving creator, a relationship that is freely offered regardless of whether an elder has attained gerotranscendence.

Undoing the Imaginative Moments

Imagination creates, but it also destroys, or to use the language of psychology, "doing" is always countered with "undoing." What might undo the moment when the old ladies in the church basement gather to witness the unveiling of their creation and feel God's light shining on the moment? Social norms! Public art usually evokes some kind of controversy, and faith communities are no exception. The bonds of community—of relationality—can be shattered by disagreement over what constitutes "good art" or "real art." Human communities, including religious groups, are frequently riled by contention about "religious" and "secular" art (beginning, we speculate, with cave dwellers).

Not only the value of art, but also art as a holy experience, is in the eye of the beholder. We imagined the numinous in Lloyd Herrold's quiet response to the painting. It was there for us as we viewed that scene, but we acknowledge the possibility that Herrold experienced no such thing. In imagining his inner landscape, we risk undoing the moment. Or, we can inquire whether we also perceive the presence of the numinous when he viewed another, more jarring composition and commented that it looked like "someone has had a bad lunch." Is that honest response really so different from his response to the lion? Finally, we can also undo the scene by thinking of all the elders—with and without cognitive impairment—who never will have a chance to go to an art museum because there is no one available to help them get there or because their community has no museum. In this act of undoing, we move from the subjective to the social, from questioning our projections of the numinous into someone else's experience to critiquing our failure to observe the intersection of art with the highly unpleasant subject of social inequality—in education, in economics, in cultural opportunity.

And what can undo Alfred Tibor's moment? The agonies of Europe in the mid-twentieth century almost ended his life. His personal resilience and artistic talent, along with the kindness of strangers and the opportunities he had to create and sell his work, all brought him to that proud moment in the studio. Still, today many factors could have undone Tibor's moment, including the lack of opportunity described above. In his eighties, Tibor is healthy, married, financially secure, and respected. He also has the energy and opportunity to make art that expresses his spiritual values. Many elders have neither.

We engaged in this exercise of doing and undoing because honest writing about aging, religion, and art must acknowledge important complexities, lest we slip into romantic, fuzzy visions of serene older people simultaneously experiencing God and art. First, as Kastenbaum reminds us repeatedly, we are often tempted to domesticate older adults in order to protect ourselves from the suffering and dark nights of the soul revealed in their creative acts and their complex artistic responses. Another complication arises in the debate over what constitutes "religious art." This debate can derail the entire discussion of aging, religion, and art, because there are such varied responses to this question.

One way of conceptualizing this subjective, evaluative process was provided by Heggen (2000), who described Paul Tillich's four categories for thinking about religious art. They are produced by combining the presence or absence of religious content (specific images connected to particular religious traditions) with the presence or absence of religious style (expression of a transforming encounter with the divine). But returning to our imagining of the church basement banner, we are left wondering into which category this product would fall. More important, how much does it matter to the women who created it or to their congregation?

Our pathway out of this labyrinth is the same one we followed when we entered—the thread of relationality. This strand, like Theseus's ball of thread, keeps us from wandering endlessly in self-made circles. It leads away from self and toward the sacred heart of religion and the arts. It leads past cultural stereotypes about solitary artists into shared experiences between creators and audiences, and within audiences themselves. And it avoids the most dreadful monster of all: the ageism that frightens potential older artists and keeps them from expressing themselves with originality and power.

Our own acts of doing and undoing imaginative moments of elders extracting something spiritual from the arts are also motivated by our personal sense of relationality, our own spiritual biases. We perform these acts here not as art critics evaluating elders' creations or artistic preferences, nor as religious judges evaluating piety. Rather, confessing our own limitations, we attempt to enter the intersubjective space of mutual recognition with other aging human beings who, like us, seek to know God and grasp meaning amidst the sometimes sublime, sometimes horrifying exigencies of human life. It is easy to see how we might behold the numinous in this space by gazing at great artworks, such as Masaccio's painting of *The Holy Trinity*, or by listening to Bach's Mass in B Minor. But our relational approach to this topic also permits us to sense the holy in the moment when a person with dementia shows us a painting of a few red flowers and, with a broad smile, talks about her mother's garden.

Visions of Relationality in the Arts and Religion

At the outset of this chapter, we stated that we wanted to bring the arts into conversation with religion. Obviously, this is an ancient conversation carried on for many centuries and across diverse cultures. Although this inquiry has, at times, lifted up the highest and best ideals of both religion and the arts, it has also dragged them through the depths of discord and fractious dissention. Fruitless arguments have been made, for example, over who conveys the truest insights about the nature of God and humanity. Our inquiry veers away from these bitter conflicts between the arts and religion toward an attempt to understand what might be gained if researchers and practitioners in gerontology entered into a deeper conversation with leaders of faith communities using the language of relationality and avoiding the more typical focus on evaluation of "substance," namely, the individual artistic product, or the level of a person's spiritual development.

Wuthnow's (2001) work on creative individuals' spirituality represents a starting point for this further study, although it must be noted that he did not approach his research with a developmental perspective or a focus on later life. Given all the research of the past quarter century on the contribution of religion and spirituality to older adults' physical and mental well-being (Idler, 2006; Krause, 2006), it would be good to know whether these findings could be applied to elder artists who understand their artistic expression as revealing their spiritual beliefs and experiences. We also need to learn more about how elder artists relate to other people. For example, having wrestled with the polarities of human life, are they more likely to show love and forgiveness? There is a long tradition of studying late-life creativity, aging artists, and the nature of "old-age style" (Lindauer, 2003), but we also need greater insight into the moral and spiritual implications for those older adults who claim some dimension of the arts as part of their core identity.

In addition, gerontologists working in applied settings should pay attention to the emotional and social sequelae of older adults' participation in the arts. In this sense, participation means active engagement by either making art or being given the opportunity to respond to it. Against the idea of parking people in wheelchairs to be passively "entertained" while paid caregivers take a break, we wonder about implications for the older adults themselves, including those in long-term care settings. The work of Gene Cohen and his colleagues (Cohen et al., 2007) is demonstrating the health outcomes of active arts participation. Could artist participation not also result in greater social interaction, a deeper sense of meaning for one's life, and, for the religious person, a clearer realization of being loved by God?

In religious circles, there is also much work to be done. Religious people believe that faith invites transformation of individuals and societies, but they seldom focus on the elimination of ageism, both internal and external, as an example of this needed transformation. The arts offer an antidote to ageism in many ways. Consider, for example, the national publicity for "Meet Me at MOMA," a program at the Museum of Modern Art in New York City that gathers groups of people with dementia every week to experience and talk about art. News articles about this program (e.g., Kennedy, 2005) are educating the public about the remarkable artistic insights of these ordinary people with cognitive impairment. Congregations could easily organize similar programs to give older people—both those who are "well" and those with dementia—opportunities to create and experience the arts and, by integrating these programs into the whole life of the congregation, begin to challenge ageist ideas about older adults, particularly those that are held by older people themselves. Arts discussions and arts creation have been shown to increase social interaction among independent living elders (Wikström, 2002) and hopefulness among hospice patients (Kennett, 2000). By attending to the arts, and by giving older people opportunities to be engaged with them, faith communities could foster elder spiritual development, encourage meaningful interpersonal relationships, and offer a resource for hope in the face of late-life challenges.

We cannot conclude this chapter about encountering the numinous through the arts without commenting on an issue of social justice, one that faith communities and arts organizations together might address. Many older people live in environments that are truly "arts deprived." Despite the efforts of organizations like the Society for the Arts in Health Care, far too many long-term care facilities still pay no attention to the arts, either by integrating them into the environment or by fostering the creative process in older people. We suspect that these organizations may also be more likely to "outsource" pastoral care to community clergy who may lack the time, interest, or training to meet the spiritual needs of residents.

On the other hand, some nursing homes are exemplars of how paintings, sculptures, fabric artworks, musical and dramatic performances, and other forms of the arts can be integrated into the daily life of residents and staff. Nursing homes with roots in the Jewish community, such as the Hebrew Home at Riverdale (New York) and Baycrest (formerly the Toronto Jewish Old Folks Home), offer outstanding models of incorporating the arts into long-term care. These facilities are also more likely to attend to how religion can structure time for frail elders through regular services and pastoral care by full-time chaplains. Exciting opportunities for collaboration between arts organizations and faith communities could emerge from conversations about how they might advocate together for high-quality, multifaceted spiritual care for older people.

We are acutely aware of the many topics we have not addressed in this chapter, but we consider this to be only the beginning of an important conversation about the arts, religion, and aging. The conversation itself taps creative thinking about opportunities for theoretical and empirical work by gerontologists, artists, and psychologists. It has crucial implications for program development by faith communities and for advocacy for more just ways of thinking and doing by all who care about older people. The conversation itself is complex and requires a thread that allows us to stay focused and avoid getting lost. This is best accomplished as we think together about how the arts enrich the soul and enable human beings to relate to one another and to the numinous in profound and mysterious ways.

REFERENCES

Arthurs, A. 2001. Afterword. In *Crossroads: Art and religion in American life*, ed. A. Arthurs and G. Wallach. New York: New Press.

Arthurs, A., & G. Wallach, eds. 2001. *Crossroads: Art and religion in American life.* New York: New Press.

Bakan, D. 1966. *The Duality of Human Existence: Isolation and communion in Western man.* Boston: Beacon Press.

Beghetto, R. A., and J. C. Kaufman. 2007. Toward a broader conception of creativity: A case for "mini-c" creativity. *Psychology of Aesthetics, Creativity, and the Arts* 1 (2):73–79.

Benjamin, J. 1998. *Like Subjects, Like Objects.* New Haven: Yale University Press.

Cohen, G. D., S. Perlstein, J. Chapline, J. Kelly, K. M. Firth, and S. Simmens. 2007. The impact of professionally conducted cultural programs on the physical health, mental health, and social functioning of older adults: 2 year results. *Journal of Aging, Humanities, and the Arts* 1:5–22.

Cole, T. R., R. Kastenbaum, and R. E. Ray, eds. 2000. *Handbook of the Humanities and Aging.* 2nd ed. New York: Springer.

Cole, T. R., D. Van Tassel, and R. Kastenbaum, eds. 1992. *Handbook of the Humanities and Aging.* New York: Springer.

Edwards, J. 2005. Before the threshold: Destruction, reparation, and creativity in relation to the depressive position. *Journal of Child Development* 31:317–34.

Freud, S. 2002. Inhibitions, symptoms, and anxiety. In *The Standard Edition of the Complete Psychological Works of Sigmund Freud.* New York: W. W. Norton. Original edition, 1926.

Glover, N. 2005. Freud's theory of art and creativity. In *Psychoanalytic Aesthetics: The British School.* Place Published. www.psychomedia.it/pm/culture/visarts/glover.htm (accessed June 2008).

Harris, N. 2001. Reluctant alliance: American art, American religion. In *Crossroads: Art and religion in American life,* ed. A. Arthurs and G. Wallach. New York: The New Press.

Heenan, E. F. 1972. The sociology of religion and the aged: The empirical lacunae. *Journal for the Scientific Study of Religion* 11:171–76.

Heggen, B. A. 2000. To tell the truth but tell it slant: Martin Luther's theology and poetry. In *Translucence: Religion, the arts, and imagination,* ed. C. Gilbertson and G. Muilenburg. Minneapolis: Fortress Press.

Heller, E. G. 2004. Interpreting the partnership of art and religion. In *Reluctant Partners: Art and religion in dialogue,* ed. E. G. Heller. New York: Gallery of the American Bible Society.

Idler, E. 2006. Religion and aging. In *Handbook of Aging and the Social Sciences,* ed. R. H. Binstock and L. K. George. San Diego: Academic Press.

Johnson, E. A. 1993. *She Who Is: The mystery of God in feminist theological discourse.* New York: Herder & Herder.

Jönson, H., and J. A. Magnusson. 2001. A new age of old age? Gerotranscendence and the re-enchantment of aging. *Journal of Aging Studies* 15:317–31.

Kashi, E., and J. Winokur. 2003. *Aging in America: The years ahead.* New York: PowerHouse Books.

Kastenbaum, R. 1999. Afterword. In *Religion, Belief, and Spirituality in Late Life,* ed. L. E. Thomas and S. A. Eisenhandler. New York: Springer.

———. 2000. Creativity in the arts. In *Handbook of the Humanities and Aging,* ed. T. R. Cole, R. Kastenbaum, and R. E. Ray. New York: Springer.

———. 2001. Riding the tiger: The challenge of creative renewal in the later adult years. In *Promoting Creativity across the Life Span,* ed. M. Bloom and T. P. Gullotta. Washington, D.C.: CWLA Press.

Kennedy, R. 2005. The Pablo Picasso Alzheimer's therapy. *New York Times,* October 30, 2005.

Kennett, C. E. 2000. Participation in a creative arts program can foster hope in a hospice care centre. *Palliative Medicine* 14:419–25.

Krause, N. 2006. Religion and health in later life. In *Handbook of the Psychology of Aging,* ed. J. E. Birren and K. W. Schaie. San Diego: Academic Press.

Labouvie-Vief, G. 1994. *Psyche and Eros: Mind and gender in the life course.* New York: Cambridge University Press.

———. 2000. Positive development in later life. In *Handbook of the Humanities and Aging,* ed. T. R. Cole, R. Kastenbaum, and R. E. Ray. New York: Springer.

Labouvie-Vief, G., M. Diehl, E. Jain, and F. Zhang. 2007. Six-year change in affect optimization and affect complexity across the adult life span: A further examination. *Psychology and Aging* 22 (4):738–51.

Lacugna, C. M. 1993. *God for Us: The Trinity and Christian life.* New York: Harper One.

Lindauer, M. S. 2003. *Aging, Creativity and Art: A positive perspective on late-life development.* New York: Kluwer Academic/Plenum Publishers.

Morgan, D. 2004. Toward a modern historiography of art and religion. In *Reluctant Partners:*

Art and religion in dialogue, ed. E. G. Heller. New York: Gallery of the American Bible Society.

Oliver, K. 2004. *The Colonization of Psychic Space: A psychoanalytic social theory of oppression*. Minneapolis: University of Minnesota Press.

Otto, R. 1958. *The Idea of the Holy: An inquiry into the non-rational factor in the idea of the divine and its relation to the rational*. Trans. J. W. Harvey. New York: Oxford University Press. Original edition, 1917.

Perlstein, S., ed. 2006. Aging and the Arts. *Generations* 30 (1).

Redeker, M. 1973. *Schleiermacher: Life and thought*. Trans. J. Wallhausser. Philadelphia: Fortress Press.

Schleiermacher, F. 1996. *On Religion: Speeches to its cultured despisers*. New York: Cambridge University Press. Original edition, 1799.

Shapira, N., A. Barak, and I. Gal. 2007. Promoting older adults' well-being through Internet training and use. *Aging and Mental Health* 11:477–84.

Shults, F., and S. Sandage. 2006. *Transforming Spirituality: Integrating theology and psychology*. Grand Rapids: Baker Academic.

Slife, B. D. 2004. Taking practice seriously: Toward a relational ontology. *Journal of Theoretical and Philosophical Psychology* 24:157–78.

Tornstam, L. 1999. Late-life transcendence: A new developmental perspective on aging. In *Religion, Belief, and Spirituality in Late Life*, ed. L. E. Thomas and S. A. Eisenhandler. New York: Springer.

Wikström, B. M. 2002. Social interaction associated with visual art discussions: A controlled intervention study. *Aging and Mental Health* 6 (1):82–87.

Winkler, M. G. 1992. Walking to the stars. In *Handbook of the Humanities and Aging*, ed. T. R. Cole, D. Van Tassel, and R. Kastenbaum. New York: Springer.

Wuthnow, R. 2001. *Creative Spirituality: The way of the artist*. Berkeley: University of California Press.

———. 2003. *All in Sync: How music and art are revitalizing American religion*. Berkeley: University of California Press.

CHAPTER EIGHT

Creativity and Aging

Psychological Growth, Health, and Well-Being

GENE D. COHEN, M.D., PH.D.

Creativity is built into the human species. It can be defined as bringing something new into existence that is valued, although the recognition of value may be delayed; the definition purposely does not differentiate between creativity as a tangible product, an idea, or a process, where each can be monumental. And the potential for creative expression is designed to last throughout the entire life cycle. In the process, as this chapter will amplify, it influences psychological growth, health, and well-being in the second half of life.

Howard Gardner, who informed us about "multiple intelligences" (1993b), also amplified our understanding of creativity presenting in some individuals as "big C" creativity, and in others as "little c" creativity, but in each case its creative essence is real and significant (Gardner, 1993a). This broad view of creativity is consistent with the view of it being universal—built into the species. Unfortunately, our understanding of creativity with aging has been limited as a result of a heavy legacy of negative myths and stereotypes about aging that have denied or trivialized creative capacity and accomplishment in the second half of life, despite earlier efforts by Lehman (1953), Simonton (1984), and others cited by Cohen (2000) to clarify and defend its reality and importance to society. As the historian Daniel Boorstin pointed out, "The greatest obstacle to discovery is not ignorance—it is the illusion of knowledge."

Too many in society and too many in the scientific community have had the illusion that studying aging would result in no knowledge about positive findings and potential. I aim to set things straight here, starting with a definition of creativity and then describing the varied and profound ways creativity manifests itself with aging, including creativity that commences with aging and blooms late in life. There will also be an equation presented that reflects positive influences of aging on creative capacity: C=me. I will then discuss dimensions of creativity that improve with aging. Our interest in and understanding of creativity and aging are surging in the burst of an interdisciplinary focus on this important phenomenon—from poetry to psychology, music to molecular biology, literary writing to life review, fine art to folk art.

The relation of ongoing psychological growth and creative expression with aging will also be delineated. Here, too, for too long science and society saw psychological development as the domain of the young, not the old, Erik Erikson (1980) being the main exception. As a student of Erikson, and based on more than three and a half decades of research and clinical work with more than 3,000 adults in middle age and later life, I will describe four phases of psychological growth and development in the second half of life, each mobilizing fresh psychological energy and insights, enabling new opportunities to access our inner creative selves.

Historically, we have entered a sea change in thinking about aging, where for the first time science and society alike are recognizing the existence of potential beyond problems in the second half of life. Understanding this potential, the greatest expression of which is creativity, translates into new approaches that can enhance quality of life and health with aging. The author's "Creativity and Aging Study," the first study totally focused on tapping into potential, will be reviewed (Cohen, 2006, 2007). Its results reveal improvement in overall physical and mental health among older adults actively involved in sustained activities providing opportunities for creative expression. The underlying mechanisms to explain the reasons for this improvement will be discussed.

In this context, the role of creativity in promoting health and preventing illness with aging will be described. Similarly, the role of creative engagement in improving how we cope with illness with aging will also be elaborated. Finally, even among those whose memory is failing, creative outlets that remain will be examined. As Henri Bergson put it, "To exist is to change, to change is to mature, to mature is to go on creating oneself endlessly."

Historical Context: A Sea Change in How Society Views Aging

Since the mid-1970s, we have witnessed two major sea changes in how society thinks about and understands aging (Cohen, 2000, 2005). Up until the last quarter of the twentieth century, aging was largely equated with a series of decremental, unalterable changes with the passage of time. Significant decline with advancing years was seen as inevitable—our destiny. Dementing disorders were collectively viewed as *senility*, a term than connoted the natural course of growing old. But by 1975 a fundamental conceptual change was stirring in how negative changes with aging were being interpreted. There was an emergence of new hypotheses that attempted to explain decrements that accompanied aging not as representing normal aging, but instead reflecting age-associated problems—modifiable disorders.

For the scientist, the idea that a negative change is caused by a problem, and not normal aging, creates a new sense of opportunity to modify the problem. For the policy maker, this recognition results in a new sense of responsibility to do something about the problem. This sea change in thinking about modifiable age-associated problems launched the modern federal infrastructure of research programs on aging. In 1975, the National Institute on Aging appointed its first director, while the National Institute of Mental Health established a new research center on mental health and aging—the first federal research program on aging established in any country (the author of this chapter had the opportunity to become the new center's first chief). That same year, 1975, the Veterans Administration launched their GRECC (Geriatric Research Education and Clinical Center) program. Rigorous research on aging in effect did not go into high speed until the last quarter of the twentieth century. The "Problem Focus" in turn led to the development of the field of geriatrics in the 1980s.

The transition from seeing progressive, unalterable negative changes with aging as being one's destiny with growing old to a new view of modifiable age-associated problems was a huge leap in itself. The culmination of the *problem* view of aging came with the concept of "successful aging," defined as aging that reflected the minimum number of problems—the minimum degree of decline—as opposed to "usual aging" that reflected more problems, more decline (Rowe and Kahn, 1998). While this was happening, it was too big a leap to go to the next step—to see that aging could be accompanied by potential beyond problems. But by the end of the twentieth century, the view that aging could be accompanied by potential beyond problems was emerging. The "potential" focus of aging reflected the emergence of the second major conceptual sea change about aging and is reflected in *The Creative Age*, the first book totally focused on creativity and aging, published at the end of the twentieth century (Cohen, 2000). The ultimate manifestation of potential with aging is creativity.

Defining Creativity and Recognizing It with Aging

When poet Stanley Kunitz (1995) won a National Book Award at age 90, for his book of poems *Passing Through*, another noted poet offered the following praise: "One of America's great poets. Most poets dry up at 50. For him to be writing poems at 90 is just incredible."

The view that most poets dry up at 50 certainly was not my impression in reviewing poetry representing a span of nearly 3,000 years, from the eighth-century BC Greek epic poet Homer, who wrote the *Odyssey* in his later years, to the Irish poet William Butler Yeats (1865–1939), who wrote his greatest verse between 50 and 75, including *The Winding Stair* in his 65th year, to the American poet Maya Angelou, born in 1928 and writing at the ripe—not at all dried up—age of 65 as poet laureate at

President Clinton's 1993 inauguration. In the book *The Best American Poetry of 1997* (Tate and Lehman, 1997), nearly half of the 75 poets listed were over 50 when they wrote the poetry that appeared in that anthology. Fourteen of them were over 60 and five were over 70 years old. Incidentally, one of those poems was written at age 63 by Mark Strand, the poet who suggested that the only good poet is a young poet. This faulty assumption about topping out with our talents at middle age is too frequently held among public policy officials, community leaders, and activists, as well as everyday older adults, patients, and their families. And as illustrated above by poet Mark Strand, it can be held even by individuals who exemplify vibrant and productive creative spirit in mature adult life. If the leading voices of our culture can be so mistaken about our creative potential as we grow older, it is no surprise that most of us underestimate it in everyday life.

If there is a "secret" to enriching your life through creativity, it begins with debunking these myths about creativity and about creativity and aging. The myths imply that creativity is for only the gifted few, and that even their talents dim with age. The truth is this: creativity is not just for artists. It is not just for geniuses (Andreasen, 2005). And it is not just for the young. Creativity is a universal life force, an energy source available to every one of us at every age—part of a set of drives that we are born with, built-in by evolution, that result in an "inner push" mobilizing ongoing psychological growth and creative potential throughout the life cycle (Cohen, 2004, 2005). And contrary to the idea that it dims with age, your capacity to think and live creatively only expands with age and experience (Cole, Van Tassel, and Kastenbaum, 1992; Cole and Winkler, 1994).

In her book *The Creating Brain* (2005), Nancy Andreasen discusses our natural capacity for creativity. She makes the important distinction between that part of our nature that is hereditary and that part that is built-in to all of us. Andreasen is in effect describing the inner push in a narrower sense, more in relation to creativity than the interaction between creative potential and psychological growth described here. She writes, "nature can be defined as an innate or inborn gift that drives an individual to creative achievement, without any obvious genetic contributions. We do not know yet how this kind of creative nature arises, but it appears to be more common than 'nature' that is clearly hereditary. Once this creative nature arises, nurturing it through a variety of environmental factors will further enhance it . . . Whatever the importance of 'nature,' 'nurture' is also important for creativity to flourish, and perhaps essential. The human brain is shaped by the world around it *from the time that a child is born to the end of adult life.*"

The concept of the *inner push* and Andreasen's related description of innate and inborn nature driving us to creative achievement further support the notion of creative potential being built-in, and built-in to the end of the life cycle.

Definition of Creativity

As suggested by the definition offered earlier, creativity is difficult to define because it is hard to get your head around the concept. Is it a product or a process? If it is a product, is it tangible, like a painting, or intangible, like an idea? To encompass each of these possibilities and more, the definition used here borrows on views of Rollo May (1975), Mihaly Csikszentmihalyi (1996), and Howard Gardner (1993b): *Creativity is bringing something new into existence that is valued.*

The Creativity Equation

The "creativity equation" represents a fun yet intriguing attempt to make an elusive concept—creativity—more graspable. The equation is this: $C = me^2$. It states that creativity (C) is the result of our mass (m) of knowledge, multiplied by the effects of our two dimensions of experience (e^2). The first dimension would be our inner world experience, reflecting psychological and emotional growth over the years. The second dimension would be our outer world experience, reflecting accumulating life experience and wisdom in growing older. All the elements interact in a synergy that sets the stage for creativity. The equation also reflects the positive influence of aging, where through the passage of time one is enabled to acquire more knowledge along with increased outer world experience and inner world growth. Aging is clearly an ally here. From a lighter perspective, the me^2 is what you realize in looking at the creative side of your self in the mirror—"Hey, that's *me* to a higher level!"

Types and Categories of Creativity with Aging

Keep in mind that creativity not only applies to artists but is apparent in all aspects of life, including the social realm, where over the history of civilization older adults have assumed the creative role of "keepers of the culture," transmitting accumulated knowledge and perspective.

TYPES OF CREATIVITY

Howard Gardner differentiates between "Big C" creativity and "little c" creativity. "Big C" applies to the extraordinary accomplishments of great artists, scientists, and inventors. These forms of creativity typically change fields of thought and the course of progress, as with Einstein's theory of relativity, Picasso's invention of cubism, and Edison's electrical inventions.

Creativity with a "little c" is grounded in the diversity of everyday activities and accomplishments. "Every person has certain areas in which he or she has a special interest," Gardner explains; "it could be something they do at work the way they write memos or their craftsmanship at a factory—or the way they teach a lesson or sell something. After working at it for a while they can get to be pretty good—as good as anybody whom they know in their immediate world."

Sometimes something little "c" can evolve to big "C" creativity, as with Maria Ann Smith, who during her sixties in the 1860s was experimenting in Australia with different fruit seeds. She took great satisfaction in this work, especially when something different grew—something new that she brought into existence that was valued. One of these successes was a hardy French crab-apple seedling from which developed the late ripening "Granny Smith" apple, bearing her name, which because of its outstanding taste and keeping qualities formed the bulk of Australia's apple exports for many years.

CATEGORIES OF CREATIVITY WITH AGING

In children's literature, the most common way an older character is described is with a single word—"old" (Kettering, 2002; Cohen, 2005). In general discussions of creativity and aging, to the extent that there was any acknowledgement of its existence, creative expression in later life was often trivialized as being narrow and simple in form. In reality, not only is creativity relevant and prevalent with aging, but it shows itself in a depth and breadth of forms. Consider four basic patterns of creativity in the second half of life.

• *Continuing creativity.* This was certainly the case for Herbert Block, aka "Herblock," whose nationally syndicated political cartoons informed and enriched our culture for more than 70 years. His first cartoon appeared when he was in his twenties; his last was published less than two months before he died at 91.

• *Changing creativity.* (While changing creativity can be considered a variant of continuing creativity, it is distinguished by the fundamental change in creative direction that the individual takes as he or she ages.) The great mathematician and philosopher Bertrand Russell, for instance, focused tightly on mathematics in his youth and middle age. When he was 42, he and Alfred North Whitehead published the *Principia Mathematica*, which remains a masterpiece of mathematical logic and synthesis. As he grew older, his focus shifted to deeper issues, particularly philosophy, and the many social ills of our time. At the age of 73, he published his renowned work, *A History of Western Philosophy*, for which he received the Nobel Prize in Literature, and he remained passionately involved in issues of peace and justice until he died at 98 (Russell, 1967–69).

• *Commencing creativity.* Some people first significantly tap into their creative potential around age 65; they are often referred to as "late bloomers." The author's own ideas about creativity with aging and especially about "late bloomers" blossomed after a visit to a retrospective exhibit of a half century of folk art at Washington's Corcoran Gallery of Art. The works of 20 of the best African-American folk artists from 1930 to 1980 were exhibited. Reading the artists' brief biographies revealed that of the 20 exhibitors, 16 (80%) had begun painting or reached a recognizable mature phase as artists after the age of 65. *Thirty percent* of these artists were 80 years of age or older.

The folk art story is particularly important because whenever examples are given of important art by older artists like Picasso, Titian, or Georgia O'Keeffe, many fire a reflex response that they are "outliers, exceptions from the rule, not typical of aging." But with folk art, older artists are the rule—across the racial and ethnic diversity of our culture (Hartigan, 1990). With their prominence, their work cannot be diminished as uncommon events. Whenever you can find a field, any field, dominated by older adults, like folk art, then one can no longer deny or trivialize creative potential with aging. And what a statement they make with their numbers about it truly being never too late in life to be creative; they also make the ultimate case for late blooming.

Grandma Moses, who only at 78 turned her serious attention to painting, with her work selected for 15 international exhibits over the next 23 years until she was 101, was but one of a huge crowd of older folk artists having a major impact. William Edmondson, who had been a janitor until 65 when he lost his job, turned then full-time to sculpture. A photographer, captivated by Edmondson's work, sent a portfolio of images of his sculptures to the Museum of Modern Art (MOMA) in New York. The result was that at 67, Edmondson became the first black artist in the history of the MOMA to have a solo exhibit, opening the doors to generations that followed (Livingston and Beardsley, 1982).

· *Creativity connected with loss.* There is nothing romantic about loss, but the human condition and the human spirit are such that when loss occurs, it is in our nature to try to transcend it by tapping into unknown or underdeveloped other capacities that we possess. Such is captured in the life and work of William Carlos Williams. Carlos Williams was a pediatrician who also wrote poetry. However, a stroke in his sixties left him unable to continue practicing pediatrics and sent him into a depression that required a year of hospitalization. He gradually emerged from that trauma and loss, turning full time to poetry, with the collection published in his book *Pictures from Brueghel* at 79 being awarded a Pulitzer Prize. In his later life poetry Carlos Williams wrote about "old age that adds as it takes away."

For so long, only the taken-away part of aging was focused on, not the what-is-added part. But the reality of aging that adds as it takes away is in fact universal, as can be seen in ancient Greek mythology, so rich in how its portrayals captured human nature. These great myths contain that of Tiresias, a mere mortal wandering in the woods one day, thinking deep thoughts, with his eyes aimlessly wandering and inadvertently falling on the goddess Athena bathing in the nude. Catching the eyes of a mere mortal viewing her naked threw Athena into a rage, and in her fury she blinded Tiresias. The other gods and goddesses questioned her, defending Tiresias as unwittingly being in the wrong place at the wrong time. They urged Athena to reconsider. She did, but she did not restore Tiresias's outer vision, instead granting him great inner vision. He became a great prophet and in his later years predicted the plight of Oedipus—exemplifying an old age that adds as it takes away.

Positive Changes That Occur Not Despite Aging but Because of Aging

Our understanding of the capacity of the aging mind has been revolutionized by the latest neuroscience research on positive brain changes with aging. We now know that every time we challenge the brain or have a new experience, neuroplastic changes occur that alter the anatomy (LeDoux, 2002). See Figure 8.1, which represents a schematic drawing of two brain cells (neurons) magnified under an electron microscope.

Neurons communicate at their contact points, known as synapses. The number and strength of the synapses determine the quality of communication within the brain. Every time we challenge our brains, existing neurons sprout new dendrites (like limbs of a tree), which in turn enable new synapse formation. At the synapses, chemical messengers (neurotransmitters) that facilitate communication among neurons are sent from the axon terminals of the sending cells to dendrites of the receiving cells. Challenge also induces dendritic spines (like branches from the limbs) to sprout from the dendrites; the dendritic spines also participate in forming new synapses. Moreover, challenge strengthens the synapses themselves. We have approximately 100 billion neurons in the cerebral cortex or thinking part of the brain. Each neuron has the capacity to generate more than a thousand dendrites, which, together with their spines, enable the formation of as many as a quadrillion (or as young children would say, a gazillion) synapses, illustrating the extraordinary capacity and complexity of the human brain (Kandel, 2006). The glial cells shown in Figure 8.1 also grow in number in response to mental and environmental challenge; glial cells help nourish the neurons, keeping them healthy.

By demonstrating the positive impact of mental and environmental challenge on brain neuroplasticity—as all the above structural changes involving the neuron are referred to—modern neuroscience validated folk advice to "use it or lose it." But modern neuroscience took folk advice a step further. It discovered that all of the same neuroplastic changes described above in response to challenge occur throughout the aging process—right to the end of the life cycle (Flood et al., 1985; Flood and Coleman, 1990; Katzman, 1995; Kolb and Whishaw, 1998; Kramer et al., 2004). Moreover, just before the close of the twentieth century it was discovered that, contrary to

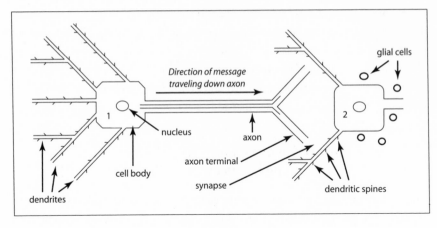

Figure 8.1 Two neurons, magnified 100,000-fold.

prevailing scientific thought, we in fact continue to produce new neurons regardless of age, and that mental challenge and environmental stimulation are critical to this ongoing process of neurogenesis (Taupin and Gage, 2002; Kempermann, Wiskott, and Gage, 2004). Hence, modern neuroscience demonstrated that it is never too late to use it to alter losing it (Diamond, 1993).

Ongoing Psychological Growth Fostering Creative Expression with Aging

The "inner push" described earlier underlies not only our capacity for ongoing creative expression, but also that for ongoing psychological growth. Ongoing psychological growth in turn affects our capacity for creative expression by helping our inner psychological climate to readjust itself, resulting in new readiness or fostering new ways to be creative. These dynamics are critical components to understanding positive changes that occur not despite aging, but because of aging. The inner push continues throughout the life cycle. Ongoing neuroplastic brain changes, affected by our experiences and challenges, subtly influence the way the inner push manifests itself at different points in the life cycle. In other words, the constantly changing brain affects the way the inner push presents over time.

In addition, ongoing life experience further alters the manifestation of the inner push, both by further altering the brain and by affecting our self-concept and understanding of ourselves. Together, these influences alter how the inner push shows itself in four different ways in the second half of life—in four different theorized psychological growth phases (Cohen, 2000, 2005). Each new developmental phase creates a new inner climate within us that allows us to reevaluate our lives and experiment with new strategies. This ongoing process results in new opportunities for us to access and activate untapped strengths, as well as new and creative sides of ourselves, enabling positive change. These four new phases of psychological development in the second half of life represent positive changes because of aging, not despite aging.

THE MIDLIFE REEVALUATION PHASE

This phase generally occurs during one's early forties to late fifties. Plans and actions are shaped by a sense of crisis or quest, although considerably more by quest. Midlife is a powerful time for the expression of human potential because it combines the capacity for insightful reflection with a powerful desire to create meaning in life. This quest is catalyzed in midlife by one seriously confronting for the first time their sense of mortality; one contemplates time left instead of time gone by on passing the midpoint in the life cycle. This dynamic new inner climate becomes a catalyst for uncovering unrealized creative sides of ourselves.

THE LIBERATION PHASE

This phase usually emerges from one's mid-fifties to mid-seventies. Plans and actions are shaped by a new sense of personal freedom to speak one's mind and to do what needs to be done. There are often mounting feelings of "if not now, when?" "Why not?" and "What can they do to me?" which foster a sense of inner liberation. With retirement or partial retirement, common during these years, comes a new experience of external liberation and a feeling of finally having time to experiment with something different. The new sense of comfort, confidence, and courage translates into creative expression for many.

THE SUMMING-UP PHASE

This phase unfolds most frequently during our late sixties and into our eighties—or beyond. Plans and actions are shaped by the desire to find larger meaning in the story of one's life as individuals look back, reexamine, and sum up what has happened. This process motivates people to give of the wisdom they have accrued throughout their lives. In the role of keepers of the culture, people who reach this phase begin to share their lessons and fortunes through autobiography and personal storytelling, philanthropy, community activism, volunteerism, and other forms of giving back. In the case of Martha Graham, it was through choreography from her mid-seventies to mid-nineties. It is also a time to deal with unresolved conflicts and unfinished business in manners that motivate us to develop creative new strategies.

THE ENCORE PHASE

This phase can develop from one's late seventies to the end of our years. Plans and actions are shaped by the desire to restate and reaffirm major themes in one's life, but also to explore novel variations on those themes and to further attend to unfinished business or unresolved conflicts. The desire to live well to the very end has a positive impact on family and community and often influences decisions to have family reunions and other events. The Delaney sisters, after a filled century of life, wrote *The Delaney Sisters: The first 100 years.* The title implies stage setting for encores. Their book became a best seller and a Broadway musical—impressive creative accomplishments.

Moving to All-Wheel Drive

Not only is the brain through neuroplasticity broadening its capacity to process and store information as we age, but also after about a half century of favoring the left side of the brain for some tasks and the right side for others, it is finally ready to put them both to work on the same task. Cabeza (2002) discovered that around middle age, we begin to use both sides of the brain simultaneously—in effect moving to all-wheel drive. He determined this by using functional MRI brain imaging to assess how young adults and middle-aged adults use their brain while engaging in the same task; their right and left hemispheres lit up differently.

This phenomenon is described as the HAROLD Model (HAROLD is an acronym for Hemispheric Asymmetry Reduction in Older Adults). Rather than asymmetric (using one hemisphere at a time), adults in the second half of life more often use both hemispheres at the same time. This process throws light on other research findings of a better integration of right- and left-brain capacities with aging. It is a remarkable illustration of the adaptive mobilization of brain reserve with aging, as well as the manifestation of new capacities (Cabeza et al., 2002).

In middle age, we observe a better integration of analytic and synthetic reasoning, the objective and the subjective, the well defined and the intuitive—the heart and the mind, so to speak. Our brain is making optimal use of both hemispheres operating together; we experience a deepening capacity for left-brain/right-brain integration, heart-and-mind thinking. This type of thinking, in Piagetian terms, is referred to as *postformal thinking* (Richards and Commons, 1990).

To the extent that the symmetrical use of the hemispheres facilitates postformal thought, it results in a different and more mature way of looking at the world that can lead to constructive reevaluation characteristic of the midlife reevaluation phase and creative new perspectives on the relationships and endeavors one is involved with, as well as potential new paths that may be followed.

Postformal thought itself often results in new insights and creative problem solving. It allows us to examine in new ways information we have had or situations we have been in for some time, bringing new perspectives and understanding into our awareness. In this sense, it can promote creativity with aging—bringing something new into existence that is valued. It can lead to new breakthroughs in thinking—not despite aging, but because of aging. The following example illustrates these points.

From the age of 22 to 27, a young naturalist in nineteenth-century England traveled the world collecting thousands of plant and animal specimens and recording his observations in dozens of notebooks. He completed his collection of data at age 27, knew he had something significant, but could not put it all together. He continually revisited this data throughout his thirties and into his forties. Gradually, he made new connections, resolving the last remaining obstacle to completing the big picture understanding of what the data meant at 45. He realized that the significance of his findings would be controversial and generate major protest, so he waited another five years until feeling comfortable about publishing the results. The naturalist was Charles Darwin, and his book was *On the Origin of Species.*

Like Chocolate to the Brain

Drawing on the unique attributes of both sides of the brain at the same time is like tapping a new capacity. It is suggested here that any activity that optimally uses both sides of the brain at the same time is like *chocolate to the brain*—an activity in effect savored by the brain. This phenomenon may offer a further explanation for the surge of late blooming in folk art with aging, for art forms draw on each side of the brain, and when this process becomes optimally synchronized in the second half of life, it is like chocolate to the brain.

Autobiography Emerging as a Major Form of Creative Expression with Aging

The desire to write one's memoir or autobiography grows significantly as individuals approach their seventh and eighth decades. Along with storytelling and reminiscing, these experiences developmentally become appealing ways of giving back—sharing what we have learned. They reflect the summing-up phase of psychological growth and development.

In a further fascinating study using functional MRI brain imaging, autobiographical storytelling was compared between 30-year-olds and 70-year-olds (Maguire and Frith, 2003). It was found that the 30-year-olds lit up predominantly the left hippocampus, whereas the 70-year-olds lit up both hippocampi—left and right together. The hippocampus is the part of the brain that processes new information coming in and sets the stage for memory storage. Both groups told their stories equally well, even though the older adults had considerably more information that they had to process.

But 70-year-olds are much more motivated to tell their story—again a developmental phenomenon that is part of the summing-up phase. Among the factors that may be operating here is that the involvement of the right hippocampus in the second half of life means that generic attributes of the right brain come into play. The right brain is more the hub of curiosity and intellectual passion, which may explain the heightened motivation of older adults to work passionately on their personal story as a creative act. Here, too, is another example of an activity that optimally uses both sides of the brain. Hence, autobiography, as well, is like chocolate to the brain with aging, stirring creative imagination.

Pragmatic Creativity and the New Senior Moment

Researchers in the field of aging have identified a growing capacity in the second half of life that is referred to as pragmatic creativity or practical intelligence. It will be explained here by a combination of two factors that are attributed to positive changes with aging, one social, the other psychological: (1) the growth of social intelligence, and (2) the emergence of the liberation phase. It is illustrated in the following example from the author's own family.

My in-laws, Howard and Gisele Miller, were stuck. They had just emerged from the Washington, D.C., subway system into a driving snowstorm. Both in their seventies, they were coming to our house for dinner and needed a cab because it was too far to walk. But it was rush hour and no cabs stopped. Howard tried calling us to get a lift, but both my wife Wendy and I were tied up in traffic and weren't home yet, and it was before we all had cell phones.

As his fingers began to turn numb from the cold, Howard noticed the steamy windows of a pizza shop across the street, and a smile came on his face. He and Giselle walked through the slush to the shop, stepped up to the counter, and ordered a large pizza for home delivery. When the cashier asked where to deliver it, Howard gave him our address, and added, "Oh, there's one more thing." "What's that?" the cashier asked. "We want you to deliver us with it," Howard said. And that's how they arrived—pizza in hand—for dinner that night.

This favorite family story perfectly illustrates the sort of agile creativity that can accompany the aging mind. Would a younger person have thought of this solution? Possibly. Creativity knows no age limits. But this kind of "out of the box" thinking is a learned trait that improves with age. It is known as "pragmatic creativity" in everyday problem solving, a capacity that research has found to be strong in later life (Cohen, 2005). Age allows our brains to accumulate a repertoire of strategies developed from a lifetime of experience—part of what has been referred to by other researchers as crystallized intelligence. Not that Howard had done the pizza parlor routine before, but the accumulated experience of other successful strategies helped stimulate the thinking that produced his creative solution. This was the social intelligence factor that builds over time with aging.

Along with the experience of years and an agility of thought, Howard's solution reflects a mature psychological development that is prominent among those in their sixties and seventies. With age can come a new feeling of inner freedom, self-confidence, and liberation from social constraints that allows for novel or bold behavior—the liberation phase. Characterized by that nudging inner voice posing, "What can they do to me?" a new sense of comfort and courage moves us to action and creative solutions. Howard, himself in the liberation phase, was not afraid to make an unusual request of perfect strangers, which was a key part of his success that night—*part of the positive capacity that comes with aging*—not *despite* aging, but *because* of it. Pragmatic creativity in essence represents *the new senior moment* that comes with aging—the creative context in which opportunity is recognized, in conjunction with a new psychological readiness for action necessary to seize the moment.

Unfinished Business in the Summing-Up Phase as an Impetus for Creative Expression

Many marvel that Giuseppe Verdi was in his 80th year when he composed his celebrated opera *Falstaff*. But why did Verdi choose to compose *Falstaff*, as opposed to a different opera? The dynamics of the "summing-up" psychological growth phase offer an explanation. As alluded to above, a number of older people going through their summing-up phase look back at any unfinished business. Verdi had unfinished business that gnawed at him for more than half a century.

When Verdi was 25, he attempted to compose an opera buffa—a comic opera—*Un Giorno di Regno* (*King for a Day*). It opened in the famous theater La Scala, in 1840, but was received so poorly that it was canceled after one performance. Verdi had recently lost his wife and a year earlier his infant son, and he became overcome with despair, vowing never to write another opera. The director of La Scala tactfully and sensitively released Verdi from his contract, but when he felt Verdi's emotional wound was healing, he gently encouraged him to compose a new opera. The result was *Nebucco* in 1842, which established Verdi's reputation in Italy.

Fifty-five years after *King for a Day* flopped, Verdi, in his summing-up phase and at the top of his field, looked back at unfinished business—his failure to compose a successful comic opera. He decided it was time to set the picture straight, to provide the missing chapter. He composed a great comic libretto, *Falstaff*. And to leave no blemish unremoved, he arranged to have *Falstaff* open in the same theater where the earlier sad disappointment occurred—at La Scala. *Falstaff*, of course, was greeted at La

Scala as a resounding success, one of the finest operas ever written. Verdi then continued with the creation of further operas as he moved toward his "encore" phase.

Perspective on the Above Biopsychosocial Connections

Part of our review of the domain of creativity and aging has been to examine its biopsychosocial underpinnings. In the process of so doing a number of connections have been described or suggested. These syntheses include connecting theory with established findings. For example, postformal thought is a phenomenon that numerous investigators have described over a period of decades (Arlin, 1975; Sinnott, 1991, 1999; Marchand, 2001); similarly, the HAROLD Model describing the brain utilizing its two hemispheres in a symmetrical manner has been replicated by a range of investigators. The relationship described between these two phenomena is a theorized one, supported, if not propelled, by what appears to be a compelling connection between them.

This also applies to the discussion of autobiography (Birren and Cochran, 2001) and aging. There has been an enormous literature about autobiography (Atkinson, 1995), reminiscing (Kunz and Soltys, 2007), and life review (Butler, 1963) in later life. The qualities of the right brain in distinction from the left were identified in the Nobel Prize–winning research of Roger Sperry. The differences in the involvement of the hippocampi between young adults and older adults in telling their life stories have been documented in methodical functional MRI brain imaging research. Again, the relationship described among these phenomena is a theorized one, supported by the apparent strong connections among them.

The four psychological growth phases described are themselves theoretical constructs. But this author's research over more than three and a half decades continues to find them. Moreover, over the past decade, hundreds of presentations to thousands of individuals in the second half of life have overwhelmingly elicited audience responses of the phase depictions ringing true, with countless comments by these individuals exclaiming that the descriptions of the four phases and the examples presented to illustrate them represent their story—their personal experience.

The Creativity and Aging Study

The Creativity and Aging Study is the descriptive title of the multisite national research project on *The Impact of Professionally Conducted Cultural Programs on Older Adults* (Cohen, 2005, 2006; Cohen et al., 2006, 2007). The study was conducted to explore the relation between creative engagement and the health of older adults. What was learned was that efforts at health promotion and prevention among older adults can only go so far when restricted to targeting problems. Ultimately, promoting health with aging is perhaps best realized when potential with aging is tapped through creative engagement, while problems are also addressed.

The Creativity and Aging Study was the first formal study, using an experimental or quasi-experimental design involving a comparison group, examining the influence of professionally conducted, participatory art programs on the general health, mental health, and social activities of older people (Cohen, 2006; Cohen et al., 2006, 2007). It was designed to draw on the underlying mechanisms that have been shown to influence positive health outcomes in older people. Results reveal significant positive differences in the intervention group (those involved in intensive participatory art programs) as compared to a comparison group not involved in intensive cultural programs. Its primary investigator was Gene D. Cohen, M.D., Ph.D., and the coordinating site was the Center on Aging, Health and Humanities at the George Washington University.

The study began in 2001 with a grant from the National Endowment for the Arts, in coordination with five other federal and nonfederal sponsors, including the National Institutes of Health and the National Retired Teachers Association/AARP, to conduct a rigorous national study examining the effects of community-based art programs on the health and functioning of older adults. The study compares the physical and mental health and social functioning of 150 older adults involved in the arts programs to a control group of 150 adults *not* in such programs. All the participants are age 65 or older, most were living independently when the study started, and both groups were comparable in their health and functioning at the start of the study. The adults who were not in the arts group were free to socialize, attend classes, or do any of their normal activities, including art (although none in the control group became involved in rigorous and sustained participatory art programs). The aim was to see if it was the *creativity* involved in the arts programs that made a difference, rather than the mere fact that these participants were engaged in a regular, structured social situation.

The arts groups met for 35 weekly meetings, analogous to a college course. There were also between-session assignments, as well as exhibitions and concerts. For example, a chorale at one site gave some 10 concerts a year in addition to their regular weekly practice sessions.

Each person's health and social functioning was evaluated with comprehensive questionnaires at the beginning of the programs, at the halfway mark, and again at the end, two years after starting. The hypothesis was that the people participating in the arts programs (the intervention group) would show *less decline* than those in the control group, who did not participate in those programs. In fact, the initial results exceeded these expectations. Many people in the arts groups *stabilized* their health—not declining at all. And some *improved* their health—this in a group of people with an *average* age of 80, which is greater than the current life expectancy!

Here are the major findings from the first phase of the study, which was conducted in the Washington, D.C., area, where the singing groups were directed by Jeanne Kelly, from the Levine School of Music. (Similar paired study groups were researched in Brooklyn at Elders Share the Arts, under the direction of Susan Perlstein, and in San Francisco at the Center for Elders and Youth in the Arts, under the direction of Jeff Chapline, and data still under analysis in these two sites reflect results moving in the same direction as the D.C. findings.) All the results were statistically significant, reflecting real differences between the two study groups that were matched in all the measures being assessed at the start of the study. Compared to the control group, those who participated in the community arts program reported the following:

- had better health after one year (those in the control group reported that their health *was not as good* after the same elapsed time);
- had fewer doctor visits (although both groups had more visits compared to a year earlier);
- used fewer medications (although both groups increased their medication usage);
- felt less depressed;
- were less lonely;
- had higher morale;
- were more socially active, and were more active than at the start of the study (those in the control group were less socially active compared to a year earlier).

Historical Context of the Study

We are at the second major turning point in the contemporary focus on aging—that of looking at potential beyond problems. This focus on potential has profound possibilities for advancing health maintenance and health promotion efforts. Societal interest in potential in later life is soaring, and it is in this context that a project studying how cultural programs affect older people could not be more timely.

Theoretical Background for the Study

The theoretical background for this study built on several major bodies of gerontological research addressing underlying mechanisms that promote health with aging

—especially those of (1) sense of control and (2) social engagement. Studies on aging show that when older people experience a sense of control (e.g., a sense of mastery in what they are doing), positive health outcomes are observed (Rodin, 1986, 1989). Similarly, when older individuals are in situations with meaningful social engagement with others, positive health outcomes are also observed (Avlund, Damsgaard, and Holstein, 1998; Glass et al., 1999; Bennett, 2002).

Biological studies reveal the involvement of mind–immune system pathways playing a protective role here, as described in research on psychoneuroimmunology (Pert, Dreher, and Ruff, 1998; Lutgendorf et al., 1999; Kiecolt-Glaser et al., 2002; Lutgendorf and Costanzo, 2003). In this study, both of these dimensions—individual sense of control and social engagement—were combined. Each time one attends an art class, one experiences a renewed sense of control—ongoing individual mastery. Because all the art programs involved participation and interpersonal interaction with others, social engagement was high.

In all three sites where we have conducted the study, there have been numerous qualitative reports of individuals who participated in the arts programs describing a sense of satisfaction and exhilaration because their performance exceeded their expectations and improved. Their growing sense of control was readily apparent. The artists involved with the various groups reported how the repeated success of the various participants profoundly affected their motivation and desire to continue; they consistently reported high self-esteem and mood as their involvement continued. This was well reflected by a 94-year-old woman in the Washington, D.C., chorale, who shared the following:

> I'm 94 years old, and wasn't sure I could sing, and was even less sure that I could follow the notes. [Becoming increasingly animated] But I found that I could sing! In fact, I'm improving! And, I can't believe it, but I'm finding it easier and easier to read the notes! I am so glad I decided to take a chance and join the chorale. This has been one of the most important experiences of my life. I hope it will never stop. My daughter feels the same way about it.

The significance of the art programs per se is that they foster sustained involvement because of their beauty and productivity. They keep the participants involved week after week, compounding positive effects being achieved. Many general activities and physical exercises do not have this high engaging, and thereby sustaining, quality.

Conclusions from the Creativity and Aging Study

These remarkable preliminary results have attracted attention in both scientific and lay circles. Clearly the community-based art programs are having a real effect on health promotion and disease prevention. These, in turn, support the independence of the individuals and their ability to live in their communities and appear to be reducing risk factors driving the need for long-term care.

The Positive Impact of Creativity on Illness and Aging
Art as Therapy for Illness among Older Adults

There is a long history of case reports and observational studies on the impact of art and art therapy on alleviating or coping with illness in later life (Harrison, 1980; Ferguson and Goosman, 1991; Callanan, 1994; Achterberg, 1995; Ashida, 2000; Cohen, 2000; Cadigan et al., 2001; Hilliard, 2003). A classic illustration is the experience of Elizabeth Layton. Until her late sixties, Layton had experienced a long chronic history of debilitating depression, going back to her young adulthood. She had received considerable medical and psychiatric treatment, but still her depression was unremitting. Then, at age 68, in her *liberation phase,* she enrolled in an art course, examined herself in her looking glass, and wondered if she could draw a self-portrait. To her surprise and elation, she was able to draw with excellence. This launched a 20-year painting career and associated fame, and her self-applied art therapy put her depression in complete remission.

In literature, the role of creative interventions in altering the course of illness is captured in the case history of Ebenezer Scrooge. Suffering from an undiagnosed chronic depression, the aging Scrooge was the beneficiary of help from an inter-disciplinary outreach team making a home visit to Scrooge in 1843—more than 100 years before the community outreach programs of the twentieth century. The team of three art therapists took advantage of Scrooge's increased capacity for conflict resolution by virtue of developmentally being in the *summing-up phase.* They applied psychodynamic dream work and creative guided imaging techniques, more than 50 years before Freud's classic work *The Interpretation of Dreams.* The outcome was a breakthrough that enabled Scrooge to be released from his depression and to use his freed-up energy to help the Cratchit family and Tiny Tim. *A Christmas Carol* is a classic portrayal of the role of creative engagement in allowing us to cope with adversity, find a new way of dealing with the world, and get out of a rut regardless of age.

Creativity and Dementia

The role for creative opportunities and interventions is now being recognized even in the area of dementing illnesses, disorders considered the antithesis of creativity (Cohen, 2006). Willem de Kooning illustrated this well. Despite having Alzheimer's disease, de Kooning demonstrated the important phenomenon of possessing an area of preserved skill. All of us have certain skills or interests that we have more highly developed than others—usually an area in which we have been creatively engaged. The challenge is to help affected individuals find those areas and have an opportunity to tap then; the result is increased quality of life from the satisfaction of being able to use that residual capacity. Although diagnosed and impaired with Alzheimer's disease, de Kooning retained some reserve creative capacity to paint, allowing him for a few years to continue to produce work sought after by museums; he then continued painting for several years beyond that, nearly up to the time he died.

Memory versus Imagination

Perhaps the ultimate illustration of the universal capacity and resiliency of creative expression can be seen with dementia, where when memory fails in a major way the creative process of imagination can still be mobilized. The satisfaction of being able to access one's imagination, even when limited, compensates in part for the frustration associated with failing memory. Anne Basting's research with her creative storytelling project, TimeSlips, poignantly demonstrates the persistence of imagination triggered by evocative narrative in the face of failing memory (Basting, 2003).

The following is a dialogue that illustrates the presence and creative role of imagination in dementia in coping with memory loss. It takes place between the author and his mother shortly after she had a series of small strokes that decimated her memory. The conversation takes place the day after her 90th birthday, which had been a wonderful and successful family event. The author's mother had had a great time.

SON: How was your 90th birthday party?

MOTHER: I'm sorry; I have no recall of it. But I heard I had a good time.

(The son switches the structure of the conversation from memory mode to imagination mode.)

SON: What would having a good time at your birthday be like?

MOTHER: Having a lot of family there.

SON: Would you have a birthday cake?

MOTHER: Sure.

SON: Would the cake have 90 candles?

MOTHER: I hope not.

Not being able to recall the party had given the mother distress. Being able to respond to imagination-prompting questions gave her a sense of satisfaction to be creatively engaged.

A New Metaphor for Aging: *Blue Sky above Clouds*

Because expectations so powerfully shape our experience, we need to replace the outdated stereotypes and language of old age with new metaphors for aging. So many of the present metaphors about aging are patronizing, but they have persisted because they are poetic: "It's the fall of your life—the leaves are dropping from your tree." "It's the winter of your years—it's cold, the ground is barren, covered with snow." How do you think baby boomers relate to these metaphors? It is time for new, more accurate metaphors—not politically correct metaphors, but *correct* metaphors, realistically and accurately capturing the experience of aging. The story of the artist Georgia O'Keeffe is especially inspiring and congruent with the life experience of aging we witness today.

Various O'Keeffe biographers have described different anxieties she experienced, one of them being a fear of flying (Robinson, 1989). As she grew more famous and as she had increasing demands to appear for shows and presentations around the world, her need to fly increased. One day, when she was in her late seventies, O'Keeffe gazed admiringly out the window of a plane at a formation of the clouds below. She recalled later that she suddenly realized at that moment that her fear of flying had disappeared. She was exhilarated. The experience provided a new direction for her art, and the end result was a huge exhibit—the biggest in her lifetime—consisting of 96 works. Among them was a large-format series, with paintings as large as 8 by 24 feet. The images in this series were inspired by the view from her airplane window; they were beautiful, semiabstract paintings of huge clouds in a blue sky. She titled them *Sky above Clouds.* Old age was no "winter of life" for O'Keeffe; her art was not crippled by her age. Rather, her age, experience, and openness to new ideas allowed her to see the blue sky above the clouds. Aging in the twenty-first century promises increasingly to be a scenario of *blue sky above clouds* in the expression of human potential, despite age-associated problems.

Do Not Go Gently

A different poetry about old age was that of Dylan Thomas: "Do not go gentle into the night; Old Age should burn and rave at close of day; Rage, Rage, Rage, against the dying of the light." This has the feeling of an encore phase (the fourth of the psychological growth phases in the second half of life) perspective. But Dylan Thomas lived only until 39 (1914–53); he made these comments as a relatively young man. Meanwhile, nearly 20 years earlier than Dylan Thomas's poem, Oliver Wendell Holmes, Jr., on retiring from the Supreme Court at 92 to have more time to read Plato, reflected in his *encore phase*, with an uncannily similar do-not-go-gentle orientation: "I cannot say farewell to life and you in formal words. Life seems to me like a Japanese picture which our imagination does not allow to end with the margin. We aim at the infinite, and when our arrow falls to earth it is in flames."

Concluding Perspectives

In the past few years, I have made a thrilling discovery . . . that until one is over sixty, one can never really learn the secret of living. One can then begin to live, not simply with the intense part of oneself, but with one's entire being.

—*Pulitzer Prize–winning novelist Ellen Glasgow*

Odd how the creative power at once brings the whole universe to order.   —*Virginia Woolf*

REFERENCES

Achterberg, J. 1995. *Imagery in Healing*. Boston: New Science Library.

Andreasen, N. C. 2005. *The Creating Brain*. Washington, D.C.: Dana Press.

Arlin, P. K. 1975. Cognitive development in adulthood: A fifth stage? *Developmental Psychology* 11 (5):602–6.

Ashida, S. 2000. The effect of reminiscence music therapy sessions on changes in depressive symptoms in elderly persons with dementia. *Journal of Music Therapy* 37 (3):170–82.

Atkinson, R. 1995. *The Gift of Stories: Practical and spiritual applications of autobiography, life stories, and personal mythmaking*. Westport: Bergan and Garvey.

Avlund, K., M. T. Damsgaard, and E. E. Holstein. 1998. Social relations and mortality: An eleven year follow-up study of 70-year-old men and women in Denmark. *Social Science and Medicine* 47 (5):635–43.

Basting, A. 2003. Dare to imagine: Exploring the creative potential of people with Alzheimer's disease and related dementia. In *Mental Wellness and Aging: Strength-based approaches*, ed. J. Ronch and J. Goldfield. Baltimore: Health Professions Press.

Bennet, K. M. 2002. Low level social engagement as precursor of mortality among people in later life. *Age and Ageing* 31 (3):165–68.

Birren, J. E., and K. N. Cochran. 2001. *Telling the Stories of Life through Guided Autobiography Groups*. Baltimore: Johns Hopkins University Press.

Butler, R. N. 1963. The life review: An interpretation of reminiscence in the aged. *Psychiatry* 26:65–76.

Cabeza, R. 2002. Hemispheric asymmetry reduction in older adults: The HAROLD model. *Psychology and Aging* 17 (1):85–100.

Cabeza, R., et al. 2002. Aging gracefully: Compensatory brain activity in high-performing older adults. *NeuroImage* 17 (3):1394–1402.

Cadigan, M. E., et al. 2001. The effects of music on cardiac patients on bed rest. *Progress in Cardiovascular Nursing* 61 (1):5–13.

Callanan, B. O. 1994. Art therapy with the frail elderly. *Journal of Long Term Home Health Care* 13 (2):20–23.

Cohen, G. D. 2000. *The Creative Age: Awakening human potential in the second half of life.* New York: Avon Books/HarperCollins.

——. 2004. *United the Heart and Mind: Human development in the second half of life.* San Francisco: American Society on Aging *Mind Alert* Publications.

——. 2005. *The Mature Mind: The positive power of the aging brain.* New York: Basic Books.

——. 2006. Research on creativity and aging: The positive impact of the arts on health and illness. *Generations* 30 (1):7–15.

Cohen, G. D., S. Perlstein, J. Chapline, J. Kelly, K. M. Firth, and S. Simmens. 2006. The impact of professionally conducted cultural programs on the physical health, mental health, and social functioning of older adults. *Gerontologist* 46 (6):726–34.

——. 2007. The impact of professionally conducted cultural programs on the physical health, mental health, and social functioning of older adults: 2 year results. *Journal of Aging, Humanities, and the Arts* 1 (1–2):5–22.

Cole, T. R., D. Van Tassel, and R. Kastenbaum, eds. 1992. *Handbook of the Humanities and Aging.* New York: Springer.

Cole, T. R., and M. G. Winkler, eds. 1994. *The Oxford Book of Aging: Reflections on the journey of life.* New York: Oxford University Press.

Csikszentmihalyi, M. 1996. *Creativity.* New York: HarperCollins.

Diamond, M. C. 1993. An optimistic view of the aging brain. In *Mental Health and Aging*, ed. M. A. Smyer. New York: Springer.

Erikson, E. 1980. *Identity and the Life Cycle.* New York: W. W. Norton.

Ferguson, W. J., and E. A. Goosman. 1991. Foot in the door: Art therapy in the nursing home. *American Journal of Art Therapy* 30 (1):2–3.

Flood, D. G., and P. D. Coleman. 1990. Hippocampal plasticity in normal aging and decreased plasticity in Alzheimer's disease. *Progress in Brain Research* 83:435–43.

Flood, D. G., et al. 1985. Age related dendritic growth in dentate gyrus of human brain is followed by regression in the 'oldest old.' *Brain Research* 345 (2):366–68.

Gardner, H. 1993a. *Creating Minds.* New York: Basic Books.

——. 1993b. *Frames of Mind: The theory of multiple intelligences.* New York: Basic Books.

Glass, T. A., et al. 1999. Population based study of social and productive activities as predictors of survival among elderly Americans. *British Medical Journal* 319:478–83.

Harrison, C. L. 1980. Creative arts for older people in the community. *American Journal of Art Therapy* 19 (4):99–101.

Hartigan, L. R., ed. 1990. *'Made with passion': The Hemphill folk art collection.* Washington, D.C.: Smithsonian Institution Press.

Hilliard, R. E. 2003. The effects of music therapy on the quality and length of life of people diagnosed with terminal cancer. *Journal of Music Therapy* 40 (2):113–37.

Kandel, E. R. 2006. *In Search of Memory.* New York: W. W. Norton.

Katzman, R. 1995. Can late life social or leisure activities delay the onset of dementia? *Journal of the American Geriatrics Society* 45 (5):583–84.

Kempermann, G., L. Wiskott, and F. H. Gage. 2004. Functional significance of adult neuro-genesis. *Current Opinion in Neurobiology* 14 (2):186–91.

Kettering, C. 2008. *National Academy for Teaching and Learning about Aging.* University of North Texas 2002 (cited July 15, 2008). Available from www.cps.unt.edu/natla/.

Kiecolt-Glaser, J. K., et al. 2002. Emotions, morbidity, and mortality: New perspectives from psychoneuroimmunology. *Annual Review of Psychology* 53:83–107.

Kolb, B., and I. Q. Whishaw. 1998. Brain plasticity and behavior. *Annual Review of Psychology* 49:43–64.

Kramer, A. F., et al. 2004. Environmental influences on cognitive and brain plasticity during aging. *Journal of Gerontology: Medical Sciences* 59A (9):940–57.

Kunitz, S. 1995. *Passing Through: The later poems, new and selected.* New York: W. W. Norton.

Kunz, J. A., and F. G. Soltys, eds. 2007. *Transformational Reminiscence: Life story work.* New York: Springer.

LeDoux, J. 2002. *Synaptic Self: How our brains become who we are.* New York: Viking.

Lehman, H. 1953. *Age and Achievement.* Princeton, NJ: Princeton University Press.

Livingston, J., and J. Beardsley, eds. 1982. *Black Folk Art in America.* Jackson: University of Mississippi Press.

Lutgendorf, S. K., and E. S. Costanzo. 2003. Psychoneuroimmunology and health psychology: An integrative model. *Brain, Behavior, and Immunity* 17 (4):225–32.

Lutgendorf, S. K., et al. 1999. Sense of coherence moderates the relationship between life stress and the natural killer cell activity in healthy older adults. *Psychology and Aging* 14 (4):552–63.

Maguire, E. A., and C. D. Frith. 2003. Aging affects the engagement of the hippocampus during autobiographical memory retrieval. *Brain: A Journal of Neurology* 126 (7):1511–23.

Marchand, H. 2001. Some reflections on postformal thought. *Genetic Epistemologist* 29 (3):2–9.

May, R. 1975. *The Courage to Create.* New York: Bantam Books.

Pert, C., H. E. Dreher, and R. Ruff. 1998. The psychosomatic network: Foundations of mind-body medicine. *Alternative Therapies* 4 (4):30–41.

Richards, F., and M. Commons. 1990. Postformal cognitive-developmental theory and research: A review of its current status. In *Higher Stages of Human Development*, ed. C. Alexander and E. Langer. New York: Oxford University Press.

Robinson, R. 1989. *Georgia O'Keeffe.* Hanover: University Press of New England.

Rodin, J. 1986. Aging and health: Effects of the sense of control. *Science* 233 (4770):1271–76.

———. 1989. Sense of control: Potentials for intervention. *Annals of the American Academy of Policy and Social Science* 503:29–42.

Rowe, J. W., and R. L. Kahn. 1998. *Successful Aging.* New York: Pantheon.

Russell, R. 1967–69. *The Autobiography of Betrand Russell.* 3 vols. London: George Allen and Unwin.

Simonton, D. K. 1984. Creative productivity and age: A mathematical model based on a two-step cognitive process. *Developmental Review* 4:77–111.

Sinnott, J. D. 1991. Limits to problem solving: Emotion, intention, goal, clarity, health, and other factors in postformal thought. In *Bridging Paradigms: Positive development in adulthood and cognitive aging*, ed. J. D. Sinnott and J. C. Cavanaugh. New York: Praeger.

———. 1999. Creativity and postformal thought: Why the last stage is the creative stage. In *Creativity and Successful Aging*, ed. C. E. Adams-Price. New York: Springer.

Tate, J., and D. Lehman, eds. 1997. *The Best American Poetry of 1997.* New York: Scribner.

Taupin, P., and F. H. Gage. 2002. Mini-review: Adult neurogenesis and the neural stem cells of the central nervous system in mammals. *Journal of Neuroscience Research* 69:745–49.

CHAPTER NINE

The Five People You Meet in Retirement

RONALD J. MANHEIMER, PH.D.

Philosophical Encounters of the Third Age

Arthur Schopenhauer, the nineteenth-century German philosopher, had a penchant for metaphor. About aging, he opined, "during the first half of life we delight in the richly patterned quilt of our experiences. The second half allows us a peek at the other side—how the quilt was made." He went on to liken the first half of life to the text of a weighty book and the second to its footnotes—the sources. On a roll, he exclaimed that "in our younger days we yearn for excitement and romance. The second half finds us puzzling over what meanings those experiences and relationships reveal" (Schopenhauer, 1890).

While he held forth on the stages of life, the gloomy Schopenhauer ("all life is vanity") had nothing to say about disengagement from the work force, retirement. In this he shares the company of those few philosophers who deigned to comment on old age such as Aristotle, Confucius, Cicero, Montaigne, and Simone de Beauvoir (Manheimer, 2000). The reason? Until the middle of the twentieth century, only a small minority, the healthy and wealthy, could enjoy the economic security, discretionary leisure time, and wide array of activity choices that British political thinker Peter Laslett characterized as the benefits of a "third age" (Laslett, 1991). Now that a large segment of the population of developed countries has entered this new domain, it is drawing as many guides and gurus as did the discovery of another modern life stage, adolescence, around the turn of the previous century (Hall, 1904).

What could be a more philosophical topic than a new life stage in which decisions concerning leaving the workforce, experiences of changes in one's body, and the effects of diminished family responsibilities trigger concerns about identity, selfhood, mortality, purpose, relationships, meaning, freedom, and even wisdom, to name some of the most prominent? Apart from contemporary academic philosophers who have contributed to the field of bioethics and aging, few modern philosophers have turned their craft on this new life stage and on such ontologically tantalizing notions as the popular exhortation to "reinvent yourself." The academic experts who have addressed philosophical questions about aging and later life tend to be psychologists, anthropologists, and sociologists, not philosophers (Manheimer, 1989).

Exemplary contributors include anthropologist Sharon Kaufman, who showed us that within each aging person's life narrative there dwells an enduring or "ageless self" (Kaufman, 1995). Noted psychologist James Birren and his collaborators, using observation and survey instruments, revealed that wisdom in the later years depended on "the integration of general cognitive, affective, and reflective qualities." Wisdom, they conjectured, had socially and biologically adaptive value (Birren and Fisher, 1990). Developmental psychologist Paul Baltes and his collaborators gave scientific credence to the great literary theme of the aging athlete, warrior, or musician who, continuing to compete despite lost strength and agility, taps into compensatory strategies drawn from well-tested experiences (Baltes and Baltes, 1990). And Swedish gerontologist Lars Tornstam drew from extensive surveys and interviews of aging Scandinavians to announce a universal life perspective shift that he termed "gerotranscendence." His research showed how an earlier narrow piety and rigidity of moral judgment could turn into a Zen-like acceptance of the paradoxes and contradictions of life as the individual gained a view of him- or herself as belonging to a benign natural order and cosmic wholeness (Tornstam, 1997).

In addition to these social scientists, there is a cadre of students of the humanities (many included in this volume) who have found their way and helped to define the contemporary field of aging interpreted through the lenses of the humanistic disciplines (Cole, Van Tassel, and Kastenbaum, 1992; Cole, Kastenbaum, and Ray, 2000). Many entered through passages that were off the beaten paths of their academic disciplines (for a collection of such accounts, see the *Journal of Aging Studies*, April 2008). They include cultural and social historians, philosophers of postmodernism and critical theory, literature experts, and students of comparative religion. Thanks to their contributions, we discover the complexities of aging through older characters of novels, poems, dramas, and cinema; we recognize the socially and culturally constructed aspects of aging and elderly people that may underlie discourse in the natural sciences; and we learn to appreciate the multidimensional richness of older lives that continue to unfold in autobiographical narratives and in painted or etched self-portraits. Collectively, their explorations are both a search for meaning as revealed in life's second half and a critical probing of hidden ideologies and unexamined assumptions rampant throughout the gerontological field. I count myself as fortunate to be among these wayfarers.

As to my own pathway (relevant to this essay), I was educated in philosophy and the product of a graduate program with the unabashed title, History of Consciousness. My doctoral thesis concerned how philosophers viewed human development (Manheimer, 1977). Not surprisingly, as a young man, I focused on the transition from youth to adulthood and the process of "self-becoming" that led from a life of sporadic enthusiasms and fleeting responsibilities (what Kierkegaard called the "aesthetic stage") to one of commitment, focused passion, and personal and communal belonging (Kierkegaard's "ethical stage") (Kierkegaard, 1968). In 1976, I took the opportunity to volunteer to lead a philosophy class at a senior center. With my entry into the world of adult education, my orientation shifted to what lay ahead—midlife and old age. My decision to contribute to the bicentennial by placing myself among older adults and exploring their hard-earned wisdom and cultural legacy altered my career and changed my life.

Since then, my involvement in the aging field has been simultaneously theoretical and applied as I have worked directly with people who were at one time "my elders" (and are now my peers) to help create community-based lifelong learning programs and organizations. During the last 20 years, I have served as director of an educational program devoted to lifelong learning, leadership service, and research—the North Carolina Center for Creative Retirement (NCCCR), an institute of the University of North Carolina at Asheville. My post has given me extensive opportunities to work with hundreds of people at different stages of retirement.

Because NCCCR has for more than six years offered a life transition seminar for midlife adults seeking to explore and plan the next stages of their lives, I have had the privilege of getting to know people as they worked through some intensely personal issues about career, family and friendship, sense of meaning, and concerns about risk and security (i.e., wealth). I have also had the pleasure of working closely with a multitude of volunteer leaders. In some cases, I have collaborated with the same individuals for close to two decades. We have grown older together.

Because of my orientation, I have instinctively perked up my ears when philosophical issues and themes were introduced in conversation (Manheimer, 1999). Not that the speakers were self-consciously aware of the philosophical content of their utterances—in most cases they did not possess the analytical tools or formal vocabulary of philosophy. Yet what they had to say and the questions they posed to themselves and others fit appropriately into the history of speculation and the quest for meaning that once belonged almost exclusively to the realm of philosophical (and theological) discourse.

To show what philosophy has to offer those about to make or having made the leap into retirement, let's see what happens when we delve into the metaphysics of, to use an old-fashioned term, the "superannuated" (gone beyond the threshold year). While no one is a "typical" retiree, some more dramatically exemplify the issues than others. Here, then, are five people you might meet in retirement, individuals whose stories offer philosophical enrichment. But, you may ask, why just five people?

The Heavenly Five

The title of this essay is a play on novelist and journalist Mitch Albom's bestseller and subsequent movie, *The Five People You Meet in Heaven* (2003). The premise of that work of the popular imagination—which *Publisher's Weekly* dubbed a "contemporary American fable"—is that after you die you pass into a transitional or limbo state (the novel's "heaven") in which certain tasks must be completed. The hero of Albom's story is Eddie, an 83-year-old, newly deceased amusement park maintenance man, who must conduct an exchange with five other deceased individuals also residing in limbo. Successful exchange will gain Eddie passage to a place yet further removed from earthly life.

Eddie's task requires that he assemble certain pieces of biographical information possessed by others, some of whom are complete strangers. The stories they tell are about how Eddie influenced or what he meant to them, even in instances in which he could not be aware unless he were omniscient. The point of this moralistic tale is that our good qualities, our virtues, however meager and unself-conscious, have greater impact in the world than we might have believed. We must come to understand this and also find forgiveness in ourselves and in others for our sins of both omission and commission. The purpose of these five meetings is to achieve enough self-understanding that, once we know the whole story, we can fully accept and value our lives.

Suggestively, Albom's tale parallels the journey-of-encounters theme from mythology, such as the four tasks Aphrodite sets forth for Psyche to accomplish, the soul's sojourn through the afterlife as depicted in the *Tibetan Book of the Dead*, and Dr. Borg's life review road trip in Bergman's *Wild Strawberries*. Japanese director Kore Eda's poignant 1998 film, *Afterlife*, explores a similar theme. The souls of the newly departed enter an abandoned building, where they are assisted by a group of counselors who, also, are no longer living. They instruct the newcomers that they have only a few days to choose one memory that will be restaged and recorded on film, a single recalled experience they will then take with them into the eternal beyond. What moment would you choose?

These mythical, spiritual, and cinematic heavenly journeys have a parable-like character that redirects our attention to the life we lead in the finitude of space and time. If our lives are fragmented, incomplete, how do we make them whole, comprehensible? Albom knows that accounts of the afterlife in various faith traditions also mirror the values and attitudes of terrestrial existence. He touches this universal instinct that beckons us to not only achieve self-awareness but experience wholeness of being and union with what is qualitatively timeless—the divine, the natural order, or perhaps some kind of cosmic consciousness. Were it not triggering some universal longing for completeness, the book would find few sympathetic readers.

If Albom's story sounds a bit dubious to those of a more secular humanist persuasion, he stands with the majority. A recent survey of 1,011 Americans 50 or older conducted on behalf of *AARP The Magazine* found that 73 percent of our fellow citizens believe in life after death, a conviction that only gets stronger with age. Furthermore, 86 percent of "believers" affirmed that "there is a Heaven" (Newcott, 2007).

The reader may wonder whether an analogy is intended here between passage into the afterlife and passage into retirement. As simply disengaging from the workforce and initiation of Social Security and (for some) pension benefits, retirement is certainly not one's death. And yet, for most people, retirement foreshadows life's termination in that it is inextricably connected to the transition from midlife to old age and our eventual "passing away." Retirement is a major rite of passage, often from a more to a less known stage of life, a transition frequently accompanied by a sense of loss (e.g., of work identity, productivity, social networks), although this may be matched by excitement about the possibilities of a newly attained freedom. Retirement frequently triggers a life review as we adjust to new routines and must accommodate new sources of meaning.

Here, then, are five people whose portraits (modified for confidentiality), in miniature, contain philosophical messages. Each sounds a theme that reverberates with one or more philosophical thinkers.

Three of the subjects attended our center's Paths to Creative Retirement program. Paths, for short, is a three-day event that brings complete strangers together from various parts of the country, individuals and couples who seek to explore how to make the most of their new life stage, even when that involves continued pursuit of a career or movement into a next vocation, whether for pay or as volunteers. By design, the seminar causes participants to reflect on the changes and choices that have brought them to the present moment, and it elicits the persistent values that have influenced their lives. The other two subjects are members of the center whom I have known and worked with for many years. One of them is now deceased.

Finding the Way

As if taking a cue from Chancellor Bismarck, who influenced the U.S. Social Security system's choice of the magic number, Betsy retired last year just a few months after her 65th birthday. "When I became president of the agency at age 55, I decided I'd put ten more years into this job and then call it quits," said Betsy of her post at a New England–based social service organization. During her 25-year tenure as an employee, Betsy saw the fast expanding, 42-agency nonprofit go from an annual budget of $3 million to $53 million. Of her scheduled retirement, she says, "I chose that age because I wanted to be able to start over."

Betsy figured that she would still have the health and energy to add a new chapter to her life story. With an undergraduate degree in history and a knack for writing, she decided before she left the agency that she would chronicle its history. "I started interviewing long time employees about three months before I turned in my keys." The project served as a great transition and a way to commemorate her departure while bestowing a gift on the agency. Despite this preparation, said Betsy, "I felt like I had walked off the edge of a cliff."

It wasn't the financial uncertainty that made this cliff walker experience vertigo. Betsy, a widow, was fortunate to have an inheritance to supplement her small pension and Social Security income. "I'm an introvert," she commented, "and my work was my support group." Not only did she find it daunting to make new friends, but also Betsy worried about the same things that other newly retired people confront—how to choose and structure daily activities, avoid boredom and isolation, and find meaning and purpose in life's second half when a career and child rearing are no longer the main focus.

As a person who had lived through some "horrendous" experiences earlier in life, Betsy knew she'd survive the transition. Still, relinquishing her professional identity and daily work habits took away her reasons for getting up in the morning and left her feeling "at sea."

To steady herself, Betsy chose another "soft landing" technique. She started keeping a journal to observe herself going through the transition. She wrote short essays on things that happened during the previous week and about anxious thoughts. She also started a small consulting business to help other nonprofit organization leaders. And she decided to spend more time in her garden.

"The gardening became my main metaphor," she said. "I'd picture myself in early May with lots of empty beds and a stack of seed and plant catalogs. I couldn't plant everything that looked inviting. Didn't have enough space. So which ones?"

Betsy had dim memories of reading Kierkegaard as an undergraduate, but she recalled and embraced one of the Danish existentialist's main tenets. About finding our path in life he said, "the way is not the problem, the problem is the way." Betsy recognized that unique opportunities often announce themselves in the form of obstacles, dilemmas, and difficulties. Betsy also remembered Kierkegaard's famous assertion that life can only be lived "forward" and understood "backward." Each of our actions and decisions, no matter how well thought through, still involves an act of faith as we encounter uncertainties and make what are sometimes irreversible choices. In what might seem a paradoxical formulation, Kierkegaard argued that an individual's task is to "choose one's self," that is, be faithful to one's destiny, one's calling.

At the heart of Kierkegaard's religious psychology lies the paradox of an underlying discord between a person's sense of sheer possibility (of actions, goals, relationships) and what belongs truly to each person (i.e., that for which he or she was brought into the world). Each life is lived toward the completion of its inner drama and the resolution of a seemingly irreconcilable duality—the finite (mortal) and infinite (immortal or immutable) aspects of self. Kierkegaard's formulation would later be adopted by Heidegger, who would secularize the terminology, preferring to characterize the individual as searching for his or her "ownmost possibilities" as he or she experienced what Heidegger termed "thrownness" (*geworfenheit*), temporal momentum toward the horizon of the future.

Between cliff walking and seed planting, metaphors of a perilous fall and joyful rebirth, Betsy described herself as in a state of suspended animation—"at sea," floating. Her floatation was not without forward momentum as, willfully, she swam on, testing her fortitude in preparing for the next phase of her life. She didn't try to defuse the tension of the unknowable by staying busy, signing up for lots of volunteer work, checking out stacks of detective novels, or rushing back to full-time employment. In a sense, she waited for the signals of what unique path would open to her.

Still, a highly pragmatic person with a distaste for passivity, she took some practical steps to ensure that she'd meet new people and keep her mind sharp by enrolling in the area's lifelong learning program (she's studying Medieval Spanish history). She did a little consulting to share her wealth of knowledge and served on the local arts commission to stay tuned to the latest "culture jolts." And she made sure she stayed physically active by continuing to walk her dog a mile and a half each morning and joining an "Over the Hill" group of avid mountain trekkers. Keeping her journal enabled Betsy to embrace her discomfort about the uncertainties that lay ahead. Betsy actively waited. She let the problem, what to do next that felt right, work itself out. She trusted that the process would bring her insight and fresh perspective and, in turn, would yield a new pattern of daily activity.

Where Betsy seems to have departed from the individualist-oriented Kierkegaardian approach was in her decision to write an institutional history. She not only wanted to understand this part of her life in retrospect, but she wanted to locate herself in the larger context of the "becoming" of an organization and group of people with whom she had worked. She felt that she belonged to this community and that its history was a part of her life story. The values and aspirations she shared with others would remain an important part of her future life, something she could take with her.

One day, almost exactly a year from when she started it, Betsy reread her retirement transition journal while traveling in a Boeing 727 at 39,000 feet. She noticed that a recent entry sounded familiar. Sure enough, she had penned a short essay on the same subject many months earlier. Noting a sharp decrease in the emotional intensity this same subject drew the second time around, she reached a conclusion. The transition crisis was over. With that, she closed the journal and put it away.

"It's not that everything had fallen into place. I was still searching," said Betsy. "I was hoping to narrow my range of options and not be scattered over too many activities." Still, she was more comfortable, more at ease with the cycle of her days. She knew what she wanted to plant, and if a few things didn't come up as she'd hoped, well, she could live with that.

Quest for Redemption

Not everyone in our town knew Dave by name, but a great many recognized the trim, fast-paced figure in jeans and a college sweatshirt, his tanned, smiling face shaded by the visor of a New York Yankees baseball cap from under which a few strands of gray hair might protrude. The Yankees? Here in the south? The guy had some nerve.

Dave and his wife Dorothy moved from Brooklyn to Asheville, North Carolina, in the early 1990s. Dave retired from the highly competitive business world of women's fashion and Dorothy from professional choreography. Dave became involved in some intergenerational classes at our center that brought mature adults and university undergraduates together in small seminars. And Dorothy volunteered to teach tap dancing in the College for Seniors. Her class was a big hit, and soon her "Rascals" tap dance troupe was performing at nursing homes, senior centers, and outdoor festivals. Dave had once considered a career in journalism but was deterred at college registration. "I'd just gotten out of the army and even though it was the GI Bill, I still wasn't going to stand in any more long lines." Instead, he chose a shorter line, signing up for NYU's School of Business. Forty years later and a newcomer to retirement, he stood in a short line to sign up for those writing courses in a lifelong learning program.

Dave achieved three important goals within the few years after he and Dorothy arrived in Asheville. First, claiming he identified with the disenfranchised, he volunteered to serve on a board working to organize an annual Native American festival called Kituah. Second, he became a Big Brother, taking on 11-year-old Chris who lived with his grandparents and who was reading at a second grade level. And third, he eventually wrote a play about his experiences with Chris.

Of Kituah, he said, "I learned that if I kept my mouth shut and stopped trying to be number one, eventually they would call on me for advice." Of his little brother Chris, he said, "Helping Chris with school, Dorothy and I tutoring him in reading, and taking him to minor league ball games, gave me a chance to do for him what I hadn't done for my own kids." And of his play, which he hoped to see produced, he said, "I finally got back to creative writing, my first love."

Although he was raised in the Jewish tradition, Dave was not especially observant. Yet his unself-conscious quest to embrace humility, undo the mistakes of earlier parenting, and give literary shape to his new life with Chris have what I have elsewhere called a pattern of "secular redemption" (Manheimer, 1989). This theme runs through a number of novels, films, and theories about growing old. In the Judeo-Christian tradition, redemption means calling on the deity to remove the blot of sin on one's soul. Redemption may be pursued through prayer and/or corrective deeds. In Dave's case, redemption meant righting the wrongs of the past and rediscovering the road not taken.

Dave was still somewhat haunted by his failed first marriage and his inattention to his children, which led to a degree of alienation from his daughter and an often tense relationship with his son. While he ran a successful business, it did not give him the creative fulfillment he imagined associated with a career in journalism. Dave did not find a comfortable place in Jewish religious practices and yearned for a way to belong to a community. Although to most people he could seem like a jovial fellow with few cares in the world, Dave had a powerful sense of incompleteness that nagged at him.

Unlike in the general Jewish tradition, where redemption is of the Jewish people as a whole, twentieth-century Jewish philosopher Franz Rosenzweig gave redemption an existential meaning—release from a self-centered, detached disposition in readiness to experience the love of both God and one's fellow human beings (Rosenzweig, 2005). For Rosenzweig, this personal redemption was intimately connected to creation and revelation, three parts of a triad that, with redemption, provided release of the fetters of the soul. Dave probably never read a word written by Rosenzweig, yet he made of his later life a similar triad. His creative pursuit through play writing enabled him to realize the dream of self-expression through striving to master an art form. The lessons of humility he learned in association with Native Americans came as a revelation about the less developed side of his personality. Dave's mentoring and tutoring Chris were ways he could assuage his remorse over past shortcomings and, at least in part, make up for or redeem his role as a parent.

Dave took advantage of learning opportunities in later life to rectify past mistakes and disappointments and to make his life whole. He used education, both academic and experiential, as the vehicle of self-change. Dave died in the summer of 1997 and was buried in the nearby Veterans Cemetery. Only a few months stood between the diagnosis of pancreatic cancer and his death. Dave was a young 72, so the brevity of his retirement life made his accomplishments all the more poignant. It was as if he knew time was short and he had much to do to earn his redemption. Although his efforts brought him a measure of peace and contentment, still he could not completely undo the past. I remember standing by Dave's hospital bed where he lay heavily sedated and breathing laboriously. His son stood across the hall pleading into his cell phone, telling his sister, Dave's daughter, that she must come at once as their father was in his last days. Although reluctantly, she did arrive in time to be with her father in his last moments.

The Purposeless Life

The concept of the absurd has multiple meanings. From the early church father Tertullian we have the famous "*creo quia absurdum*," "I believe because it is absurd." The "it" is the incarnation of the divine into the mortal, Jesus, a paradoxical man-God. Something more than human reason is required to embrace a belief in a doctrine as hard to fathom as the coexistence of the temporal and eternal. The absurd took on different meanings in the minds of twentieth-century French literary thinkers Jean-Paul Sartre and Albert Camus. In Sartre's case, because, as he asserts, "existence precedes essence," we find ourselves thrown into a world without intrinsic meaning but discover our radical freedom to give birth to ourselves as bearers of meaning and value through our actions. His lifelong colleague Simone de Beauvoir beautifully summarized this view when she said, "I was born to fulfill the great need I had of myself" (de Beauvoir, 1962). Many of us remember Camus' character, Meursault, the antihero of the novel *The Stranger*, who murders an anonymous Arab man on a beach in Algeria because in a world without meaning or God, everything is permitted. For Camus, a philosopher of "extreme situations," it takes the jolt of sudden awareness through an act of seemingly capricious daring to wake up to the central value of life, pure existence and the capability to invent meaning. Unfortunately, Meursault has to pay with his life to achieve this realization.

Ned, a man in his late fifties who retired at an early age from the insurance industry after attaining moderate wealth, espoused a fondness for the absurd. His choice of career, he explained, came through a friendship with a mentor who hired him almost on a whim just to prove that he could mold a taciturn introverted personality into a highly successful salesman. But selling insurance was never Ned's passion. In fact, he did not have a passion. So he pursued this line of work and was successful, in part, because he saw it as a game. In retirement, Ned and his wife moved from the Midwest to a fashionable New England coastal town where they planned to lead an idyllic life of leisure. Instead, they became bored with the lack of cultural and social opportunities. So, a few years later, they moved to the small but culturally vibrant Asheville, North Carolina.

Ned describes his retirement activities as a series of explorative ventures into civic groups, college classes, and hobbies (woodworking, mountain biking). He feels no sense of commitment to these activities but rather "noodles along," sticking with the things that continue to hold his interest and letting go of the ones that do not. He does not want a reason to get up each morning, he says. Rather, he prefers to rise because he feels refreshed, not because he hears the call of a purpose or responsibility that would be uniquely his own. Ned, somewhat like Camus in his later works such as *The Myth of Sisyphus* and the novel *The Plague*, is leery of systems of meaning that point to the validity of ideologies, religions, or grand philosophical theories. He senses, as did Camus, that justification for domination and induced self-repression may lurk within these lofty ideals. Yet, periodically, Ned travels off to spiritual retreats that sometimes require considerable self-discipline such as a vow of silence, an austere diet, and early morning meditations.

Like Dr. Rieux in *The Plague*, Ned adheres to a tenet of the Hippocratic Oath: "Do no harm." Ned prefers to enjoy life free of fixed meaning and purpose, to take each day as it comes. He is unabashedly selfish and acknowledges that he has few friends. He is attentive to his wife and his children and grandchildren, not because he holds some culturally approved notions of parental responsibility or marital fidelity, but because he finds pleasure in these connections.

Ned has no convictions about life after death, but he is not indifferent to that mystery. He prefers to leave it a mystery. In fact, he prefers to see his life and the life of those around him as mysterious and ultimately unknowable and incomprehensible. It is in this conviction that he shows great delight. "Am I a misfit?" he sometimes wonders aloud.

Unlike the literary existentialists' antihero characters, Ned has not pursued an absurdist existence as a theme of self-liberation or rebellion against empty social conventions. Like many affluent retirees, he has sought to reward himself by building an impressive "trophy" home and buying a number of fancy sports cars. It would be easy to judge Ned as exhibiting the existentialists' famous "false consciousness," in his case self-deception through fixation on material wealth as a substitution for authenticity. Yet Ned has a foot in both camps and laughs at his own foibles while continuing to pursue them. He loves the joyful freedom of the indeterminate, the capricious, and the enigmatic. His is a classic divided consciousness.

The Unknowable Self

The popular personality typology known as the Enneagram is represented by a nine-pointed figure symbolizing nine personality types and, through connecting geometric lines, their relationship to one another. According to the theory, each type emerges from the undifferentiated "pure essence" of early childhood as the result of instances of unconscious avoidance or fear that eventually crystallize into the type's "fixations." While these might have proven successful coping mechanisms earlier in life, they become hindrances in adulthood because they limit us to habitual behaviors and responses that are no longer productive or beneficial to us.

Bess learned about the Enneagram through a seminar offered by her church, where she has a history as a leader. Retired since age 50 after an attractive IBM buyout, Bess has been a major community activist and a well-respected organizer. Groups often seek her out to join their cause because they know how effective and competent she is. Bess is a self-purported type Three, labeled "The Achiever," whose "core motivation is to be pleasing to others, admirable, successful, and the best," according to the description found in books on interpreting the Enneagram types (Riso and Hudson, 1999).

Bess's trouble began about 10 years into retirement. She began to feel that her community activism no longer kindled her passion, nor did it bring the sense of satisfaction and self-esteem it had done earlier. She couldn't figure out why the importance of activism was waning. The Enneagram workshop introduced her to the idea that her civic activism was part of her need to be liked and to gain the approval of others, especially people whom she respected. There was nothing wrong with this motive, she understood, except that it had a compensatory function that distorted a sense of self-worth that was independent of pleasing others. To move toward this experience of intrinsic self-worth, Bess would have to decrease or completely relinquish her do-gooder activities. But that meant diminishing her social identity and possibly disappointing others who "would not understand" why she was seemingly "acting out of character." Shedding the mantle of civic activist also meant encountering the demons of the unconscious, those childhood fears and avoidance formations that originally led to her personality type. Although disengaging from civic activism when regarded as no longer authentic is viewed as a positive developmental step in the Enneagram theory, the process can be a painful one.

So intense was Bess's struggle that when she did step back and take time for more leisure activities, travel, meditation, and the enjoyment of "just being alive," she would break out in hives and experience severe anxiety. A return to even a small measure of civic activism would usually blunt this anxiety and the hives would vanish.

Bess's dilemma can be viewed in Eriksonian terms as the polarity of integrity versus despair (Stage Eight) as one seeks to come to terms with a lifetime of effort and accomplishment only to question whether it has been for naught. In Erikson's view, acceptance of mortality and of one's life history as containing an intrinsic necessity or inner logic of connectivity is crucial for mental health and to attain "wisdom."

Bess had studied Erikson's epigenetic life stage theory, but she had found it too oriented to the male psyche. Wisdom, for her, was less a matter of achieving individual integrity and more how you engaged in relationships and whether you acted in such a way so as to promote social justice. Still, promoting social justice had somehow worn thin even as she retained her commitments to various causes such as racial equality and women's rights.

A frequently articulated fear expressed by those on the brink of retirement is loss of identity. While for many this identity is derived from the duties, skills, and accolades of professional life, for Bess it was more centered in her passion for social welfare and in the skills she brought to community issues and organizations. She could easily have retained this identity because it was not based on how she had earned her livelihood. Overidentification with a career does tend to submerge the multitude of other ways we know who we are (e.g., through family, friendships, cultural heritage, religious affiliation, and the core of values, dispositions, and preferences that have been with us throughout our adulthood). As people step back from their work roles, these other identity links begin to emerge out of the background, gaining in importance.

What if, as we shed the productive doer identity of our working years, we find ourselves falling into a dark chasm of passionless indifference rather than rising toward the light of sheer being? Would that not be cause for anxiety and depression? And suppose you knew that all you needed to do was to return to productive doer roles and activities that you had established during your career or in your postemployment phase? Bess's dilemma was to find the strength to practice detachment from the known in order to allow the unknown to emerge. However, the goal of this process is ambiguous and so only after one reached the point of illumination would the pathway become clear. As Bess once said, "If I have a destiny, it would be only in retrospect that I would know it."

Echoing a trend that has emerged from the school of "positive psychology," one of Bess's friends admonished her that if she put the best face on her situation and emphasized positive thoughts about what she had already accomplished, she would be able to focus on gaining tranquility and a new lease on life. The friend encouraged Bess to read up on "positive aging," as it seemed to offer the quickest and most efficacious way of finding happiness. Bess, never one to shun a possibly valuable resource, did just that. She even tried out a series of "happiness exercises" she found listed in one book (Seligman, 2004). These exercises included writing a letter of gratitude to someone whose kindness you had never adequately acknowledged, writing down three things that went well each day, and taking an online survey to assess your "signature strengths" (Peterson and Seligman, 2004).

The outcome for Bess was her feeling "double-bound." "I was supposed to avoid skepticism and embrace optimism," said Bess, "and I was supposed to see my situation as something that I could control if I just adopted the right attitude. But since I didn't find that I was all that much happier for carrying out these exercises, I felt that I had somehow failed at them and that I was to blame for my condition."

What Bess was able to rescue from her dip into positive psychology was an ancient figure to which the happiness psychologists such as Seligman and Peterson often paid obeisance, Aristotle. Serendipitously, Bess came upon Aristotle in an ethics class in which she was enrolled at the Center for Creative Retirement. Aristotle, she learned, argued in the *Nicomachean Ethics* (1962) that *eudaimonia*, usually translated as happiness but closer in meaning to "flourishing," is the highest human good. For Aristotle, *eudaimonia* is far from synonymous with pleasure; rather, it is a by-product of leading a life harmonious with the best and most complete of human virtues such as temperance, justice, and courage. These virtues, for Aristotle, demonstrate the principle of the "mean" or median between qualities of character bounded by excess and deficiency. Courage, for example, is intermediate between deficiency of bravery or timidity and excess of heroics or bravado that is untempered by reasonable fear. The truly courageous person is neither paralyzed by fear nor emboldened beyond reasonable caution. Virtues are in this sense forms of excellence toward which human beings ought to strive. To aim at fully developing our potential for excellence is to set a course for a form of happiness that requires considerable self-discipline and delayed gratification.

Bess realized that what she was struggling with could not be resolved through a framework of behavioral optimism, a "thinking makes it so" mentality, although she could see the grain of truth in the psychological theory. Aristotle, however, helped her see that finding a way to balance rather than completely abandon her social activism was a truer course to follow. She was able to hold on to the value of Aristotle's civic responsibility while acknowledging that she needed to identify new goals that better corresponded to the changes taking place in her life. This added complexity brought her considerable insight into some of the hidden paradoxes of growing older although it also brought her a persistent measure of despair.

The Other

Modern philosophy from the time of Descartes has struggled with the philosophical status of relationships. Descartes argued that an irrefutable starting point for philosophy derived from the self-interrogated bedrock of the thinker's awareness of his or her own act of thinking, the infamous "*cogito ergo sum.*" Getting a philosophical system launched is always the hardest challenge. Descartes' rooting a system of rational speculation in the mind of the subject rather than in an independent physical or conceptual reality led to some difficulties that would persist to annoy subsequent thinkers, namely, how does a person ever get outside the thinking subject to prove a connection to a world independent of the mind? Solipsism, the collapse of reality into the hallucinatory world of the thinking subject, is often considered the great failing of philosophies that start from an origin in subjectivity.

Roy had never read anything by the twentieth-century French philosopher Emmanuel Levinas or any of the works of Levinas's one-time teacher, the German philosopher Edmund Husserl, founder of the school of phenomenology. But the discovery Roy made at the end of a weekend seminar would have delighted both thinkers. Levinas studied for a short time in the 1930s under Husserl and gradually became fascinated with the so-called problem of intersubjectivity. The problem has many variations ranging from the question "how can we know the minds of other people?" to "how can our evaluation of another person as a fully autonomous being not be based on a series of derivative ideas of our own minds?" Why, you might ask, would anyone trouble themselves about such matters?

Philosophers are a troubled sort because they are inclined to suspend rational belief in certain ideas and assumptions that seem matters of common sense to most people. It's self-evident, we might argue, that other people exist as self-conscious subjects, not unlike ourselves. So of course they have inherent dignity and rights of self-determination. Why would anyone feel a need to prove this? Historically, as our own U.S. Constitution shows, there was a time that required asserting the notion of "inalienable rights" as universal even if that assertion was based on the shaky premise that a divine creator had bestowed those rights. Could one find a basis for establishing the presence of other minds and the intrinsic dignity of other people as possessing a reality that was "precognitive" or simply given to consciousness as already constituted and not just a figment of a subject's projected awareness? Levinas and Husserl thought they could do this by interrogating consciousness methodically until the shell of subjectivity was pierced by the unmediated presence of the other.

Roy had enjoyed a long and successful career as a financial advisor. He was only stepping back now in his mid-seventies. "My clients are my best friends," he announced, giving expression to his reluctant departure from the business that he sold to his associates. A few health scares and realization that it was getting more difficult to maintain his usual level of performance convinced Roy that he could no longer play the game the way he preferred. He had seen too many other CEO types hanging on despite the warning signs and didn't want to make the same mistake.

Roy's transition plan involved a new project that would take him and his wife on a lengthy driving tour of the United States. He planned to attend several academic conferences and to interview numerous academic experts in the field of aging about how older people tended to, or more typically, neglected to, plan financially for retirement. This was going to be his next field of expertise, and he had already written and published a couple of articles in professional journals on this topic.

Roy and Ramona are among the many couples for whom the pressures and scheduling limitations of careers have functioned to keep the lid on underlying marital problems. With retirement, the diminishing of external pressures and the availability of more time to be together, some couples experience a flare-up of long suppressed conflicts and differences. These flare-ups can, however, serve as an opportunity for strengthening a marriage.

It was in an exercise devised for NCCCR's Paths to Creative Retirement workshop called "Mansions of the Soul" that Roy caught a glimpse of something that surprised him. The exercise invites participants to estimate the percentage of their time they currently allocate to activities ranging from work to household maintenance to leisure activities by writing the figures within the spaces of a house floor plan. Once they have made these calculations, they do the same for the allocation of time in the projected next stage of their lives. For individuals who attend the workshop as couples, each partner shares his or her time-allocated floor plan. Some couples find their future time investments mutually harmonious, while others discover discontinuities. "She wants to travel all over the world," said one husband, "while I've been traveling for years in my work. I just want to stay home and putter around the house." Other differences can be even more major.

Hearing Roy's wife, Ramona, talk about her book clubs, her grandchildren through a previous marriage, her circle of friends, and her volunteer activities caught Roy's attention. "She has this perfect life at home where she's very happy and I'm going to be taking her away from it," he said, as if dumbfounded by the obvious. Ramona, chiming in, explained that she felt supportive of Roy's plan but had negotiated some reprieves so she could travel home by plane for several important family events. "Roy isn't big on family," said Ramona. In fact, Roy wasn't "big on" anything other than Roy's enjoyment, goals, and self-fulfillment. He was, from all evidence, a loving husband. But Ramona was more a character in Roy's self-narrative than a cocreator of that story. She was derived from his subjectivity, and although endowed with "certain inalienable rights," those rights were bestowed by her narrator, Roy.

As Roy spoke about his goals and his realization that Ramona was a separate person with her own claims on life and on him, it was as if he had just concluded, "Ramona exists!" She didn't exist because Roy speculated, "I think, therefore I exist. I think 'Ramona,' therefore Ramona exists." Now it was, "Ramona is a real person who supersedes my existence. She possesses a reality that my reality can never encompass." It is this apperception of the precognitive, nonderivative other person that Levinas dubs "alterity" (Levinas, 1969). Now what is Roy going to do with this epiphany?

New Retirements, Old Selves

The first character that Albom's Eddie meets in heaven is a carnival worker who died when Eddie was a child. Eddie discovers that the man's heart attack occurred when he swerved his car to avoid hitting the 8-year-old Eddie, who was chasing after a ball that had rolled into the street. Known because of his stained skin as the Blue Man, this character expounds on a hidden truth that reveals the subsequent purpose of the five encounters: "each of us was in your life for a reason." Heaven, according to this messenger, is the opportunity to learn from others what your life has been all about, and this, in turn, leads "to the peace you have been searching for."

Once again, Albom knows how to seduce his reader by evoking an idealized resolution of human striving. The very notion that each life is shaped by a destiny peopled with characters whose lives are woven into our every action may strike many as a species of magical thinking, while others may find this an edifying truth. The premise raises questions about the meaning of individual freedom and personal responsibility if everything has been foreordained. Many people have struggled with the impulse to read design into what earlier may have seemed accidental and incidental events. It's hard for us to accept chance.

With regard to the five people in Albom's novel, it is a sorry state of affairs to imagine that only after your life was over could you discover that your existence had some greater meaning and your actions some nobler purpose than you felt while "on earth." But Albom isn't writing for the dead, and he knows, or hopes, that his reader is thinking about his or her actions and relationships in the here and now while there is still time to have those crucial conversations, make amends, and make one's life whole.

The five tenets of Mitch Albom's moral tale are as follows: nothing that happens to us is random, life requires sacrifices, forgiveness releases us from anger, true love persists beyond the grave, and penance helps bring redemption. The five people you meet in retirement teach us the following: destiny and initiative are paradoxically related, we cannot undo the past but can better ourselves through redemptive actions, integrity is an ongoing struggle, we should never lose our ability to entertain the absurd, and a lifetime of narcissism can be shattered in a moment.

Our cast of five—Betsy, Dave, Ned, Bess, and Roy—reflects one of the central issues that emerge in decision making about retirement: control, or, to use a more fashionable philosophical term, "personal agency." The mere fact that one has a number of choices suggests that how you will lead the next part of your life is, to some degree, up to you. Betsy found ways to manage institutional succession and personal change so that the choices and uncertainties became less an impasse than a threshold to the future. To invert sadness, remorse, and disappointment into enthusiasm, atonement, and rejuvenation, Dave chose the path previously, as Frost put it, "less traveled by." Ned, something of a mythical trickster, chose a life of irony and absurdity as the expression of his freedom. Bess, seeking to find balance through her struggles with symptoms of depression, persists on the edge between the familiar and the unknown, the well-trod path and the seemingly pathless terrain that awaits her. And Roy, in allowing the other to burst the shell of his willful self, strives paradoxically both to insist on his personal projects and to give himself up to his significant other.

Each of the five narratives contains an ambiguity between willful acts of doing and of letting be. An important part of later-life wisdom is to know when to assert oneself proactively and when to exercise the refined tolerance for ambiguity and uncertainty that Keats called "negative capability."

It would be nice to think of the five stories and related philosophies described in this chapter as universal messages for anyone standing on the threshold of retirement.

You simply put the puzzle of the five lives into a single pattern and, voila, light springs forth and an illumined pathway opens. Unfortunately, our five characters are too idiosyncratic, too culture bound, and too incomplete as mere sketches of richer, more complex lives to open the portal to the realm of retirement. Their value is not to make philosophical passage through the third age easier, but to enhance that pathway by making it more thought provoking.

Like the metaphorical limbo of Albom's heaven, retirement is a kind of intermediate stage between earthly concerns and our death. Even if, like Eddie, people cannot afford to quit work or simply prefer remaining employed, the very possibility of retirement hovers over us as a persistent reminder that life is finite and that we are unwittingly racing toward its terminus. This heightened awareness of a narrowing window of time and opportunity can lead to greater deliberateness, to a desperate clinging to the familiar, to Dylan Thomas's "rage against the dying light," or to a welcomed sense of liberation. The loss of an employment-based identity may produce intimations of nonexistence that, in turn, may erode the bulwark of accomplishments we have built up over the years or trigger a shift in perspective that helps us acquire greater clarity about our lives as, with newly gained humility, we reassess our values and priorities.

For many people, the prospect of retirement resembles entering a second adolescence of dizzying possibilities and choices. Retirement, for some, might be a welcomed second chance, a kind of Heaven.

REFERENCES

Albom, M. 2003. *The Five People You Meet in Heaven*. New York: Hyperion.

Aristotle. 1962. *Nicomachean Ethics*. New York: The Library of Liberal Arts.

Baltes, P. B., and M. M. Baltes. 1990. Psychological perspectives on successful aging: The model of selective optimization with compensation. In *Successful Aging: Perspectives from the behavioral sciences*, ed. P. B. Baltes and M. M. Baltes. New York: Cambridge University Press.

Birren, J. E., and L. M. Fisher. 1990. The elements of wisdom: Overview and integration. In *Wisdom, Its Nature, Origins, and Development*, ed. R. J. Sternberg. Cambridge: Cambridge University Press.

Cole, T. R., R. Kastenbaum, and R. E. Ray, eds. 2000. *Handbook of the Humanities and Aging*. 2nd ed. New York: Springer.

Cole, T. R., D. Van Tassel, and R. Kastenbaum, eds. 1992. *Handbook of the Humanities and Aging*. New York: Springer.

de Beauvoir, S. 1962. *The Prime of Life*. Trans. P. Green. Cleveland: World Publishing Co.

Hall, G. S. 1904. *Adolescence: Its psychology and its relations to physiology, anthropology, sociology, sex, crime, religion, and education*. 2 vols. New York: Appleton.

Kaufman, S. 1995. The Ageless Self: Sources of meaning in later life. Madison: University of Wisconsin Press.

Kierkegaard, S. 1968. *Concluding Unscientific Postscript.* Trans. D. Swenson and W. Lowrie. Princeton: Princeton University Press.

Laslett, P. 1991. *A Fresh Map of Life: The emergence of the third age.* Cambridge: Harvard University Press.

Levinas, E. 1969. *Totality and Infinity: An essay on exteriority.* Pittsburgh: Duquesne University Press.

Manheimer, R. 1977. *Kierkegaard as Educator.* Berkeley: University of California Press.

———. 1989. The narrative quest in qualitative gerontology. *Journal of Aging Studies* 3 (3):231–52.

———. 1999. *A Map to the End of Time: Wayfarings with friends and philosophers.* New York: Norton.

———. 2000. Aging in the mirror of philosophy. In *Handbook of the Humanities and Aging,* ed. T. R. Cole, R. Kastenbaum, and R. E. Ray. New York: Springer.

Newcott, B. 2007. Life after death. *AARP The Magazine,* September/October.

Peterson, C., and M. E. P. Seligman. 2004. *Character Strengths and Virtues: A handbook and classification.* New York: Oxford University Press.

Riso, D. R., and R. Hudson. 1999. *The Wisdom of Enneagram.* New York: Bantam.

Rosenzweig, F. 2005. *The Star of Redemption.* Trans. B. E. Galli. Madison: University of Wisconsin Press.

Schopenhauer, A. 1890. The ages of life. In *Counsels and Maxims.* London: Swan Sonnenschein.

Seligman, M. E. P. 2004. *Authentic Happiness: Using the new positive psychology to realize your potential for lasting fulfillment.* New York: Free Press.

Tornstam, L. 1997. Gerotranscendence in a broad cross-cultural perspective. *Journal of Aging and Identity* 2:17–36.

CHAPTER TEN

The Age of Reflexive Longevity

How the Clinic and Changing Expectations of the Life Course Are Reshaping Old Age

SHARON R. KAUFMAN, PH.D.

Biomedicine, throughout the twentieth century and into our own, has thus not simply changed our relation to health and illness but has modified the things we think we might hope for and the objectives we aspire to. That is to say, it has helped make us the kinds of people we have become . . . And, I suggest, we are increasingly coming to relate to ourselves as "somatic" individuals . . . as beings whose individuality is, in part at least, grounded within our fleshly, corporeal existence, and who experience, articulate, judge, and act upon ourselves in part in the language of biomedicine.

—*Rose, 2007, pp. 25–26*

How do we know and "live" old age today? In the last few decades, many older adults in the United States (and their families) have come to understand their bodies, lives, possibilities, and futures—including what constitutes the "normal" life span—in terms of their options for medical interventions that may extend life and contribute to its quality. From the medical management of cholesterol, blood pressure, and heart disease to surgeries of all kinds; from the multitude of palliative or aggressive cancer interventions to drugs for depression, memory enhancement, and sexual dysfunction; from heroic life-extending procedures in hospital intensive care units to hospice care at home, older adults and their families have more options than ever before among standard, alternative, and experimental treatments that potentially postpone, alter, or ameliorate both the frailties that accompany late life and end-stage conditions. Those options create new ways of thinking about meaning, identity, and value in later life, and they give rise to new burdens and responsibilities for older people themselves, their families, and health care professionals. Life-extending medical treatments for those in late life open up both a world of hope (for renewal, rejuvenation, and health maintenance) and a socioethical problem space in which consideration of the worth of late life and our relationship to loved ones is, more and more, organized around the somatic, and in particular ways.

At least two developments illustrate this trend. First, clinical medicine has come to rely more and more on numbers, pictures, and results generated by a plethora of diagnostic tests and procedures that enable ever-more finely tuned interpretations of disease states and bodily conditions. Doctors, patients, their families, and the public learn to understand what constitutes standard medical care, health, and illness and learn to weigh the risks and benefits of future treatment options in terms of those results and scores. More broadly, we come to think about the "truths" of the body—and of life itself—through those numbers, scores, and scans. Blood pressure and cholesterol measurement, prostate specific antigen test numbers, kidney creatinine levels, cardiac ejection fractions, mammogram and CT findings, stages of cancer, white blood counts, and liver function scores, for example, are all *representations*—of the extent of disease and degree of health—that have come to matter to us. We organize behaviors, engage treatments, undertake the care of others, and consider the future in terms of those representations. The ubiquity of diagnostic tests and their numerical and pictorial results contributes to ways of knowing and pondering the somatic that did not exist even a decade ago.

Second, many conditions—cancers, heart failure, kidney disease, and liver disease, for example—can be managed as chronic illnesses for long periods of time, even decades, and well into very late life. Treatment regimens for those in late life, such as dialysis, chemotherapy, radiation, and surgery, can be daunting. When the effects of treatments that prolong life come up against a subjective sense of diminishing quality of life and increasing bodily suffering, the questions of how long to continue living with the illness(es) *and* with the treatments, and at what costs, arise for older adults and those who care for them. Bodily symptoms understood through medical knowledge about disease states become part of the older person's (and family's) calculus for the now ever-present choice between pursuing life-prolonging treatments and "letting go."

This chapter begins to explore the brave new world into which late-life medical treatments have led us. Individuals in "advanced liberal democracies" (Rose, 2007, p. 26) think of themselves as authors of their own life stories, active participants in the shaping of the life course through decision making of all kinds. This approach to life is accompanied by the knowledge that biology is no longer destiny; we know that we can maximize health through our own behaviors and that medicine has the tools to intervene to stop the course of serious disease. Illness prevention, health promotion, and risk reduction are ubiquitous features of middle-class life. Body- and health-oriented activities are accompanied by an additional phenomenon, an expectation and willingness to allow intervention into our own bodies—*to experiment on ourselves*

—that is exquisitely heightened today at every age. Developments in the clinic reveal how we are making ourselves into risk managers, experimental objects, and, overall, beings who must consider deeply how much value the body has in relation to the meaning of life. Thus, many today want to think of themselves not only as authors of their own life stories but also as authors of their own life trajectories. The latter authorship is enabled by standard medical practice, choice about life-prolonging treatments, and choice about the timing of death.

Drawing on my anthropological research of old age and the clinic, this chapter describes the ways in which three kinds of medical intervention are shaping an imaginative and technological enterprise in which (1) the limits to the body and the limits to life are always being pushed and (2) the boundary between prevention and life extension becomes ever more murky in an aging society. This chapter ponders our emerging ways of considering and acting on late life when the traditional truth of the predictable arc of human life (Cole, 1992) is replaced with a vision of the life course in which the body and self can be remade through clinical technique and death can be deliberately pushed out into the future.

The Treatment of Aging: The Ethical and Sociomedical Context of Life Extension

The extension of progressively older lives through medical means is occurring in a complex sociocultural context. Surgery, drugs, and devices have changed the life expectancy for many older people in American society. Centenarians are no longer uncommon. The rapid growth of the over-85 age group and better health in very late life for many people are redefining "old." For example, "60 is the new 40" and "80 is the new 60" join other popular remarks that signify a changed understanding of life-course expectations for those who can access all that medicine has to offer. An explosion in the varieties of preventive and life-saving interventions for elderly people is changing our expectations for late life and changing the practices of many medical specialties in the United States (Solomon et al., 2000).

Yet amid the unequivocally positive medical advances of recent years lies significant cultural confusion about "natural" aging and "natural" old age. Our understandings of what is *natural* about human life, including the ways we respond to illness, grow older, and die, are forever being remade, and medical treatment into ever-older age is one striking example of how medical science and practice in American society manufacture *the natural* today. Nature, "a human idea with a long and complicated cultural history" (Cronon, 1996), has always been entangled with cultural values about fate and human agency, the uses of the body in life and death, and the essential, innate quality of things, including the human being. *Nature* has been considered to be both part of us and separate from us, and our descriptions and understanding of it are linked to concepts of God, fate and human agency, culture, society, science, and the body (Merchant, 1990; Coates, 1998; McCullough et al., 2008).

Nature is perhaps most starkly revealed as a cultural construct at sites where routine medical practice and technology converge. Technologically assisted human reproduction, transplant and implant recipients, people maintained by life-extending chronic care therapies, and brain-dead bodies that are warm and breathing all exemplify how malleable *nature* and the natural body can be in the hands of clinical practice. These hybrid forms embody the most current incarnation of the indeterminacy of both *culture* and *nature*; they subvert and redefine older understandings of *natural* to include emerging inventions of culture, especially biomedical technologies and the socioeconomic structures that support their development and use.

Our notions of a "natural" old age are formed and supported by biomedicine's successes. We live in an era in which routine life prolongation through medical technique is coupled with many widely desired life-enhancement and modification interventions (e.g., designer drugs, hormone replacement therapy, hip and knee replacement, cataract surgery, cosmetic surgery). Any vision of "natural" aging becomes increasingly difficult to sustain in a society with insatiable demands for medical intervention—in more areas of life, in more of the body's vital processes, and in ever-older age—to achieve greater health, longevity, and "optimal well-being."

The confusion about "natural aging" is expressed in a century-old debate about the relationship of aging to disease. Whether aging is disease, whether "normal" aging is "pathological," and whether aging per se leads inevitably to death are all issues that have been and continue to be questioned in the medical literature and public life. Historians and others have noted that conceptions of "normal" and "natural" in relation to aging are, like all scientific knowledge, not objective or given, but rather are constituted in particular social and political contexts and are elaborated over time as scientific ideologies change (Canguilhem, 1991; Holstein, 1997; McCullough et al., 2008). The terms of the debate have shifted with the growing sophistication of biological knowledge and with changes in the politics of medical science and the delivery of health care, but the debate itself is ongoing. That debate, which manifests itself in the clinic, exists also as an ongoing undercurrent in medicine and biology. For example, biogerontologist Leonard Hayflick noted a failure among scientists, clinicians, and the broader public to distinguish between research on the fundamental mechanisms of aging and research on age-associated diseases (Hayflick, 2000).

The debate about the relationship between "natural," "normal" aging and disease opens new ways of thinking about the older body/self because it is now tied to life-extending treatments and to the explosion in biotechnological promise. The lack of clarity about what constitutes normal aging and natural decline and what distinguishes those processes from disease (which often can be treated to stave off decline) both fuels cultural desire for medical interventions into very late life and changes clinical understandings about which treatments are "standard" and appropriate at ever-older ages.

Finally, confusion about natural aging also has been expressed in the last several decades, mostly in the United States, in debates about whether decline and death can and should be avoided, that is, postponed for as long as possible with clinical technique. Beginning in the 1980s, philosophers, social scientists, and some clinicians noted that aging and death had come to be regarded as scientific "problems," amenable to technical solutions (Callahan, 1987; Estes and Binney, 1989). Callahan, particularly, reflected on how American society, including the profession of medicine, has lost a sense of the "natural," finite life span (1987, 1993). He and others observed that death has come to be considered an option (Muller and Koenig, 1988).

Most recently, developments in the biosciences have encouraged the view that aging is a treatable disease. Rapidly expanding knowledge of the human genome, together with advances in tissue engineering, the bioengineering of drugs, and the ability to manipulate cellular aging genetically, creates societal expectations about applications of genetic technologies to cure the diseases of later life, stave off death, and alter the "natural" process of aging (Wade, 2001; Hall, 2003). These goals have become intertwined and largely inseparable.

Research emerging from the biotechnology revolution, especially research on the cloning of tissues and organs and the arrest of cellular aging through the manipulation of telomerase, deepens rather than ends the debates because it equates normal aging with disease and allows both clinicians and the public to consider new possibilities for a standard-of-care medicine in which "normal" aging is treatable. Genetic knowledge; ever-more sophisticated transplant techniques; smaller, safer, and more effective implantable cardiac devices; and specifically targeted drugs for cancers and other diseases are some of the recent innovations that drive hope for individual longevity, make the promises of the biotechnology revolution appear to be real, and, importantly, create expectations about existing treatments for the extension of late life.

There is a growing literature on the justification and benefits of performing many kinds of procedures on people older than age 80 (Kaufman, Russ, and Shim, 2006). Together with the promise of more technologies, the present availability of interventions for elderly people and the normalization of life-extending, life-enhancing treatments at ever-older ages promote the notion that aging and death are not inevitable and that one can "grow older without aging" (Katz and Marshall, 2003). These promises and options also foster the assumption that one can, and should, choose to intervene. (The "good" of intervention in late life is not as pervasive in Europe, where limitations to health care resources are widely acknowledged. See, for example, Dey and Fraser, 2000.) There are no longer steadfast clinical assumptions, in the United States, about technological or biological limits to what one can do for older people. Furthermore, intervention leads to more intervention because "natural" age limitations for procedures are no longer thought to be inevitable by health professionals. Many patients, for their part, have become proactive health care consumers responsible for questing after their own health, longevity, and even "good" death. And all of us become patients, or potential patients, as we age.

A deep concern among some philosophers, physicians, social theorists, and observers of biomedicine about manipulating mortality and "the natural" at all ages—as though "the natural" were a stable, unchanging object and category of knowledge—stimulated the thoughtful report issued by the President's Council on Bioethics in 2003 titled "Beyond Therapy: Biotechnology and the Pursuit of Happiness." The authors of that report noted the strong societal preoccupation with longevity, optimal health in advanced age, the expectation that "old age" can be treated, and the taken-for-granted malleability of the body and self at all ages, including into late life. That report also noted that the boundaries between medicine's focus on cure and its concern with life enhancement are becoming increasingly blurred. As the practices of the biomedical sciences continue to move beyond the confines of disease entities and whole individuals to investigate life itself rather than disease, they are ushering in a new genre of medicine, now known as regenerative medicine, which is part cure, part prevention, and part experimental science. The altered gaze that accompanies this new kind of medicine permits the old body to be viewed as simultaneously a diseased entity, a site for restoration, and a space for improvement.

This new way of thinking about the old body has direct implications for clinical intervention and thus for the experience of growing older and being old, which are only beginning to be explored. Nuland called the social phenomenon that accompanies the new scientific developments (especially those using stem cell and cloning technologies for potential therapeutic cloning) a "rush to promise" and "an uncritical embrace of medical advancement" in which public expectations outpace medical application of laboratory discovery (Nuland, 1998). Callahan (1993), Habermas (2003), Kass (2004), Sandel (2004), and others ponder the fate of "dignity," intergenerational relations, and the traditional meanings of the life cycle and life-course development in the face of the array of technologies for enhancing life, postponing senescence, and staving off death that are now normalized and standard. From selecting the sex of babies to manipulating the growth of children, from altering mood and behavior with drugs at every age to creating superior athletes and clearer thinkers, and finally, from prolonging life at ever-older ages to authorizing the timing of our own deaths, the techniques of contemporary medicine have enabled us to consider all these interventions—at all ages and life stages—as *normal,* as standard medical practice.

Thus, we are led to think that we can influence the kind of aging, and end of life, that we have come to hope for and idealize. The quest for health in late life "has become central to the telos of living" (Rose, 2007, p. 28) for so many.

There are enormous pressures from multiple societal sources—older people themselves, their families, the "technological imperative" in medicine, the structure of health care financing, the excitement surrounding new interventions, and specialist and subspecialist training and practice—to prolong the lives of the very old who face serious or critical illness. Those pressures often collide with coexisting, conflicting values that stress a minimum of medical intervention at advanced ages and at the end of life, an honoring of patient autonomy to forego death-prolonging measures, and an awareness of the suffering, pain, and reduced functional ability and quality of life that some life-prolonging procedures impose. The coexistence of these competing cultural trends and values becomes evident in older individuals' (and family) dilemmas and angst about whether to proceed with potentially life-extending therapies (such as renal dialysis, cardiac interventions, organ transplant, feeding tubes); in the widely shared, wrenching stories about starting, ending, or attempting to stop heroic, death-defying procedures for a loved one in intensive care units (Kaufman, 2005); and in ongoing medical, bioethical, and cultural debate—about enhancement for the healthy versus medical treatment for the sick, about self-fulfillment versus social justice, and about the possible ways in which identity, consumerism, and technology could be disentangled. There is no doubt that choices for intervention in late life have socio-ethical ramifications.

The Freedom of Options

Enacting one's own freedom—through one's obligation and commitment to health and long life—is a complex and demanding enterprise. That commitment takes at least three forms today. First, health promotion has become a meaningful social practice (Crawford, 2006) connecting identity and ethical comportment. As individuals, we must *decide* on prevention and health maintenance strategies for ourselves and our family members. Failure to care for the self is, without question, understood as a moral transgression (Crawford, 2004). Because we regard the body as open to manipulation at every age, because we desire to intervene and can, and because health care consumption, throughout life, is valued for its ability to maximize the authentic self (Elliott, 2003) and maximize *life* itself, developments in the realm of geriatric intervention influence our understandings of late-life somatic ideals, as well as our responsibilities toward the old body/self, in ways that could not have been predicted even 15 years ago. "Selfhood has become intrinsically somatic—ethical practices increasingly take the body as a key site for work on the self" (Rose, 2007, p. 18).

Second, our self-regulating prevention and promotion strategies are based on risk awareness and emergent biomedical knowledge that organize our actions and anxieties vis-à-vis risk. Beck (1992, 2006), Giddens (1990, 1991), and others have described the ways in which *risk* as a way of knowing and risk assessment as a technique for living constitute the structural conditions of life in postindustrial society. There is no doubt that risk awareness drives much health care delivery today, and both health and health care are largely understood as risk reduction through individual risk assessment (Dumit, 2005; Rose, 2007). We manage risk proactively *as individuals*. For example, screening (for high cholesterol, diabetes, heart disease, cancer of the breast, prostate, colon, etc.) is important because it enables us to calculate our individual risk numerically, and risk scores become the grounds for treatment (Armstrong, 1995). Indeed, Woodward (1999), in her essay titled "Statistical Panic," provides a cogent analysis of the ways in which our "society of statistics" provokes panic by engaging the experience of always being at risk, mostly through knowing the numerical scores of our corporeal conditions. Clinicians in some fields work to treat risk itself (Shim, Russ, and Kaufman, 2006; Grady, 2007), and some individuals with family histories of cancer or genetic disease desire presymptomatic, subclinical identification of risks in order to preempt the manifestation of disease (Rose, 2007). Health risks are conceptualized as individuals' problems whose solutions reside, therefore, in individual strategies for behavior change or clinical intervention.

Third, we are responsible consumers. We demand to know what is in our medicines. A plethora of health and wellness newsletters and Web sites give advice about drugs and drug interactions and the pros and cons of treatments and behaviors. Above all, individuals have become responsible for knowing, and then for deciding. Yet more information and increased surveillance of the body lead to enhanced risk acuity in a seemingly endless feedback loop, in the demand for more intervention. Practices of risk avoidance and reduction organize, in great part, the quest for health promotion, life extension, and enhanced "quality of life." Yet that quest depends on an ethical balancing act between competing desires—how to live longer yet not past the moment when suffering exceeds "meaning."

In sum, not only are the practices of biomedical science and of clinical medicine shaping the way we understand the self, the old body, aging, and our interpersonal commitments (Estes and Binney, 1989), but also the multiple (and even contradictory) ways we understand aging and old age are changing clinical practices and the sense of responsibility toward the self and others that underlies those practices (Kaufman, Shim, and Russ, 2004). One result of this reciprocal sociomedical process is that societal expectations about longevity and medical care come together in a *shifting ethics of normalcy*, in which life extension often receives priority, sometimes regardless of the state of "life," and in which caregiving and love are explicitly tied both to the bodily conditions of older adults and to clinical acts that either extend life in advanced age or allow "letting go." The ramifications of this shift—for expressions of the meaning and value of late life and for interpersonal relationships—have hardly been explored.

Reflexive Longevity: Three Clinical Interventions

In my ongoing anthropological investigation of the expanding use of life-extending medical interventions for older individuals, I am concerned with the reciprocal effects of clinical practices and meanings of old age *on how we quest for and practice longevity.* While there is no doubt that for many older adults organ transplantation, cardiac procedures, and cancer treatments, for example, "add both years to life and life to years," treatment effects are not always perceived as entirely life-affirming by older adults, their family members, or their health professionals. Some treatments are fraught with dilemmas about suffering, quality of life, and the "worth" of added weeks, months, or years. In addition, older people and their families remain linked to the tools of the clinic (Russ, Shim, and Kaufman, 2005; Shim, Russ, and Kaufman, 2007) regardless of the physical, emotional, and social burdens, or side effects, of late-life medical intervention. Debate about "the good" of these interventions into ever-later life will continue. My interest in them is to explore who we are becoming in the context of medical technique, that is, the ways in which we engage the question of how to live in, and into, advanced age.

What follows is a rapid tour of three examples of the uses of medicine in an aging society.[1] All are emblematic of the rising age for interventions of all kinds. They point to the ways in which medicine is shaping life in old age, including some of our anxieties, and they illustrate how the goal of open-ended longevity influences medical care and the desires of health professionals, families, and older adults for more intervention. Each of the three interventions described below gives rise to what we might call a specific form of "*quality of life.*" That is, cardiac procedures may heighten perceptions of living with individual risk. Living donor kidney transplant enables a way of thinking that connects mortality and longevity with interpersonal obligation. Chronic renal dialysis exemplifies a condition that some describe as between life and death. Perhaps these "*qualities of life*" are coming to inform late-life identity (for those who can access medicine's tools) in ways that are unprecedented.

Treating Risk: Cardiac Procedures

With increasing frequency, the oldest members of U.S. society are undergoing cardiac interventions aimed at prolonging life. Coronary artery bypass surgery is now commonplace for people in their eighties and is not unusual for people in their nineties. There has been tremendous growth in the use of stents to open clogged arteries in the past decade as well. Physicians implant automatic cardiac defibrillators (to stop and correct a potentially lethal hearth rhythm) into approximately 40,000 patients annually, many of them in their eighties and nineties.

Overall, the growing normalization of cardiac treatments to the very old is made possible by the decreasing risks of the procedures themselves. As devices such as stents and defibrillators become smaller, as techniques for implanting them become safer, and as less invasive procedures are being used with greater frequency and success, physicians and the public have learned to view them as standard interventions that are justified and that one does not, easily, refuse. Reduced risks associated with these cardiac procedures produce a sense that life extension is open-ended *as long as one treats risk* (Shim, Russ, and Kaufman, 2006).

Physicians interviewed in my study of the uses and effects of life-extending technologies discussed the fact that noninvasive treatments almost always pave the way for additional, often more aggressive, procedures and that aggressive procedures pave the way for less aggressive ones. They described both types of intervention as a "technology parade," in which cardiologists, then cardiac surgeons, and finally electrophysiologists (who implant automatic defibrillators) each provide a life-extending procedure that is, in part, facilitated by the one that came before and that is designed both to manage existing disease and to ameliorate future risk. As growing numbers of elders receive more kinds of interventions, the "extravaganza of cardiology," as one doctor put it, becomes an increasingly accepted and "natural" part of old age. For practitioners and patients alike, that trend influences the absence of deliberation about whether to treat. Instead, treatments become standard practice among elderly adults, and standard practice trumps individual choice (Shim, Russ, and Kaufman, 2006). For example, an 83-year-old man, who recalled being told he needed bypass surgery, remarked:

> When I went to see the cardiologist after the stress text, and he said, "You've got a problem. And it's gonna have to be fixed. It's not a choice of whether you want to go through it or not. If you want to live, it's just going to get worse and you'll have a heart attack, and that'll be it." And to me it was not that hard a decision to make. Because when you're faced with that kind of choice, your decision, I think, is made for you.

While debates in clinical medicine are emerging about whether the use of the automatic implantable cardiac defibrillator in very old individuals is appropriate therapy (de Lissovoy, 2007), physicians agree that use of this device is on the rise, and it is considered more and more "standard" among physicians and patients in their eighties and beyond. Recently expanded medical criteria developed during clinical trials allow thousands of older Medicare recipients to qualify for the implantable cardiac defibrillator, a device that, in regulating a chaotic heart rhythm, prevents sudden death from a heart attack, the kind of death many (perhaps most) of us actually want in late life. Although some physicians ponder the ethics and practical appropriateness of implanting this device in patients in their nineties, several cardiologists echoed the statement of one who reported,

> I don't even blink when I have a patient that comes up that's 80-something, because the 75–78 year old is sort of the standard. I'd say the number I think twice about is 90 or above. But we have many patients over the age of 90 now.

Clinicians who implant these devices speak about "actually treating for risk, not just looking for risk." Some frame accountability to themselves and their patients in terms of proactively treating risk. For example, one cardiologist spoke for others when he said,

> Now we've come all the way to the point where we realize, scientifically, that you can put an ICD in someone who's never had an event at all, without doing any other testing, but just bring them in from the office and put it in. Because at some point, they may face this arrhythmia risk, and, scientifically, they'll be better if they have this than someone who doesn't have it. We've all grown to accept that. So I think I've changed in terms of my thinking about what's treatable or when it should be treated.

The logic and growing ease of risk reduction support the imperative to intervene later and later in life with this device and other procedures, as well as a reconceptualization of ever-older age as a stage of life when risks can and should be managed and averted (Shim, Russ, and Kaufman, 2006).

Implantable cardiac devices are big business—one of the fastest-growing and highest-profit-margin medical devices. Companies that manufacture these devices are looking at defibrillators as a new area of growth, and already sales are growing 20 percent annually (Meier and Sorkin, 2005). Even more sophisticated heart-regulating devices are available and coming onto the market. Together these devices form part of the landscape, the moral socioscape, in which aggressive medical options are increasingly made available to very old people. Older adults and their families, then, are forced to ponder an individual ethic of life extension and to imagine both the goal of the device (Does it extend "natural" life?) and the kind of care that would accompany the longer life it potentially enables (By averting sudden death does it allow other diseases to emerge later on?).

In the cardiac fields overall, physicians, as specialists and technicians, provide a preventive or risk-averting safety net to patients via the techniques available. The notion of risk powerfully dictates clinical responsibility; thus, deciding to treat risk is a doctor's responsibility. Because mortality and morbidity are often low risks with these procedures, even in advanced age, physicians and patients both have come to see them as "natural choices" when faced with symptoms that may be, or are, life threatening (Shim, Russ, and Kaufman, 2006).

Bodily Obligation toward Self and Other: Kidney Transplant

There is growing demand for transplantation among older people with kidney disease. The number of kidneys transplanted to people over age 65, from both living and cadaver donors, has increased steadily in the past two decades in the United States. For example, in 2003 more than 11 percent of total kidney transplants went to individuals age 65 or older; in 2006 almost 14 percent went to that age group (Organ Procurement and Transplantation Network, 2007). Transplants are no longer unusual in the seventh decade of life and are sometimes performed into the early eighties. There is a substantial amount of adult child–to–older parent living kidney donation and a substantial amount of older living spouse kidney donation as well (Kaufman, Russ, and Shim, 2006). Older members of many ethnic groups and all socioeconomic statuses are transplant recipients—this is not a procedure only for the affluent.

While there is an enormous range of patient and family response regarding the desire for a kidney transplant if one has end-stage kidney disease, most patients in their seventies would rather have a transplant than remain on dialysis, even if it means remaining on a years-long waiting list for a cadaveric organ. There is also a wide range of patient and family responses regarding the pursuit of a living kidney donor. Some older adults (and their family members) are extremely active in soliciting prospective living donors or are willing to accept potential donor volunteers:

> When I learned that I wouldn't have to wait around on dialysis if I had a live donor, my wife lined up 14 people who would donate. You have to be proactive. You can't just sit around, or you'll die waiting.

Others refuse family, friend, or coworker offers for a living donor and wait for four to five years for a cadaveric kidney:

> The only thing they asked me in the clinic was, did I have anyone in the family who was willing to donate a kidney for the transplant? My nephew was willing to donate, and I said, no way, I wouldn't do it. If his other kidney failed, he would have been in trouble. It's not worth saving my own life to take on that moral burden. I waited for a cadaver kidney, and I waited five years.

> Let's face it. I'm not that young. I only have so much to go. I don't want to put someone else in jeopardy. I've got to go sometime.

A new category of older cadaveric kidneys was created in 2001 to ease the organ shortage and make kidneys more readily available to older adults (Ojo, 2005). It is comprised of kidneys from older deceased people (over age 50 or 55) that are not quite "perfect" and may have carried some diseases. In other words, they have "lived" longer and more fully than younger cadaveric kidneys, which are usually procured following lethal trauma, rather than years-long disease. At the time of this writing patients over age 65 have the option of remaining on the United Network for Organ Sharing (UNOS) waiting list four to seven years for a "younger" kidney, waiting fewer years for an "older" kidney, or taking a kidney from a living person—with virtually no waiting time. Older patients and their families quickly learn that their "choice" must take into consideration time and age because the older you are, the more precarious your health may become in a few years, ruling out medical suitability for a transplant, thus the greater the urgency for a transplant sooner rather than later. Time is of the essence, if one is older, regarding the source of the kidney for transplant.

Among living donors, the number of adult children donating kidneys to their parents is increasing. Younger adults are donating to their relatively young parents, middle-aged children are donating to their parents over age 70, and grandchildren are donating to their grandparents. These practices open the sites of bodily debt, the tyranny of the gift (Fox and Swazey, 1992), and the sociomedical commitment to longevity to new dimensions of somatic responsibility and obligation (Kaufman, Russ, and Shim, 2006). For example, the responsibility to pursue greater health and longer life merges into the obligation people have for one another. Living donor kidney recipients narrated variations of the following theme: My family needs and wants me to live because it is possible for me to do so, and I want to live. Therefore, because I need to live, they (or some of them) will offer to donate a kidney for me, and, although it may not seem right, I must accept it.

Everyone who engages the world of transplant medicine makes moves to include and exclude, to name and rank those who will be considered worthy of giving and receiving. For example, from a daughter who donated to her father:

> We all have different roles in the family. My brother is married and has two young children. And I think if the chips had really come down, he might have stepped forward. My sister is married. I'm single. I had nobody else to consider. I didn't have to consult anyone. So that's just the way it was.

A husband who donated to his wife remarked:

> Naturally the kids said, "Take me." That was a given. They automatically offered. But we didn't want the kids. They're young; they have their own lives, and they may need their kidney later on. We both felt that if I was compatible, I would do it. I was

really worried, during the testing, that they would find something, or that I would be too old, and I wouldn't be able to give. And it didn't happen and we were very pleased. And I'm sure the kids were relieved.

Kidney transplantation is one standard medical treatment for end-stage renal disease. Love, obligation, and the ability to save the life of another become compelling reasons to offer and give while one is alive. This is the starkest example of the way in which interpersonal commitment comes to be expressed through a clinical intervention that is, simultaneously, an end-stage disease management strategy; a restorative, regenerative technique; and a therapy to enhance both physical function and quality of life.

Death Brought into Life? Kidney Dialysis

Perhaps nowhere is the relationship between living and quality of life, on the one hand, and dying and the awareness of death, on the other, made more troublesome than in the example of chronic kidney dialysis. The normalization of long-term renal dialysis has its origin in the 1972 law extending Medicare benefits for dialysis to all individuals with end-stage renal disease. Since then, advances in dialysis care mean that physicians are successful at dialyzing patients with complicated diseases, including the very old. One result of this normalization is that health professionals now feel that it is unethical not to offer dialysis to anyone with end-stage disease; thus, the dialysis population is graying. But the goals of treatment have not changed from a half century ago to reflect an aging society, and the idea of "end-stage" is mostly not discussed in treatment (Russ, Shim, and Kaufman, 2005). For example, a social worker described how dialysis culture has changed:

> Everyone has the right to dialyze. Nothing disqualifies patients today. When dialysis first started in the 1960s it was selective medicine. Now there is a drive to keep people alive longer. Period. They are just placed on dialysis and told that this is what we need to do. It is automatically assumed that a patient wants dialysis. "No" is never presented as an option.

In the outpatient clinic, which is the most common pathway through which dialysis is initiated, patients typically resign themselves to the small steps and procedures that lead to dialysis, without actually "choosing" to start the life-saving and life-prolonging therapy. For instance, patients agree to blood tests that track the loss of kidney function. They are fitted with a fistula for dialysis access. Those unremarkable actions anticipate and justify the start of treatment. Proactive patient decision making, when it occurs at all once dialysis starts, often focuses on balancing desired longevity with diminished quality of life due to multiple chronic diseases of later life and the dialysis treatments themselves (Russ, Shim, and Kaufman, 2005).

Unlike other clinical treatments, kidney dialysis is a nonteleological endeavor. Death is avoided by intensive, ongoing treatment, but no cure is available. Thus, patients on chronic dialysis live outside the notion of medical progress. The central paradox for older people on dialysis is that in order to extend time, to have more of it, one has to "give it away" to the hours and days on the dialysis machine. Some older adults interviewed articulated a strong sense of being between life and death, the feeling that death comes to occupy considerable experiential space. Some feel themselves to be in a desperate situation, for example, "Why am I still here?" or, "I'm stranded." Others feel that they have already departed—in the sense that they are already promised to death and their time on dialysis is simply awaiting fulfillment of that promise, for instance, "Dialysis is a shadow life, that takes you away from real life." Yet few talk about proactive discontinuation, although many ask when and under what conditions can they stop treatments. For long-term dialysis patients who are old, life is purchased with "quality of life" because the chronic conditions that accompany the need for dialysis often worsen with time, causing loss of function, existential suffering, or both (Russ, Shim, and Kaufman, 2005).

Taken together, four powerful sociocultural engines drive a great deal of medical treatment to elderly people in the United States and influence our expectations about late life. Clinicians are aware that treatments, for the very old, can be a double-edged endeavor, yet they want and feel obligated to provide life-extending options, sometimes regardless of a patient's extreme frailty. Older people, some of whom are ambivalent about living on and on with deteriorating health and functional abilities, do not usually want to authorize their own death by proactively stopping or rejecting a life-saving therapy. Families do not want the responsibility of saying "No" to life-extending therapies for their loved ones, and, of course, they are hopeful that treatments can extend meaningful life. Finally, our procedure-driven health care finance arrangements guide everyone toward treatments—because they are standard, normalized, and expected. Importantly, it is through the lens of the clinic—the range of medical interventions offered—that more and more of us experience and practice *hope* when we imagine longevity.

Conclusion

Has age disappeared as a meaningful, central characteristic of bioidentity? Life, health, age, illness, and death have become objects to be acted on via the instrumental techniques that clinical medicine and the biological sciences offer (Rabinow, 2000).

One's own biological destiny is no longer fixed, immutable. Prevention and intervention are possible even into advanced age. We are made to embrace the idea that it is our responsibility to choose clinical intervention because biomedical technique has extended choice to every aspect of existence (Rose, 2001, p. 22), including the extension of ever-longer lives and the timing of death.

Yet while autonomous "choice" about therapies remains a powerful ideal in medical and consumer discourse in American society, choice is organized and constrained by at least three features of the health care delivery system. First, health professionals limit the choices patients can make by the treatments they offer. These offerings, in turn, are determined by Medicare reimbursement regulations to hospitals and physicians, the structure of specialist medical practice and clinical practice guidelines, the patient's particular insurance coverage, and the physician's own priorities about what needs to be done. Next, in many cases, standard treatment subverts choice because options are rarely equally weighted. For example, procedures considered low-risk (stents, dialysis) quickly become standard practice, thereby eliminating clinical choice about whether to refuse those procedures. Third, many people, perhaps most, do not know what to want in the way of specific treatments, especially if they are at risk of death. Neither do they always understand distinctions among and risks of different medical options. Furthermore, in many instances we are "eager for medicalization" (Becker and Nachtigall, 1992), eager for medicine to define the parameters of and solutions to our problems (Shim, Russ, and Kaufman, 2007). Thus, it is difficult, at every age, to say "No" to medical technique.

The tension between our desire to make the old body ever-more malleable and to extend life because we can and the desire for a death without technological interference will not disappear. In fact, that tension will become more pronounced, in part because of the open-ended promises of bioscience to increase longevity, and in part because the recent emphasis in academic medical centers on translational research links the promises of the laboratory with clinical practice more directly than ever before, thus highlighting the somatic way of "knowing" old age and focusing attention on the somatic as the crux of meaning. Together, research and intervention shape an imaginative enterprise in which the limits to corporeal malleability are always being pushed; the future of the life course is idealistically mapped; and obligation and indeed love are understood through bodily substance in relation to clinical offerings, the demands we place on the clinic, and the demands the clinic makes on us. We have entered the age of reflexive longevity, and "how to live"—which includes our reliance on and desire for medical intervention—is very much at stake in questions about the nature of old age.

ACKNOWLEDGMENTS

The research on which this chapter is based was funded by the National Institute on Aging under grants AG20962 and AG028426 to Sharon R. Kaufman, principal investigator. I am indebted to the health professionals and patients who made these studies possible.

NOTE

1. The findings on cardiac procedures, transplant, and dialysis described here are drawn from anthropological research conducted by Sharon Kaufman, principal investigator, in collaboration with Ann Russ and Janet Shim. Sharon Kaufman led the investigation, collected most of the data on kidney transplantation, and was responsible for interpretation of all findings. Ann Russ gathered the ethnographic data on kidney dialysis. I draw from work in which she was the first author (Russ, Shim, and Kaufman, 2005). Janet Shim collected the data on cardiac procedures and some of the data on kidney transplants. I draw from work in which she was the first author (Shim, Russ, and Kaufman, 2006, 2007). Findings that emerged about the impacts of those three types of intervention on the self, the family, and the changing face of medical intervention were developed in collaborative discussion and are published elsewhere.

REFERENCES

Armstrong, D. 1995. The rise of surveillance medicine. *Sociology of Health and Illness* 17 (3):393–404.

Beck, U. 1992. *Risk Society: Towards a new modernity.* London: Sage.

———. 2006. Living in the world risk society. In *Hobhouse Memorial Public Lecture.* London: London School of Economics.

Becker, G., and N. D. Nachtigall. 1992. Eager for medicalisation: The social production of infertility as a disease. *Sociology of Health and Illness* 14:456–71.

Callahan, D. 1987. *Setting Limits: Medical goals in an aging society.* New York: Simon and Schuster.

———. 1993. *The Troubled Dream of Life: In search of peaceful death.* New York: Simon and Schuster.

Canguilhem, G. 1991. *The Normal and the Pathological.* New York: Zone Books.

Coates, P. 1998. *Nature: Western attitudes since ancient times.* Berkeley: University of California Press.

Cole, T. R. 1992. *The Journey of Life: A cultural history of aging in America.* Cambridge: Cambridge University Press.

Crawford, R. 2004. Risk ritual and the management of control and anxiety in medical culture. *Health (London)* 8 (4):505–28.

———. 2006. Health as a meaningful social practice. *Health (London)* 10 (4):401–20.

Cronon, W. 1996. In *Uncommon Ground: Rethinking the human place in nature*, ed. W. Cronon. New York: Norton.

de Lissovoy, G. 2007. The implantable cardiac defibrillator: Is the glass half empty or half full? *Medical Care* 45 (5):371–73.

Dey, I., and N. Fraser. 2000. Age-based rationing in the allocation of health care. *Journal of Aging and Health* 12:511–37.

Dumit, J. 2005. The depsychiatrisation of mental illness. *Journal of Public Mental Health* 3:8–13.

Elliot, C. 2003. *Better than Well: American medicine meets the American dream.* New York: W. W. Norton.

Estes, C. L., and E. A. Binney. 1989. The biomedicalization of aging: Dangers and dilemmas. *Gerontologist* 29 (5):587–96.

Fox, R. C., and J. P. Swazey. 1992. *Spare Parts: Organ replacement in American society.* New York: Oxford University Press.

Giddens, A. 1990. *The Consequences of Modernity.* Stanford: Stanford University Press.

———. 1991. *Modernity and Self-Identity: Self and society in the late modern age.* Stanford: Stanford University Press.

Grady, D. 2007. Deadly inheritance, desperate trade-off. *New York Times,* August 7, p. F1.

Habermas, J. 2003. *The Future of Human Nature.* Cambridge, UK: Polity.

Hall, S. S. 2003. *Merchants of Immortality: Chasing the dream of human life extension.* Boston: Houghton Mifflin.

Hayflick, L. 2000. The future of ageing. *Nature* 408 (6809):267–69.

Holstein, M. 1997. Alzheimer's disease and senile dementia, 1885–1920: An interpretive history of disease negotiation. *Journal of Aging Studies* 11:1–13.

Kass, L. 2004. L'Chaim and its limits: Why not immortality? In *The Fountain of Youth: Cultural, scientific, and ethical perspectives on a biomedical goal,* ed. S. G. Post and R. H. Binstock. New York: Oxford University Press.

Katz, S., and B. Marshall. 2003. New sex for old: Lifestyle, consumerism, and the ethics of aging well. *Journal of Aging Studies* 17 (1):3–16.

Kaufman, S. R. 2005. *And a Time to Die: How American hospitals shape the end of life.* New York: Scribner.

Kaufman, S. R., A. J. Russ, and J. K. Shim. 2006. Aged bodies and kinship matters: The ethical field of kidney transplant. *American Ethnologist* 33 (1):81–99.

Kaufman, S. R., J. K. Shim, and A. J. Russ. 2004. Revisiting the biomedicalization of aging: Clinical trends and ethical challenges. *Gerontologist* 44 (6):731–38.

McCullough, L. B., J. Caskey, T. R. Cole, and A. Weir. 2008. Scientific and medical concepts of nature in the modern period in Europe and North America. In *Altering Nature.* Vol. 1: *Concepts of "Nature" and "The Natural" in Biotechnology Debates,* ed. A. B. Lustig, G. P. McKinney, and B. Brody. New York: Springer.

Meier, B., and A. R. Sorkin. 2005. New suitor makes higher bid for troubled heart device maker. *New York Times,* December 6, p. C1.

Merchant, C. 1990. *The Death of Nature.* New York: HarperCollins.

Muller, J., and B. Koenig. 1988. On the boundary of life and death: The definition of dying by medical residents. In *Biomedicine Examined,* ed. M. M. Lock and D. Gordon. Dordrecht; Boston: Kluwer Academic Publishers.

Nuland, S. B. 1998. Medicine isn't just for the sick anymore. *New York Times,* May 10, p. WK1.

Ojo, A. O. 2005. Expanded criteria donors: Process and outcomes. *Semin Dial* 18 (6):463–68.

Organ Procurement and Transplantation Network. 2007. Data. http://optn.org/data.

Rabinow, P. 2000. Epochs, presents, events. In *Living and Working with the New Medical*

Technologies: Intersections of inquiry, ed. M. M. Lock, A. Young, and M. M. Cambrosio. Cambridge: Cambridge University Press.

Rose, N. 2001. The politics of life itself. *Theory, Culture and Society* 18 (6):1–30.

———. 2007. *The Politics of Life Itself: Biomedicine, power, and subjectivity in the twenty-first century*. Princeton: Princeton University Press.

Russ, A. J., J. K. Shim, and S. R. Kaufman. 2005. Is there life on dialysis? Time and aging in a clinically sustained existence. *Medical Anthropology* 24 (4):297–324.

Sandel, M. J. 2004. The case against perfection. *Atlantic Monthly* 293 (3):50.

Shim, J. K., A. J. Russ, and S. R. Kaufman. 2006. Risk, life extension and the pursuit of medical possibility. *Sociology of Health and Illness* 28 (4):479–502.

———. 2007. Clinical life: Expectation and the double edge of medical promise. *Health (London)* 11 (2):245–64.

Solomon, D. H., J. R. Burton, N. E. Lundebjerg, and J. Eisner. 2000. The new frontier: Increasing geriatrics expertise in surgical and medical specialties. *Journal of the American Geriatrics Society* 48 (6):702–4.

Wade, N. 2001. *Life Script: How the human genome discoveries will transform medicine and enhance your health*. New York: Simon & Schuster.

Woodward, K. 1999. Statistical panic. *Differences: A Journal of Feminist Cultural Studies* 11 (2):177–203.

CHAPTER ELEVEN

Ethics and Aging,
Retrospectively and Prospectively

MARTHA B. HOLSTEIN, PH.D.

As individuals and members of families, in work environments, communities, and nations, we develop moral understandings that inform how we ought to be and act. These understandings are most often implicit, requiring attention only when they cease working effectively (Walker, 1998). They are deeply influenced by culture, power relationships, values, and professional norms that are often taken for granted if noticed at all. At times, however, new situations, issues, and problems arise for which we have few, if any, moral understandings. At other times, scholars or practitioners bring different experiences and training to an area, leading to alternative perceptions and responses to what once may have appeared unproblematic. Such changes provide opportunities for rethinking and lead to what has been called the critical turn in ethics (McCullough, 2005). In gerontology and ethics, for example, the evolution of feminist thinking called attention to the ways in which gender operates in our moral practices and beliefs so that "generalizations and idealizations" most often reflected conditions that certain people are more likely to meet than others (Walker, 2003, p. xiv). Feminists and other scholars have also introduced ways to think about ethics that are based less on theory and abstract rules and principles than on, in Walker's (1998) terms, an "expressive-collaborative" model of decision making that is context sensitive.

Most often, ethical dilemmas can be framed in "right versus right" terms when one can defend two or more choices on the basis of held values (Kidder, 2003). Problems such as those posed by chronic illness, for example, are painful to face and even harder to resolve. How shall we care for an aging parent who has Alzheimer's disease while also caring for our immediate family and ourselves? How ought responsibilities for such care to be distributed among individuals, families, and the public sector? End-of-life care is another such example. While respecting a person's right to make treatment choices, when do cognitive changes so impair judgment that others must decide? How might biases influence such decisions? How ought safety and risk to be balanced when an old woman lives alone in a dangerous neighborhood but insists on leaving the door unlocked so neighbors can drop in? Questions such as these, which are just a small sample of the pressing concerns that we face, call for ethical analyses that yield justifiable actions when we can't do everything and when no answers are perfect.

Because ethics is a disciplined and systematized reflection on our moral practices (Walker, 2003), it can raise questions about our conventional moral values and judgments and also reveal how relationships of power influence moral practices. Who does what for whom and on what basis? The gendered nature of caregiving, often effaced by the language of "family care," is one example. Similarly, the historic subject matter of ethics—relationships among equal strangers in the public sphere—is suggestive of the hidden power that has determined what ethical issues received attention. Moral philosophy, until the past 20 years or so, paid almost no attention to the private sphere and so to issues that directly affected the lives of women and legitimate relationships of dependency (Walker, 2003).

In what follows, I will defend an approach to ethics that is intersubjective, interdisciplinary, and methodologically diverse; that takes emotions seriously as sources of moral knowledge and moral value; that is not the sole purview of "experts"; and that embeds ethics in the everyday social worlds in which we live and work. "Moral experience," in the words of philosopher Barry Hoffmaster (2001), "does not have the clarity, precision, and rigor, or the constancy and consistency that a moral theory requires, and those demands cannot be imposed on moral experience without substantial loss and distortion" (p. 223). We learn about the moral values we esteem in the practices of individuals and communities and can then use these to help ground further reflections (Walker, 1992; Kuczewski, 1999). In other words, "doing" ethics is a whole lot messier than abstract principles and theories would suggest, which doesn't make ethical analysis less important or our actions taken as the result of such analysis less justifiable. As practical ethics evolves, we are discovering the importance of understanding the "is" as well as the "ought" and turning to older people and their life worlds as important sources of moral information, a lesson that Brian Hofland (2001), who led the Retirement Research Foundation's major initiative in "Autonomy and Long-term Care," takes from the foundation's four-year, $2 million initiative.

Following a background sketch of ethics and aging, I will consider the areas, primarily around decision making, where apparent general agreement about values and obligations has been achieved. These areas include autonomy, as expressed in informed consent; a procedural, principle-based approach to decision making; and advance care planning. As shall become quickly clear, however, almost from the start even apparent agreements were challenged. I will use long-term care, where many of the practical ethical problems arise, to suggest how conceptual changes, if put into practice, directly affect the lives of individuals and families. These changing ideas about autonomy, safety, and the role of families and considerations of human dependency, vulnerability, and embodiment, for example, are still at the fringes of practice. I will draw the chapter to a close by reflecting on the continued gap between concept and practice and how these changes in conceptual understandings can lead to different ways of thinking about our moral obligations and our ways of caring in the community. While resources will be a barrier to some changes, that constraint should not be the reason to fail to address them—how do we know where we are if we do not know where we are going?

Ethics and Aging: The Background

While explorations into the moral dimensions of aging have roots as far back as Ecclesiastes, "ethics and aging" in its contemporary version emerged far more recently (see *Gerontologist*, 1988; Jecker, 1991; Moody, 1992; McCullough and Wilson, 1995a; Cole and Holstein, 1996). In 1973, an isolated publication reported on a project addressing the ethical grounding of public policy for older people (Neugarten and Havighurst, 1973), a topic that has been too little addressed in the intervening years (see Holstein, 2005; Fahey, 2007). In a field still dominated by theologians, the "edges of life" received the most attention (Ramsey, 1970) until the late 1970s and early 1980s, when a deepening interest in the ethical problems of medicine led to what Jonsen (1998) described as the "birth of bioethics." In 1979, the Belmont Commission (1979), established to determine ethical principles to guide research on human subjects, issued its report that identified three principles—respect for persons, beneficence, and social justice—as the core values for such research. In roughly similar fashion, these principles were embodied in the first edition of what has become almost a canonical text in biomedical ethics, Beauchamp and Childress's book, *The Principles of Biomedical Ethics* (2001), now in its sixth edition. This text added nonmaleficence (or do no harm) and changed respect for persons to respect for autonomy, a significant if often unnoticed redefinition of moral obligation (Lysaught, 2005).

Procedurally, in the now dominant model, these principles were to be weighed and balanced when physicians and other health care professionals encountered ethical conundrums. Quandaries were to be resolved by ordering or reconciling the relevant moral principles and following the appropriate action guide or rule. In practice, as we shall see below, informed consent, as a practical manifestation of autonomy, quickly came to be the first principle among equals. It also became the basis for advance care planning, carrying the commitment to personal autonomy beyond individuals' ability to speak for themselves. Introduced in acute care settings, the commitment to autonomy and its expression in informed consent was then transferred to nursing homes and community care, where it works less well.

Ordering, weighing, or reconciling the differing values and interests of morally autonomous, rational, and competent individuals became <u>the</u> way of "doing" bio-ethics. As we shall soon see, however, this method may have gained acceptability in hospitals, medical schools, and nursing homes, but, almost from the beginning, ethicists and others began to question its applicability in long-term care and other morally problematic situations that involved older people. The challenge to autonomy, as captured in informed consent procedures, also faced more general challenges for ignoring, for example, institutional power or compromised autonomy (Dodds, 2000). Often described as an ethics of strangers, this approach to ethics fit poorly with the situation of long-term care, a situation involving intimates or near intimates rather than an ethics of strangers, most often focused on preserving space for self-directing actions. What it offered, however, was both a specific content in terms of midlevel principles and rules and a procedural approach to resolving ethical dilemmas first in medicine and then extended to other health and social service arenas.

Core Values

When we use the phrase "ethics and aging," we are talking about both process and content. The content, based on familiar principles and rules, reflects generally held values across professions. These values, although not without criticism for their starkness and limits (McCullough and Wilson, 1995a; Kuczewski, 1999), form a minimalist core of what is expected of professionals in the field of aging. These values include rules about confidentiality and privacy, autonomy or self-determination, boundaries, and respect, but also beneficence or best interests, values that frequently clash. How does one honor self-determination at the same time that one acts in someone's best interests? What is the role for professional judgment amidst prescriptive rules and principles? One can also see how some values are more open to interpretation than others. What does respect require of us? How well does a concept of autonomy that focuses on making decisions and best represented by standard informed consent procedures reflect an older person's deeper values and needs? Is self-direction the most important value to protect? Is supporting that value the extent of our public obligation?

Yet, as feminists, communitarians, and others have pointed out, even if we honor these values in all our practices, they do not reflect the whole of morality. Hence, there have been recent efforts to add to or modify the principles that ought to guide our thinking about ethics and long-term care (Kuczewski, 1999; Eckenwiler, 2007), the wide range of services that are offered to people who need assistance with day-to-day tasks. For those less committed to identifying new or different principles, there was a search for a deeper conceptual understanding of what matters when rendering care, especially long-term care, to older people (Tronto, 1993, 2001; Clement, 1996). Context, relationships, and the particular features of individual lives, especially vulnerability and dependency, became important considerations (Walker, 1992; Tronto, 1993; Parks, 2003; Lloyd, 2004; Hoffmaster, 2006). Feminist philosopher Margaret Walker (2003), for example, claims that standard forms of moral thinking make assumptions about "independence and full reciprocity in human relationships" (p. xvi) that leave out people who are involved in caregiving or responding in other ways to human vulnerability and frailty. As a result, too little ethical attention has focused on unavoidably dependent relationships. Concern about ethics and aging also involves the moral implications of ageism and norms that idealize certain actions and expectations that seem to suit some people far more than others (Holstein and Minkler, 2003; Walker, 2003) and the ethical implication of public policy (Holstein, 2005). While a detailed look at these issues is beyond the scope of this chapter, they are part of the essential subject matter of a thoroughgoing examination of ethics and aging.

Autonomy and Decision Making

The primacy of autonomy, although running counter to historical medical paternalism, was relatively straightforward to implement in the medical care setting, in part because it did not require major shifts in the organization of medical care. Limited to the doctor-patient relationship, it did not demand attention to those excluded from this relationship. Nor did it address existing power relationships—between doctors and nurses, doctors and patients, or insurers and patients—that operated in medical care settings. Autonomy, as enacted, meant decision making. Informed consent established a competent patient's right to accept or refuse medical treatment, including the provision of food and water even if the result was death. Informed consent (or refusal) assumed relationships among equals in which a quasi-contractual agreement is reached. This individualistic focus did not have to address the kind of choices available to individuals depending, for example, on their insurance status, gender, or race and the ways in which choices were structured (Sherwin, 1992; Dodds, 2000).

Advance Care Planning

In the mid-1980s, ethicists and legislators attempted to extend this model of informed consent to decision making for people no longer able to decide for themselves. Individualistic in keeping with the commonly held view of autonomy, the dual goals were to "optimize the rights of individual patients to refuse treatment and to protect physicians and other surrogate decision-makers from liability" (High, 1991, p. 612). A living will or a durable power of attorney for health care (generically referred to as advance directives) became the legal instruments (the Patient Self Determination Act was passed in November 1990) to meet these goals. They allow individuals to decide, in advance of incapacitation, how they wish to be treated and whom they prefer to make decisions. For patients without directives, law and/or moral guidelines instructed surrogates (most often family members) to decide, in ranked order: as the patient would have chosen (substituted judgment), or as in the patient's best interests (Cole and Holstein, 1996). Advance directives are probably the most familiar element in end-of-life care for people working in the field of aging and continue to be the subject of considerable research attention. A recent keyword search for advance directives turned up more than 150 references, many very recent.

Ironically, the drive to spread the word about directives and to improve these instruments may not be the most important route to improved care at the end of life. A recent *Hastings Center Report* posed this question: why has it been so difficult to improve end-of-life care? Directives addressed treatment choices and so placed autonomy as the "cornerstone of our approach to decisions near the end of life" (Jennings, Kaebnick, and Murray, 2005, p. S53), a fragile foundation on which to rest this humanly difficult time. A recent study by Teno et al. (2007) revealed that "the signing of an advance directive, which designated a proxy, led to greater use of hospice and fewer reported concerns with communication" (p. 189) among family members, but the researchers cautioned that "singly focused public health interventions, such as the PSDA and its reliance on AD completion, will not improve the quality of end-of-life care. Rather, multifaceted and sustainable interventions are needed to truly improve the care of the dying and those around them" (p. 194). Like informed consent, directives do not demand much of the medical care system, and they emphasize individualism, rationalism, and detached decision making that suit some people some of the time and many people none of the time.

Reevaluation of advance directives has led to new instruments and related activities that rely on "advance care planning in a system with specially trained personnel" using forms that are highly visible, standardized, and immediately actionable (Hickman et al., 2005, p. S30). One example, among several, is the well-studied "Physician Orders for Life-Sustaining Treatment" (POLST) paradigm. POLST uses a brightly colored medical order form with the patient's wishes stated as physician orders. The form accompanies patients across settings and reflects conversations among the medical team, the patient, and the family. It is actionable, specific, and effective immediately (Hickman et al., 2005). This last element sets POLST apart from other advance planning instruments. Rather than an expression of patient's wishes only, it is written as physician orders. Given the power structure in medical settings, orders have strength that expressed wishes or proxy decisions may not. Moreover, its simplicity and bright colors make it immediately visible. While not adopted in all states as a proxy instrument, for people who care deeply about having their wishes honored, POLST is a powerful ally.

For proxy decision makers, a chilly label for families or other loved ones trying to make hard choices, Murray and Jennings (2005) advise offering information, counseling, and support so that they can make good decisions in often evolving situations, suggesting that to see "surrogacy as simply an information processing task is to miss most of its human angst and drama" (p. S57). For older people who are institutionalized, Kuczewski (1999) advises a more communal engagement with decision making so that choices at the end of life can support narrative integrity. Nursing home staff "have a responsibility to monitor the decision-making process . . . to assure that the process upholds the integrity of the person, the integrity of who that person is and what her life means" (p. 25). Johnson (2005) observed that compensated caregivers are moral agents and so "their voices should be considered in decision-making about individual patients" (pp. S40–41). Narrative integrity means seeing what ought to come next for the older person in the light of his or her values and lifestyle that may transcend written communications.

A Focus on Long-Term Care

The Retirement Research Foundation's critically important four-year initiative on "Autonomy and Long-Term Care," launched in the mid-1980s, turned empirical and philosophical attention to how long-term care practices and settings made the exercise of autonomy virtually impossible (Ambrogi and Leonard, 1988; Agich, 1990; Lidz, Fischer, and Arnold, 1992), while Bart Collopy (1988) contributed a fine-grained, conceptual analysis of autonomy particularly recognizing that the inability to act on our choices does not mean denying the right to choose. In what remains a classic account, he also called attention to issues that remain unresolved: How should the relationships between competency, the possibility of incapacitated choice, and autonomy be negotiated? How might a family or a paid care provider balance the person's right to be left alone with the possibility that positive action might make real choice possible? How might a care provider address the distinction between short-term and long-term autonomy (Collopy, 1988) or his or her professional obligation to mitigate harm but also to respect autonomy (Kane and Levin, 2001)? How might these unresolved issues, for example, directly relate to the problem of elder "self-neglect," an issue that has yet to be adequately explored through the prism of ethics?

American nursing homes now post a "Patient Bill of Rights." They less often facilitate an autonomous expression of selfhood (Lidz, Fischer, and Arnold, 1992) or find ways to act as microcommunities that support both collective aims and individual needs. Given the facts of institutional life—highly regulated, heavily financed by Medicaid, market-driven, and often operated by distant corporations for a profit, along with frequent staff turnover—enhancement of the interstitial autonomy that

Agich (1995) proposed and I discuss below will always be difficult. Most simply put, if a decisionally capable resident cannot have any say about when she has her shower or who is her caregiver or what or when she shall eat, her autonomy is restricted even if the no-code order is clearly marked on her chart (Agich, 1990; Hofland, 1990). In the nursing home, such mundane things as making private phone calls are dramatically affected by regulations, organizational policies and procedures, and financing mechanisms. What noninstitutionalized people take for granted—coffee at 3 p.m. or a shower at 7 a.m.—assume an importance that may be difficult for outsiders to perceive (Kane and Caplan, 1990). In a nursing home, residents must try to live a "private life in a public place" (Collopy, Boyle, and Jennings, 1991, p. 7) where their roots are dissolved and their frailty means relying on others often in vastly unequal power relationships. Threatened by dementia, vulnerability, and ageist social values, nursing home patients must assert what more physically and mentally able people assume in their moral universe: reciprocity, rough equality, and the opportunity to make real choices about things that matter to them (Shield, 1988; Diamond, 1992; Lidz, Fischer, and Arnold, 1992). Further, as Lidz, Fischer, and Arnold (1992) noted, nursing home patients are considered to be receivers and not givers. Yet, full membership in the moral community entails responsibility to others and to the community at whatever level such responsibility can be displayed (May, 1986; Jameton, 1988). Responsibility entails involvement in fostering the well-being of the entire community as well as personal responsibilities for shaping one's own life. Feminist ethics, characterized by a relational ontology, suggests that because the self exists only "through and with others" (Sevenhuijsen, 2000, p. 9), this concept of responsibility, while receiving far less emphasis than rights, might be more fitting for the dominant population of nursing homes—old women.

Contextual features of nursing home life, now undergoing modifications as the result of the culture change movement, have generally limited what is possible. Until these contextual features (e.g., minimal staffing and wages, institutional imperatives, regulatory expectations, unequal power because of hierarchical structures, irregular physician and ancillary medical personnel presence) are addressed, improvements can only be modest. Admissions agreements (Ambrogi and Leonard, 1988), for example, are improved, and as a result of OBRA '87 (Omnibus Budget Reconciliation Act), patients are invited to participate in "care planning" and nursing homes are evaluated at how well they do this. Yet, nursing homes remain the most regulated of health care institutions (in part the result of abuses uncovered in the 1960s and 1970s), meaning that the room to maneuver is limited. They are also generally governed by a market mentality, which means that when people are the most vulnerable, they are also placed in the position of being customers governed by the philosophy of buyer beware (Collopy, 1995). These needs put an enormous responsibility on facilities to balance community and individual, to use resources prudently, and to respond to legal and regulatory requirements (Collopy, Boyle, and Jennings, 1991).

Some nursing homes have responded to criticisms by joining in what is called the movement for "culture change" (e.g., the Eden Alternative, Pioneer Practices, the Greenhouses). As these movements are more systematically evaluated, we should gain a better understanding of how real the possibilities for change are. A likely constraint, however, is the fact that about three-quarters of nursing homes in this country are for-profit entities, meaning that relatively modest Medicaid payments to nursing homes must generate a return to external stakeholders.

Another positive sign has been the increased attention to dying in nursing homes. While we are quick to deny that nursing homes are the way station before death, "over 20% of older Americans meet their deaths in a nursing home" (Johnson, 2005), a fact that begs for improving how nursing homes support dying residents. Ironically, the resistance to seeing nursing homes as places where people decline and die had meant that nursing homes feared citations if patients lost weight or showed other signs that death was approaching. Regulatory scrutiny, intended to weed out bad facilities and to assure that residents are not maltreated, can, inadvertently, interfere with good care for the dying. One symbol of this problem is the transfer of the resident to the hospital where a new team takes over, making the patient's values and wishes less likely to be known when death is imminent. Above all, as Johnson (2005) points out, dying in nursing homes is incremental; hence, the focus on dramatic decisions such as the provision of food and water to a person in a persistent vegetative state may be less important than keeping the person safe, warm, and fed.

Regulations are a generally neglected area of ethical analysis. Accepting that regulations must protect and prevent harm, what other purposes should they serve and what moral values ought they to support? Can regulations be devised that strike a balance between standards of care and professional discretion to "respond to their [the professionals] own particular problems of care as they make creative use of the dependency that is an essential fact of nursing home life" (Collopy, Boyle, and Jennings, 1991, p. 13)? How can professionals in nursing homes help other staff members, who are motivated to do the right thing, respond ethically to vulnerable residents? It will not be easy to change regulations, which developed as a result of the long history of abuse and inadequate care (Holstein and Cole, 1995). Regulatory change requires trust. It also calls for developing a vision of what we want nursing homes to be, an end best reached by bringing together regulators, caregivers, families, and residents to talk together about what regulatory changes and other social responses, like education and training, might lead to fulfillment of the vision.

Interestingly, assisted living, which has burgeoned in the past 20 years, has received far less ethical scrutiny than nursing homes, perhaps because of the almost singular focus on autonomy, which is the prevailing value for residents who have their own apartments and often drive their own cars. As with any congregate living, however, individual needs and values can easily clash with the needs of the community and other residents; for example, as people age in place in assisted living, what is the right and good action if they develop dementia and disrupt meals but the family insists that they not be moved? What obligations does the facility have to people who argue that they entered the assisted living facility in the belief that they would live among people who were like them—relatively independent and without advanced dementia? How ought the facility to balance these conflicting needs? What if some residents need more medical help than the facility can offer but don't want to leave? What if families insist that they will step into the breach and help even if mother falls regularly and gets lost once she walks out the front door?

Holes in the Dike

The problems that occur in long-term care are ambiguous and elude easy definition (Hofland, 1990; McCullough and Wilson, 1995a). Perspectives are multiple. Even decisions that may, on the surface, appear straightforward, such as "code" or "no-code," often become painfully difficult. What about the person with Alzheimer's disease who still smiles and laughs and seems at ease with her now diminished life (Dworkin, 1993; Dresser, 1994)? Is she still the same person she was when she executed the directive, or can directives be overridden based on the quality of her current life? Patients themselves may have a hard time weighing benefits and harms; a treatment that may seem temporarily too burdensome may have a positive long-range result. How is competency determined so that gender and other biases don't lead to pre-sumptive decisions about a person's capacity to be involved in decision making? How can we increase the chances that the loss of decision-making capacity does not inter-fere with facilitating the person's ability to live in habitual ways? How do we create responses to the fluidity of most decision making in LTC (for a discussion about preventive ethics see McCullough and Wilson, 1995b)? I raise these many questions—without having answers—to suggest why ethicists, often joined by practitioners, have been, over the past decade or so, revisiting old questions and introducing newer ways to think about both old and new issues.

A potpourri of reasons may account for shifts in thinking. One cause was empirical research. How were decisions made (Kaufman, 2001)? What problems did case man-agers (Kane and Caplan, 1993) or home care aides (Holstein, 1999b) face? Who provided most of the care to older people in the community, and what were the ethical implications of such caregiving (Hooyman and Gonyea, 1995; Holstein, 1999a, 2007; Kittay, 1999)? This research alerted us not only to problems but also to an understanding of what ethical behaviors worked in practice as individuals, families, and care providers sought a "common habitable moral world" (Walker, 1992). In long-term care, a deductive, "bottom-up" identification of ethical problems seems more appropriate than top-down, inductive approaches (Kuczewski, 1999; Hoffmaster, 2001; Lindemann, 2006) that decreed, in advance, what moral values counted. Case-based ethics or casuistry and feminist ethics of care, for example, demonstrate the usefulness of practical reasoning that takes context, relationships, and the unique features of situations into account (Jonsen and Toulmin, 1988; Tronto, 1993; Held, 2006). Moral thinking that was particularistic rather than universal and relied less on principles than on conversation and communication also helped to shape what was emerging as a newer and more flexible form of moral thinking (Moody, 1992). Perhaps this form of thinking, involving give and take, negotiation, compromise, and sensitivity to relationships, best reflected the ways in which people went about making moral sense of their lives.

The need to seek a comfortable, mutually supportive moral world seems to be most imperative in the home care setting, where multiple actors—client or patient, family, formal caregivers, care coordinators, to name a few—each had a moral stake in what occurs (Collopy, Dubler, and Zuckerman, 1990; McCullough and Wilson, 1995a; Wetle, 1995). The almost single-minded focus on the client, which has governed common enactments of autonomy, obscures the relationships that both formed and continue to shape who we are as individuals and are central to community living. Arras (1995) convincingly defends the interests of family members as morally significant and not evidence of a to-be-avoided conflict of interest. While he starts from the premise that the older person's interests ought to come first, he argues that families have legitimate interests of their own that ought not to be demoted or bypassed. As we see in numerous family situations, the client's wishes to stay at home and accept no outside services might mean that his daughter has to choose between working full-time and caring for her father. To further complicate the situation, that "choice" evaporates if he does not qualify for public benefits and neither father nor daughter has the resources to pay privately for the care he needs. Caring for the caregiver means better care (Kittay, 1999; Parks, 2003) and is a ripe area for continued analysis on justice-based grounds (Holstein, 1999a, 2007). Balancing care and justice is a potent moral aim.

Similarly, the consistent evocation of independence as the end state of care obviates the need to morally attend to matters of dependency and vulnerability. These fundamental human conditions can rarely be avoided; yet, only recently have they received moral scrutiny (Agich, 1990, 1995; Collopy, Dubler, and Zuckerman, 1990; Kittay, 1999; Hoffmaster, 2006). In home care, where loss and frailty are so present, the task is not only about "independence," however thin that becomes, but also integration of illness into daily life and self-identity (Jennings, Callahan, and Caplan, 1988). To acknowledge frailty and vulnerability and to feel with the person help us to see that norms of respect and dignity extend beyond decision making, and that caring bestows a "life-sustaining web" of connections among people (Tronto, 1993, p. 103). To acknowledge dependency also frees one to focus on other things in life that have real personal value.

Vulnerability also reveals what many feminist philosophers have called "relational autonomy" (MacKenzie and Stoljar, 2000), an expression that conveys multiple messages, but for long-term care it serves as a reminder that care is the "product or outcome of the relationship between two or more people" (Fine and Glendinning, 2005, p. 616). Close attention to the caring relationship as a mutually constructed activity opens opportunities for rethinking dependencies and for empowering both caregiver and care receiver. If we think about caregiving in this way, we can begin to construct an ethic for long-term care that acknowledges and responds to the exploitation that care workers and family caregivers often experience while acknowledging that frailty and vulnerability cannot be thought away. These conditions offer strong ethical warrants for a response that is based on feeling with as well as doing for (Hoffmaster, 2006; Fahey, 2007). Thus, how different the fact of dependency could be if it were endowed with its own accounts of practices and virtues—like gratitude— unique to the experience of dependency. Such an account would add to our knowledge of what it means to live a fully human life (Tronto, 2001). Yet, American culture can accept dependency only among the very young; it cannot easily integrate the dependent older person into a system of valuing that elevates youth, action, zestful living, success, and productivity. While I do not want to revert to a lachrymose view of aging as represented in the decline-and-loss paradigm, I also do not want to herald an overly rosy picture of advanced age. Thus, in long-term care many factors other than the patient's "right" to make a decision assume importance.

Long-Term Care: Further Reflections
Changing Ideas about Autonomy

Having touched on the growing concern about the ways in which autonomy is conceptualized and enacted, I would like to explore how new ways of thinking about this protean concept can significantly expand our understanding of long-term care ethics. As noted above, in its common understanding autonomy continues to mean self-directing action, encapsulated in informed consent procedures. This view, however, is far "thinner" than what long-term care practice requires. It is, for example, often reduced to making choices in the absence of attention to the conditions that make real choice possible (availability of choices; ability to pay for them; meaningful for one's life), or it is narrowly defined so that it does not oblige us to actively cooperate with an older person's efforts to "reorient themselves" as they seek to "remake their world" (Agich, 1995, p. 124). It thus means more than removing barriers to and honoring choice. It is a long way from the paradigmatic Kantian rational "man" to the 88-year-old woman with congestive heart failure, mild cognitive impairment, and osteoporosis. With an understanding of autonomy that emphasizes the chance to live in both habitual and meaningful ways, autonomy becomes concrete. It commits us to foster the development of the self and the expression of individuality (Agich, 1990) as positive duties. It also suggests that concrete expressions of autonomy —life as a career, self-direction, exercising only chosen obligations—do not reflect the circumstances in which most older people (or most of us more generally) live (see Walker, 2003, for an extended critique of how concrete expressions of autonomy fit poorly with many older people's lives).

Hence, is that sort of autonomy really the preeminent value for a very old woman in a nursing home? Or is "actual autonomy" more about older people being able to live in "accord with whom they really are" (Agich, 1995, p. 121), and less about making a choice in the moment than about living in ways that are meaningful instantiations of identity? This claim is not to suggest that paternalistic interventions are desirable, but rather that we must enrich our understanding of autonomy so that it accounts for the kinds of selves we are, or are struggling to be, when loss impedes what might otherwise be taken for granted. The right to choose means little when it simply suggests the absence of coercion. It gains meaning when the older person is given the space and the conditions to help him or her answer the question of "who am I?" as the former conditions that gave shape to his or her "horizons of meaning" (Taylor, 1989) dissipate. That we live our lives coherently and purposefully matters at any age.

It is possible that home care may be a laboratory for rethinking the everyday meanings of autonomy. Examination of a central problem—that of safety—is one place to begin. In a microcosm, it reflects the issues brought about by the uneasy combination of the need for care and the wish for independence. At home people may take risks that seem deeply troubling to caregivers. Labeled "emboldened autonomy," clients assert choices that require caregivers to determine "whether risky choices are adequately informed, voluntary, and truly competent" (Collopy, Dubler, and Zuckerman, 1990, p. 8). For the client, however, safety, as conventionally understood, is one of many values and needs to be weighed in terms of "concrete benefits and harms" (Collopy, 1995, p. 142). Collopy (1995) advises caregivers to see the question of safety and risk as open to revision over time. This longitudinal view permits greater freedom to make temporary and sometimes fragile trade-offs between safety and independence. Above all, Collopy (1995) asks us to value psychosocial safety, which allows people to live in ways that promote a "safe harbor," a zone that alleviates the suffering that emerges from threats to one's personal identity (Cassell, 1991). Collopy's effort to redefine safety in terms of maintaining one's sense of harmony, personal identify, and meaning in the face of loss fits well with Agich's (1990, 1995) notions about autonomy, while also underlining McCullough and Wilson's (1995a) reminder that in long-term care there is rarely a single narrative that defines the "problem" as there often is in acute care.

Sadly, however, in home care, more often encountered than "emboldened autonomy" is the condition of "eroded autonomy." Empirical research (Aronson, 2002) is suggestive. Clients who receive home care start out with the determination to take charge. They minimize exposure to harmful judgments and assert their personal boundaries often by shrouding "their needs and limitations" (Aronson, 2002, p. 405). But such control is usually fragile as they face constant needs to revise their sense of self as their physical and mental capacities change. Because community care systems are rarely adequate to respond to changes, clients are "pushed over the edge" (pp. 407–10). They feel "diminished and disrespected" (p. 407) as strangers become their source of care, especially strangers who have instrumental tasks that they are obliged to do. Caregiving by the clock can be depersonalizing and minimalist. Barely holding themselves together, they withdraw further from outside contacts and keeping up appearances. For these older people resignation becomes their way of coping. They could no longer be in charge; they knowingly let go of "past preferences and wishes" (p. 410). While grateful for what they receive, they also ask for little and adopt the singular goal of avoiding institutionalization. In these situations, we see how minimalist typical views of autonomy are. A richer conception of autonomy demands a richer notion of justice and human flourishing. Yet, these systems of care often describe themselves as "person-centered" and autonomy-based.

Caregiving

Caregiving, especially the issue of caregiver burden, is central to the gerontological research agenda. It is also a significant problem of justice, the moral value that is easier to praise than to enact. Without family support, provided mostly by women, the costs to the public sector would be more than $400 billion annually (Arno, Levine, and Memmot, 1999). The twin assumptions—that public policies can be constructed around the availability of informal caregivers and low-wage nursing assistants—are not ethically neutral (Abel, 1991). They raise critical questions about distributive justice within the family (Okin, 1989; Jecker, 1995; Holstein, 2007) and among people depending on race and class. This reliance on family care further reminds us how parts of the medical and social care system relate to one another. Thus, Diagnostic Related Groups (DRGs) and other medical care system reforms, while saving dollars for the Medicare program, increase the burden on informal caregivers, generally wives and female spouses (England et al., 1991).

The persistence of gender-based inequalities in caregiving increases women's economic disadvantage and risks for poverty in old age. These accumulate over time and "intensify with changes in marital, health, and employment status" (Wakabayashi and Donato, 2006). Yet, social expectations are so powerful that women have fewer "excuses" than men not to give care, and given the wage discrepancies between men and women, it makes economic sense for women to leave the workforce or reduce working hours to engage in caregiving. Thus, for men domestic labor is a choice, but for women it is an obligation (Clement, 1996; Calasanti and Slevin, 2001). Interrupted work histories and part-time work affect lifetime earnings, Social Security, and pension benefits if any are available. Further, out-of-pocket costs, for example, for elder care, are rarely discussed, yet they erode the income of adult daughters who are providing the care. Whether it is Depend incontinence products or detergent or over-the-counter drugs, these costs are high, especially when income is already marginal. A report (Gross, 2007) in the *New York Times* places out-of-pocket costs at about $5,500 a year. People earning less than $25,000 spent 20 percent of their income on caregiving. These out-of-pocket costs often mean that individuals dip into savings, or postpone saving for their own retirement, thereby compounding the effects of lost wages and benefits. Class is thus deeply implicated in caregiving because "economic privilege [or lack of it] determines the degree to which families are strained by the demands of home care" (Parks, 2003, p. 52). As Parks further observes, the working poor bear the greatest costs because they must leave work or reduce working hours and lack the flexibility that so many professional women have. This is one price paid for America's consistent reluctance to embrace more socially oriented solutions to problems of dependency, such as supporting it through the Medicare program balanced in some way with continued contributions from individuals and families.

However, the President's Council on Bioethics (2005), while acknowledging that families, in particular women, faced enormous caregiving responsibilities, did not call for a deeper and more sustained public commitment. Instead, the essential message of the report to caregivers was to not abandon their older members even when the difficulties appeared to be insurmountable. In the effort to make certain that such abandonment did not occur, the council strongly critiqued living wills not because they were not strong enough but because they might lead to such abandonment. The council may consider family caregivers saintly, but it did not offer them any chance of the kind of equality that feminist philosophers and gerontologists have called for. Such equality might include continued accumulation of Social Security benefits and any pensions for which the caregiver might be eligible. It might include generous respite care, an annual "vacation" from caregiving, and, as noted above, assistance with the out-of-pocket costs. More significantly, by removing the boundaries between morality and politics, care can be made an element of what is expected of citizens (Tronto, 1993).

The gender issue is not only relevant for the informal care provider. When we look at the formal sector of paid caregivers, we see a comparable pattern of inequality and potential exploitation. An almost all-female workforce, which is most often African-American or ethnic minorities, has responsibility for overwhelmingly female recipients of care. Both are vulnerable. Care work is socially devalued, income is limited, and benefits are almost nonexistent. If the worker is employed by a provider agency, she is relatively powerless to set the conditions of her own work or to choose to whom she gives care. She is also relatively powerless in the face of disrespectful treatment by the care receiver or her employer (Kittay, 1999).

Thus, while the buzz word in long-term care today is "rebalancing," that is, bringing more care into the home and the community rather than providing it in institutions, there is a moral price that is paid. The exploitation of women and the "co-optation of their sense of responsibility to others," both paid and unpaid, cannot be defended on ethical grounds (Parks, 2003). A more generous response to family members—help with out-of-pocket costs, continued earning of Social Security credits —and more resources to support a collective response to need would be a beginning. Good care in the community cannot be given without programs that are adequately funded to meet care needs and to relieve the often overwhelming responsibilities of family members.

Another form of damage to caregiving relationships is the limitations imposed by the action-guide approaches—that is, the weighing and balancing of abstract principles such as autonomy and beneficence—to ethics. As feminist philosopher Margaret Urban Walker (1992) points out, this way of thinking "does not fit well in contexts of personal relationships or responsive care-taking, situations that require sensitivity, flexibility, discretion, and improvisation to find precisely what responds to very particular cases" (p. 28). She adds that "such contexts require awareness of histories of relationships and understandings specific to these histories, for these determine what responses between these particular people mean" (pp. 28–29). By concentrating only on those problems that action guides can address, we simply miss a large portion of people's moral life. Moreover, we miss the operations of power and the depth of interconnections of people involved in giving and receiving care. In practice, the ethical problems that arise in home care are mostly about who will provide care, how that care will be provided, what risks can be taken, and how better to distribute the load.

Embodiment

A less obvious but important concern in LTC and aging more generally is the body, in particular the vulnerable body. It is, as Twigg (2000) observed, strangely absent from discourses about aging. Yet, the body is the most important contact we have with the world, a source of judgments that others make about us and that we make about ourselves. Vulnerable bodies—frequently referred to as "fourth-agers"—do not fit with the "current preoccupation with autonomy and independence" (Lloyd, 2006). Marked by the appearance of serious infirmities, the fourth age is undeniably "old." As generous and kind as the caregiver may be, the older person's body is exposed in ways that emphasize differential power and beauty. The body, and what it no longer can do, becomes central to experience and to self-definition. In nursing home care and to a lesser extent in home care, where old and naked bodies dominate many interactions between professionals and older people, the aversion to the old body is enacted. Yet we expect both family members and minimally paid care workers to treat the person in this body with respect. Hence, evasion through a task orientation becomes a common strategy. Hoffmaster (2006) observes that "rather than focusing on the person for whom a task is being performed, focus [is] on the task itself." The reward, he suggests, "is distance from fear and discomfort" (p. 42). Yet, if professionals in this field do not attend to the phenomenological body, we cannot understand its moral importance. How might dignity and respect be enacted when the "visual field" is disrupted by an old body? Compare if you can the bodies that you see in ads for retirement communities and the bodies that are bathed and cleaned and fed in long-term care settings. My use of the word "bodies" rather than "people" is deliberate because I want to urge a confrontation with the attitudes that each one of us may have but not wish to face.

I raise this issue in an unavoidably sketchy form to encourage each of us to engage with the fact of embodiment. The body is material, but it is also socially constructed and thus not to be ignored as a morally significant—and modifiable—part of our lives. It is a major source of our subjectivity. We need not have vulnerable bodies to begin to experience threats to moral agency, self-esteem, and other features of our identity as we age. To return again to the notion of relational autonomy, the fact that we are embodied means that social attitudes, norms, and cultural practices that contribute to the devaluation of the aging body affect something as basic as our ability to make choices.

Conceptual Development and Practice

I have just surveyed both the areas of general agreement in ethics and aging and those areas where there is emerging conceptual clarity—in terms of autonomy, safety, obligations to families and other caregivers, and procedural approaches—but few changes in practice. The pursuit of independence has limited the moral attention devoted to vulnerability and dependency, a void that often results in emotional distancing. Many older people are receiving care but are not cared for. Jan Baars (2006) labels it the "pit-stop" model of providing care; Julia Twigg (2007, personal communication) sees it as care controlled by the clock and instrumental tasks. Managerial efficiency and putative relationships between autonomous individuals dominate these models of care.

This gap originates in substantive changes in how this country and others in the West think about and organize social welfare programs, and approaches to ethics adopted by many caring professions and described in earlier sections of this chapter also help to perpetuate this gap. The prevailing neoliberal ideology and the resulting "risk society" assume that markets, individuals, and families are and ought to be the primary sources of well-being in late life (Lloyd, 2004; Baars, 2006; Polivka and Longino, 2006). This view justifies reducing expenditures for social care. Lacking a social view that care is central to a just society (Tronto, 1993) and working within a commodified setting, professionals in aging face serious obstacles to change. These larger social obstacles are reinforced by codes of ethics, especially in social work, which are prescriptive. Even something so taken for granted as evidence-based practice can reduce professional maneuverability and constrain opportunities to use experience to guide ethical action in particular circumstances (Tronto, 2001; Parton, 2003; Banks, 2004; Lloyd, 2004). Often too, resource constraints in these fields make it difficult to attract experienced professionals to the public or private not-for-profit sectors, where so much of the work is done. The organization of work, including bureaucracies and hierarchical arrangements, further limits the willingness of line staff to raise moral uncertainties. They fear being labeled as unprofessional (Prilleltensky, Rossiter, and Walsh-Bowers, 1996).

Professionals, especially those supported by the public sector, may have the most difficulty integrating changing ideas about autonomy or family interests, for example, and the resulting moral expectations into their practices. Traditional social work ethics retains a deep commitment to individual autonomy understood as self-direction, which, when combined with time and resource constraints, makes support for Agich's (1990) concepts of nodal autonomy (single decisions about one issue at a time) as opposed to actual autonomy (the ability to live in habitual ways) central to practice. To support the latter, in today's political environment, would call for a political or collective response that deepens and widens the choices available to people and makes time commitments less clock-bound. Yet, with professionalism under threat from many directions, a more flexible, often ambiguous and particularistic approach to ethics seems out of reach, especially if one barely has the time to meet the expectations of organizations and funding sources. The possibility for reflexivity, or the chance to expose one's premises to questioning and to "alternative framings of reality in order to grapple with the potentially different outcomes arising out of different points of view" (Parton, 2003, p. 9), becomes nearly impossible. Given these constraints, algorithmic approaches to making decisions are more likely than the reflexive and democratic deliberation that many ethicists have recommended, especially for the complex and intimate world of long-term care (Moody, 1992; McCullough and Wilson, 1995; Hugman, 2005).

An intersubjective process exposes different views, develops alternative perspectives, and, in the end, can serve the client's needs more effectively. Absent the opportunity to reflect, to engage in dialogue, and to learn to live with ambiguity, care can be less than it ought to be. When the ability for helping professionals to think together about newer conceptual developments in ethics and to use their experiences as guides to ethically justifiable action is not part of day-to-day practice, then decisions may also be constrained. To understand how changes in thinking about ethics and long-term care can work in daily life also means shifting from seeing the moral actor as one who follows prescribed rules in individualistic terms to conceiving this actor as one engaged in intersubjective processes created through communication. The conditions for ethical behavior would then shift from its current preoccupation with getting the worker to internalize the rules to developing processes of ethical communication and to incorporating a relational view of ethics into practice. Yet, deliberation and its requirements—time, a safe place for discussion, equality of participants, moral imaginings, courage to say the nonconventional—are usually beyond the capacities of the underfunded long-term care environment.

Conclusion

In the past 25 years, ethics as seen through the prism of age has become part of the professional and public conversation. Yet, new ideas—some more than two decades old—do not transfer easily to practice. If this gap can be bridged, what difference would it make? I think of the change as leading to an ethics of solidarity that brings together not only caregivers and care receivers but also policy makers and leaders in relevant professions to see what commitments a just society ought to make toward its most vulnerable members. I see such a commitment as making it possible for care, compassion, and concern to pervade each encounter with another person who needs care, and involving alertness to the demands of care but also the necessity for justice. If our moral identity is always in process, evolving through and with our relationships, as feminist ethics suggests, then our moral practices as helping professionals must rest on ongoing dialogue and interpretation so that we don't adopt ethical norms and values that diverge from what may be important to the older people for whom we care.

Questions abound. If we think of ethics in terms of human flourishing and support of human capabilities (Nussbaum, 2000), a broad vision that would require significant changes in how we think about social obligations to assure economic and other forms of security, then ethics supports a vigorous political agenda. This vision means that public policy, uneasily joined to ethics, ought to be a central concern. Debate around the ideal physician-patient relationship has been a familiar subject for articles and texts, but less often is the focus on the institutions and power structures in which these relationships occur. How would ethical reflection inform our thinking about the physical changes associated with aging in their phenomenological and moral aspects? How would it assess the imposition of culturally normative standards that may suit some people far more adequately than others (Holstein and Minkler, 2003)? Now that this country is less a melting pot than a potpourri of different racial and ethnic groups, how might we integrate ideas about difference into our moral thinking? Questions such as these call for continued examination if the field of ethics and aging is to transcend the current focus on decision making.

I look to a richer morality about living as we age despite ageist and other negative attitudes. Many ethicists (Kittay, 1999; Parks, 2003; Walker, 2003; Hoffmaster, 2006; Lindemann, 2006) have expanded the subject matter of ethics to include issues of exploitation and oppression in all its forms and have recognized that dependency and vulnerability, as facts of life, call for moral analysis. Vulnerability and dependency thus call for as much moral attention as is now devoted to independence and autonomy if we are to account for the many different ways in which we grow old. These examples suggest that we need to widen our vision—what we perceive as morally important is critical. If we do not notice some act or situation as morally problematic, we will neither think about nor seek to change it. Thus, the conception of morality that seems appropriate is not limited to the resolution of interpersonal value conflicts; rather, it is a broader vision that encompasses "a conception of a good person, of mature individual personality, and of a good life, perhaps a multiplicity of social relations, which is not entirely concerned with social relations" (Flanagan, 1991, p. 17). Morality is also deeply connected to self-esteem and self-identity. We tend to easily forget about this aspect when we think of ethics as only about the resolution of dilemmas.

None of the above is to denigrate the importance of the gains that have been made over the past 25 years. Serious attention to end-of-life care means that fewer people suffer from intractable pain or have unwanted treatments foisted on them. Despite the persistence of biases about old women (Parks, 2000), decision making is increasingly a shared enterprise. The concepts captured in the terms confidentiality, dual relationships, safety and risk, and conflicts of interest have become central to the common language of health and social service professionals. But these are often seen too starkly to account for the nuances that occur, especially in long-term care, where many people and organizations are involved in caregiving, where care is tacitly rationed, and where safety and harm are in tenuous equilibrium (Collopy, 1995; McCullough and Wilson, 1995; Kane and Levin, 2001). The danger is that these concepts can become ossified, leaving little flexibility to respond to the specifics of different situations and different people. Expertise, in the form of practice parameters and evidence-based practice, often marginalizes experience (Parton, 2003; Banks, 2004), while traditional forms of ethical reasoning dominate over newer and more context-specific forms of reasoning (Kittay and Meyers, 1987; Walker, 1992; Abramson, 1996; Hoffmaster, 2001). I look toward a continued conversation.

REFERENCES

Abel, E. K. 1991. *Who Cares for the Elderly: Public policy and the experiences of adult daughters.* Philadelphia: Temple University Press.

Abramson, M. 1996. Toward a more holistic understanding of ethics in social work. *Social Work in Health Care* 23 (2):1–14.

Agich, G. 1990. Reassessing autonomy in long-term care. *Hastings Center Report* 20 (6):12–17.

———. 1995. Actual autonomy and long-term care decision making. In *Long-Term Care Decision: Ethical and conceptual dimensions*, ed. L. B. McCullough and N. L. Wilson. Baltimore: Johns Hopkins University Press.

Ambrogi, D., and F. Leonard. 1988. The impact of nursing home admissions agreements on resident autonomy. *Gerontologist* 28 (Suppl.):82–89.

Arno, P., C. Levine, and M. Memmot. 1999. The economic value of informal caregiving. *Health Affairs* 18 (2):182–88.

Aronson, J. 2002. Elderly people's account of home care rationing: Missing voices in long-term care policy debates. *Ageing and Society* 22:399–418.

Arras, J. 1995. Conflicting interests in long-term care decision making: Acknowledging, dissolving, and resolving conflicts among elders and families. In *Long-Term Care Decisions: Ethical and conceptual dimensions*, ed. L. B. McCullough and N. L. Wilson. Baltimore: Johns Hopkins University Press.

Baars, J. 2006. Beyond neomodernism, antimodernism, and postmodernism: Basic categories for contemporary critical gerontology. In *Aging, Globalization and Inequality: The new critical gerontology*, ed. J. Baars, D. Dannefer, C. Phillipson, and A. Walker. Amityville: Baywood Publishing.

Banks, S. 2004. *Ethics, Accountability and the Social Professions.* New York: Palgrave Macmillan.

Beauchamp, T., and J. Childress. 2001. *The Principles of Biomedical Ethics.* 5th ed. New York: Oxford University Press.

Belmont Commission. 1979. *Belmont Report: Ethical principles and guidelines for the protection of human subjects.* Washington, D.C.: National Commission for the Protection of Human Subjects of Biomedical and Behavioral Research.

Calasanti, T. M., and K. F. Slevin, eds. 2001. *Age Matters: Realigning feminist thinking.* New York: Routledge.

Cassell, E. 1991. *The Nature of Suffering and the Goals of Medicine.* New York: Oxford University Press.

Clement, G. 1996. *Care, Autonomy and Justice: Feminism and the ethics of care.* Boulder: Westview.

Cole, T. R., and M. Holstein. 1996. Ethics and aging. In *Handbook of Aging and the Social Sciences,* ed. R. H. Binstock and L. K. George. San Diego: Academic Press.

Collopy, B. 1988. Autonomy in long-term care: Some crucial distinctions. *Gerontologist* 28 (Suppl.):10–17.

———. 1995. Safety and independence: Rethinking some basic concepts in long-term care. In *Long-Term Care Decisions: Ethical and conceptual dimensions,* ed. L. B. McCullough and N. L. Wilson. Baltimore: Johns Hopkins University Press.

Collopy, B., P. Boyle, and B. Jennings. 1991. New directions in nursing home ethics. *Hastings Center Report* 21 (2 Suppl.): 1–16.

Collopy, B., N. Dubler, and C. Zuckerman. 1990. The ethics of home care: Autonomy and accommodation. *Hastings Center Report* 20 (Special Suppl.).

Diamond, T. 1992. *Making Gray Gold: Narratives of nursing home life.* Chicago: University of Chicago Press.

Dodds, S. 2000. Choice and control in feminist bioethics. In *Relational Autonomy: Feminist perspectives on autonomy, agency and the social self,* ed. C. Mackenzie and N. Stoljar. New York: Oxford University Press.

Dresser, R. 1994. Missing persons: Legal perceptions of incompetent patients. *Rutgers Law Review* 606: 636–47.

Dworkin, R. 1993. *Life's Dominion: An argument about abortion, euthanasia, and individual freedom.* New York: Knopf.

Eckenwiler, L. 2007. Caring about long-term care: An ethical framework for caregiving. Washington, D.C.: Center for American Progress.

England, S. E., et al. 1991. Community care policies and gender justice. In *Critical Perspectives on Aging: The political and moral economy of growing old,* ed. C. E. Estes and M. Minkler. Amityville: Baywood Publishing.

Fahey, C. J. 2007. The ethics of long-term care: Recasting the policy discourse. In *Challenges of an Aging Society: Ethical dilemmas, political issues,* ed. R. A. Pruchno and M. A. Smyer. Baltimore: Johns Hopkins University Press.

Fine, M., and C. Glendinning. 2005. Dependence, independence or interdependence? Revisiting the concepts of "care" and "dependency." *Ageing and Society* 25:602–21.

Flanagan, O. 1991. *Varieties of Moral Personality.* Cambridge: Harvard University Press.

Gerontologist. 1988. Autonomy and long-term care. *Gerontologist* 28 (Special Suppl.).

Gross, J. 2007. Study finds higher costs for caregivers of elderly. *New York Times,* November 19.

Held, V. 2006. *The Ethics of Care: Personal, political, and global.* New York: Oxford University Press.

Hickman, S. E., et al. 2005. Hope for the future: Achieving the original intent of advance directives. *Hastings Center Report* 35 (6 Suppl.):26–30.

High, D. 1991. A new myth about families of older people. *Gerontologist* 31 (5):611–18.

Hoffmaster, B., ed. 2001. *Bioethics in Social Context.* Philadelphia: Temple University Press.

———. 2006. What does vulnerability mean? *Hastings Center Report* 36 (2):38–45.

Hofland, B. F. 1990. Introduction. *Generations* 14 (Suppl.):5–8.

———. 2001. Ethics and aging: A historical perspective. In *Ethics in Community-Based Elder Care,* ed. M. Holstein and P. B. Mitzen. New York: Springer.

Holstein, M. 1999a. *From Rules to Caring Practices: Ethics and community-based care for elders.* Chicago: Park Ridge Center.

———. 1999b. Home care: A case study in injustice. In *Mother Time: Women, ethics and aging,* ed. M. U. Walker. Lanham: Rowman and Littlefield.

———. 2005. A normative defense of universal age-based policies. In *The New Politics of Old Age,* ed. R. B. Hudson. Baltimore: Johns Hopkins University Press.

———. 2007. Long-term care, feminism, and an ethics of solidarity. In *Challenges of an Aging Society: Ethical dilemmas and political issues,* ed. R. A. Pruchno and M. A. Smyer. Baltimore: Johns Hopkins University Press.

Holstein, M., and T. Cole. 1995. Long-term care: An historical reflection. In *Long-Term Care Decisions: Ethical and conceptual dimensions,* ed. L. B. McCullough and N. L. Wilson. Baltimore: Johns Hopkins University Press.

Holstein, M., and M. Minkler. 2003. Self, society, and the "new gerontology." *Gerontologist* 43 (6):787–96.

Hooyman, N., and J. Gonyea. 1995. *Feminist Perspectives on Family Care.* Thousand Oaks: Sage.

Hugman, R. 2005. *New Approaches in Ethics for the Caring Professions.* New York: Palgrave Macmillan.

Jameton, A. 1988. In the borderlands of autonomy: Responsibility in long term care facilities. *Gerontologist* 28 (Suppl.):18–23.

Jecker, N., ed. 1991. *Aging and Ethics: Philosophical problems in gerontology.* Clifton: Humana Press.

———. 1995. What do husbands and wives owe each other in old age? In *Long-Term Care Decisions: Ethical and conceptual dimensions,* ed. L. B. McCullough and N. L. Wilson. Baltimore: Johns Hopkins University Press.

Jennings, B., D. Callahan, and A. Caplan. 1988. Ethical challenges of chronic illness. *Hastings Center Report* 18 (1):1–16.

Jennings, B., G. Kaebnick, and T. Murray, eds. 2005. Improving end of life care: Why has it been so difficult? *Hastings Center Special Report* 35 (6).

Johnson, S. 2005. Making room for dying: End of life care in nursing homes. *Hastings Center Special Report* 35 (6):S37–41.

Jonsen, A. 1998. *The Birth of Bioethics.* New York: Oxford University Press.

Jonsen, A., and S. Toulmin. 1988. *The Abuse of Casuistry: A history of moral reasoning.* Berkeley: University of California Press.

Kane, R., and A. Caplan, eds. 1990. *Everyday Ethics: Resolving dilemmas in nursing home life.* New York: Springer.

———, eds. 1993. *Ethical Conflicts in the Management of Home Care: The case manager's dilemma.* New York: Springer.

Kane, R., and C. Levin. 2001. Who's safe? Who's sorry?: The duty to protect the safety of HCBS consumers. In *Ethics and Community-Based Elder Care*, ed. M. Holstein and P. B. Mitzen. New York: Springer.

Kaufman, S. 2001. Clinical narratives and ethical dilemmas in geriatrics. In *Bioethics in Social Context*, ed. B. Hoffmaster. Philadelphia: Temple University Press.

Kidder, R. 2003. *How Good People Make Tough Decisions*. New York: Simon & Schuster.

Kittay, E. F. 1999. *Love's Labor: Essays on women, equality, and dependency*. New York: Routledge.

Kittay, E. F., and D. T. Meyers. 1987. *Women and Moral Theory*. Lanham: Rowman and Littlefield.

Kuczewski, M. 1999. Ethics in long-term care? Are the principles different? *Theoretical Medicine* 20:15–29.

Lidz, C., L. Fischer, and R. Arnold. 1992. *The Erosion of Autonomy in Long-Term Care*. New York: Oxford University Press.

Lindemann, H. 2006. *An Invitation to Feminist Ethics*. Boston: McGraw Hill.

Lloyd, L. 2004. Mortality and morality: Aging and the ethics of care. *Ageing and Society* 24:235–56.

———. 2006. A caring profession? The ethics of care and social work with older people. *British Journal of Social Work* 36:1171–85.

Lysaught, M. T. 2005. Respect, or, how respect for persons became respect for autonomy. *Journal of Medicine and Philosophy* 29 (6):665–80.

MacKenzie, C, and N. Stoljar, eds. 2000. *Relational Autonomy: Feminist perspectives on autonomy, agency, and the social self*. New York: Oxford University Press.

May, W. 1986. The virtues and the vices of the elderly. In *What Does It Mean to Grow Old: Reflections from the humanities*, ed. T. R. Cole and S. Gadow. Durham: Duke University Press.

McCullough, L. B. 2005. The critical turn in clinical ethics and its continuous enhancement. *Journal of Medicine and Philosophy* 30:1–8.

McCullough, L. B., and N. L. Wilson, eds. 1995a. *Long-Term Care Decisions: Ethical and conceptual dimensions*. Baltimore: Johns Hopkins University Press.

———. 1995b. Managing the conceptual and ethical dimensions of long-term care decision making: A preventive ethics approach. In *Long-Term Care Decisions: Ethical and conceptual dimensions*, ed. L. B. McCullough and N. L. Wilson, 221–40. Baltimore: Johns Hopkins University Press.

Moody, H. 1992. *Ethics in an Aging Society*. Baltimore: Johns Hopkins University Press.

Murray, T., and B. Jennings. 2005. The quest to reform care: Rethinking assumptions and setting new directions. *Hastings Center Report* 35 (6):S52–57.

Neugarten, B., and R. Havighurst, eds. 1973. *Social Policy, Social Ethics, and the Aging Society*. Washington, D.C.: U.S. Government Printing Office.

Nussbaum, M. 2000. *Women and Human Development: The capabilities approach*. Cambridge, UK: Cambridge University Press.

Okin, S. 1989. *Justice, Gender, and the Family*. New York: Basic Books.

Parks, J. 2000. Why gender matters to the euthanasia debate: On decisional capacity and the rejection of women's death requests. *Hastings Center Report* 30 (1):30–36.

———. 2003. *No Place Like Home? Feminist ethics and home health care*. Bloomington: University of Indiana Press.

Parton, N. 2003. Rethinking professional practice: The contribution of social constructionism and feminist "ethics of care." *British Journal of Social Work* 33:1–16.

Polivka, L., and C. Longino. 2006. The emerging postmodern culture of aging and retirement security. In *Aging, Globalization, and Inequality: The new critical gerontology*, ed. J. Baars, D. Dannefer, C. Phillipson, and A. Walker. Amityville: Baywood Publishing.

President's Council on Bioethics. 2005. *Taking Care: Ethical caregiving in our aging society*. Washington, D.C.: President's Council on Bioethics.

Prilleltensky, I., A. Rossiter, and R. Walsh-Bowers. 1996. Preventing harm and prompting ethical discourse in the helping professions: Conceptual, research, analytical, and action frameworks. *Ethics and Behavior* 64 (4):287–306.

Ramsey, P. 1970. *The Patient as Person*. New Haven: Yale University Press.

Sevenhuijsen, S. 2000. Caring in the third way: The relation between obligation, responsibility and care in Third Way discourse. *Critical Social Policy* 20 (1):5–37.

Sherwin, S. 1992. *No Longer Patient: Feminist ethics and health care*. Philadelphia: Temple University Press.

Shield, R. R. 1988. *Uneasy Endings: Everyday life in an American nursing home*. Ithaca: Cornell University Press.

Taylor, C. 1989. *Sources of the Self: The making of modern identity*. Cambridge: Harvard University Press.

Teno, J. M., et al. 2007. Association between advance directives and quality of end-of-life care: A national study. *Journal of the American Geriatrics Society* 55:189–94.

Tronto, J. 1993. *Moral Boundaries: A political argument for an ethics of care*. New York: Routledge.

———. 2001. An ethic of care. In *Ethics in Community-Based Elder Care*, ed. M. Holstein and P. B. Mitzen. New York: Springer.

Twigg, J. 2000. Carework as a form of bodywork. *Ageing and Society* 20:389–411.

Wakabayashi, C., and K. M. Donato. 2006. Does caregiving increase poverty among women in later life? Evidence from the health and retirement survey. *Journal of Health and Social Behavior* 47 (3):258–74.

Walker, M. U. 1992. Feminist ethics and the question of theory. *Hypatia* 7 (3):23–39.

———. 1998. *Moral Understandings: A feminist study in ethics*. New York: Routledge.

———. 2003. *Moral Contexts*. Lanham: Rowman and Littlefield.

Wetle, T. 1995. Ethical issues and value conflicts facing case managers of frail elderly people living at home. In *Long-Term Care Decisions: Ethical and conceptual dimensions*, ed. L. B. McCullough and N. L. Wilson. Baltimore: Johns Hopkins University Press.

PART III

AGE STUDIES IN THE
PUBLIC SPHERE

CHAPTER TWELVE

Age, Meaning, and Place

Cultural Narratives and Retirement Communities

STEPHEN KATZ, PH.D., AND KEVIN MCHUGH, PH.D.

Humanistic studies of aging have elaborated biography, narrative, and life course as important interpretive tools to explore the human experience of living in time. This chapter contributes to this endeavor by looking at habitation as a meaning-making process in the relationship between person and place. Our examples are retirement communities and the ways in which the constitution of their spatial structures, migrational flows, symbolic landscapes, and public imagery represents wider cultural narratives about aging and identity. We argue that such narratives can be contradictory. Today as older adults build life-sustaining environments to challenge age-denigrating or age-denying spatial orders, they also face the dictates of post-traditional aging in the twentieth and twenty-first centuries. The differentiating cultural features of post-traditional aging have been theorized in various contexts by writers such as Mike Featherstone, Mike Hepworth, Andrew Blaikie, Kathleen Woodward, and Simon Biggs. These features include the fragmentation and blurring of traditional chronological stages and roles, advances in longevity technologies and life expectancy, expansion of lifestyle consumerism oriented to older groups, and new work and retirement arrangements. As Gilleard and Higgs note, "post-traditional culture extends equally to life after retirement as well as before" (2000, p. 25). Hence, while post-traditional aging can offer older individuals new opportunities for self-identity, community, and mobility, it is often promoted through "positive aging" cultures that stretch middle age into a troubling celebration of growing older as an ageless, timeless enterprise.

The dilemmas of post-traditional aging and the contradictions of its narratives form the background to our discussion of retirement spaces. Specifically, Stephen Katz focuses on Canadian snowbird retirement culture in Florida and how retirement "flow" adds to our understanding of retirement "time." Kevin McHugh follows with an interpretive analysis of retirement communities in Arizona, home of the Del Webb Sun City phenomenon and some new trends targeted to empty nesters and pre-retirees. In both cases, we ask how people and places change and age together in such communities, where the nexus of discourse, landscape, and place speaks to us about the new possibilities and mobility of aging in Sunbelt America despite its utopian aura. The idea of a utopian gerontopolis is raised in the concluding section. We begin with an overview of spatial gerontology and its relevance to the gerontological humanities.

Part I: Spatial Gerontology and Canadian Snowbirds (by Stephen Katz)
Spatial Gerontology

Spatial gerontology is an interdisciplinary component of aging studies comprising three subfields: ethnographic microsociology, environmental gerontology, and migrational-global analysis. These areas share common ground where their research examines the residential arrangements and adaptational resources that facilitate (or limit) an individual's adjustment to aging. Ethnographic microsociology draws on social constructivist and interactionist models to elucidate the subjective and symbolic qualities of built environments. For example, Jaber Gubrium's (1975, 1993) approach to nursing homes frames them as microcomplexes of architectural, administrative, and familial emotional interactions and power relations. Similarly, Frida Furman (1997) finds a vibrant interactive world among older women and their community within their local hair salon. Even the lobby of an apartment building where older residents meet, if observed as an ethnographic site, becomes rich in meaning about the making of age identities in everyday life (Gamliel, 2000). Qualitative ethnographies can also explain how historical changes to the economic and symbolic values of large urban spaces can affect the personal experiences of aging inhabitants (see Vesperi, 1985).

The discoveries of ethnographic research provide an important inside perspective on aging-in-place debates, which are a major element of the second subfield, environmental gerontology (EG). As Wahl and Weisman (2003) show, EG has a long history (see also Andrews and Phillips, 2004). However, EG became well represented in gerontological scholarship only with the work of M. Powell Lawton. Lawton, along with others (Lawton, Windley, and Byerts, 1982; Altman, Lawton, and Wohlwill, 1984), examined the relationship between competency, adaptation, context, and environment in the lives of older persons. As the researchers worked on identifying the "person-environment fit" in different situations, the data they generated were significant for understanding how people can negotiate the shifting relationship between independent and dependent conditions of their lives. Thus, much of the EG research focuses on the practicalities of housing modification and design, residential decisions, displacement and relocation, and the role of localities and neighborhoods in planning new environments. Underlying such issues are questions about "aging in place" that inform decisions about the benefits or disadvantages of living at home or in familiar surroundings for older people who face physical, cognitive, behavioral, or financial problems. Such questions also extend to ethical concerns about how residential arrangements sustain quality of life (Heywood, Oldman, and Means, 2002; Rowles and Ravdal, 2002).

EG research joins ethnographic microsociological studies where together they tackle the issue of attachment to place through the material worlds of things. Any tour of a typical home and its cherished objects evokes a lifetime of memories, stories, and creative narratives about how place and resident came to be and grow together. Likewise, any upset and change to the intimate and delicate balance between private and public spaces, especially where home care services are required, can be disruptive of the resident's identity (see Twigg, 2000). Complementing the ethnographic and EG focus on micro- and local conditions of age and place is gerontological research that explores the geodemographic features of migration and global processes. Migrational-global analysis (as we call it) is macro-oriented and constitutes a recent third subfield in spatial gerontology. Here matters concern how the mix of migrational movements, global processes, and aging populations loosens traditional spatial boundaries and opens new social territories. In the work of social theorists such as John Urry (2000) or Armand Mattelart (2000), even the concept of *society* itself is of limited value when it comes to grasping the global movements of peoples and cultures, as they operate in terms of *flows* that include diasporas, transcultural lifestyles, transnational economic networks, diverse citizenries, touristic identities, migrant labor pools, virtual webs of connectivity, and borderless transportation systems.

Chris Phillipson has further argued that globalization "has elevated aging to an issue that transcends individual societies or states" (2006, p. 47) and, as such, "disturbs and reconfigures conventional narratives about the meaning of growing older" (p. 48). Older populations are no longer static and immobile; rather, they stretch across places and environments in ways that both sacrifice normative structures of lifelong security and pursue pathways to experimental lifestyles and identities. The globalizing and fragmenting of relations between identity, community, and place have allowed more people to imagine and retell their futures through choice of place(s).

For example, in Canada, if the country's changing places, cities, and regions were mapped as a geography based on age, they would present a fascinating image of these spatial dynamics of Canadian life courses. Victoria (British Columbia) has become the nation's "retirement city," while Barrie (Ontario) is becoming one of the youngest places. Each city faces specific housing, transportation, and zoning challenges as local governments struggle to serve their different demographic groups. Some areas such as the vast suburbs of Toronto were built for young families and based on the automobile. However, as the suburban populations in Toronto age, the community planning and public services to accommodate the growing number of older residents are not in place and will be challenged in the future (Anderssen and Mick, 2007). Meanwhile, Elliot Lake, a former Ontario mining town, has been transformed into a gray-boom center for retirement living, where in the last 20 years the median age has gone from 22 to 55, with one-third of the town over 65 (White, 2007).

Phillipson also reminds us that the new mobility creates a politics of belonging that excludes people from certain environments, especially in urban settings that are being re-narrated or "rebranded" as exciting, youth-oriented centers of global consumerism and prosperity (Phillipson, 2007). Here older groups can find themselves marginalized from the very communities they helped to build and likely discover their lifelong biographical goals disrupted by new cosmopolitan environments. Further, the consumer lifestyles of global living depend on widening life-course inequalities, where wealthier parts of the world are buoyed by the stifling hierarchies and stunted life chances of people aging in poorer parts of the world (see Dannefer, 2003). These examples illustrate something of the spatial dynamics of aging in post-traditional society. As Anthony Giddens claims, in traditional cultures "most social life was localised," while in post-traditional cultures, along with migration, "the lifespan becomes separated from the externalities of place, while place itself is undermined by the expansion of disembedding mechanisms" (1991, p. 146).

Into this contradictory global landscape enter forms of individualization that accompany the degradation of universal entitlements to care. The creation and celebration of global, post-traditional aging identities also come with a moral edict to live in ways that maximize individual responsibility in the service of meeting new overarching political goals of minimizing risk and dependency. The projects of self-discovery for elder pioneers in new retirement spaces are not immune from the markets and politics of neoliberal social programs. Integral to the cultural narratives of positive aging, therefore, is its governance through the coercive individualism of global processes that erode the subsidies and services of welfare states and national economies. Hence, the geopolitics of aging today presents a double challenge: both to draw from and to resist the global reordering of those social spaces where care, continuity, generation, and community coexist.

Snowbirds and the Cultural Narratives of Sociability, Mobility, and Difference

One of the most interesting places where all three subfields of spatial gerontology and their associated geopolitical issues converge is the Sun City retirement communities and the older migrational and "snowbird" groups that inhabit them. Beginning in the 1960s and built across the Sunbelt areas of Florida, Texas, California, Arizona, and most recently in Mexico, these communities exemplify retirement lifestyles that boast active, healthy aging and mobile, transcultural networks.[1] Critics have pointed to the idealized images of ageless aging promoted by these communities. They are also seen as isolating advantaged groups into gated, naturalized enclaves represented as utopian "havens," "villages," and "estates" (Laws, 1996; McHugh, 2000; McHugh and Larson-Keagy, 2005). The exclusivity of Sun City environments means, as McHugh comments, that they "are defined as much by the absent image—old poor folks in deteriorating neighbourhoods in cold, gray northern cities and towns—as by the image presented: handsome, healthy, comfortably middle-class 'seniors,' busily filling sun-filled days" (2000, p. 113). In other words, the retirement Sunbelt is a spatial and cultural expression of accumulated social inequalities embedded in the life courses and biographies of aging individuals. These issues will be elaborated further in the following sections of the chapter.

Here we need to explore the fact that these communities, once they are built and inhabited, become human environments that link the experience of aging with cultural narratives of mobility and sociability in unique ways. In the early 1950s, sociologist G. C. Hoyt studied one of the original migrational retirement "parks" in Florida, the Bradenton Trailer Park founded in 1936. He discovered that while climate had been a big factor in attracting people to the park, it was "sociability" that kept them there (Hoyt, 1954, p. 366). And sociability continues to be the interactive force that draws mobile aging identities together. It is a keyword in the cultural narrative that suggests that retired persons gather together because of shared experience, age, and lifestyle. Sociability is especially germane in the context of Canadian snowbirds, many of whom occupy mobile park homes as well as other kinds of accommodations and communities in Florida around the area that Hoyt studied.

The term *snowbird* is a curious metaphor about sociability, because there are no such actual birds, ornithologically speaking. (There are also *sunbirds* who migrate from south to north to escape the heat of southern climates and *snowflakes* who stay for short periods of time.) Yet, *snowbird* is a perfect metaphor because it implies flight, seasonality, nesting, and flock-sociability in different locales. Snowbirds are also a case of what John Urry (2000) refers to as a "mobility" of global citizens who move across boundaries and borders without loss of rights or status. They signal a new relationship to "home" from its being a stable place to a distribution of negotiable places along with the nomadic excursions between them. The cultural narrative of mobility implies that aging identities for snowbirds are also multiple, attached to flight, flow, and flock. Hockey and James comment that groups such as snowbirds "exemplify a practice which not only challenges age-based conceptions of leisure, but in addition disrupts notions of home-based family life as an increasingly and necessary sedentary practice towards the end of the life-course" (2003, p. 176).

While it is difficult to calculate snowbird numbers, estimates often suggest that at least half a million stay in Florida for at least three months a year (see Smith and House, 2006). As Coates, Healy, and Morrison remark about snowbirds, "they are certainly responsible for bringing Canadians, Americans, and Mexicans together on a regular basis more than any other social, cultural, or economic force in North American life" (2002, p. 438).[2] Earlier research on the first large-scale survey of Canadian snowbirds in the late 1980s carried out by Richard D. Tucker, Charles Longino Jr., Larry Mullins, and Victor W. Marshall was published in a series of papers about the relationship between migration and permanence (Tucker et al., 1988, 1992; Marshall and Tucker, 1990; Longino et al., 1991). The teams also discovered that it is a matter of degree or gradient rather than a binary distinction between a "here" and a "there," thus snowbird culture provided new meaning to traditional conditions of residence, territory, distance, and portability of resources.

As part of their mobility, snowbirds form their own moveable networks that attract other snowbirds. Longino and Marshall review a study of snowbirds and report that they "were nomadic in the sense that their social ties were primarily with the same migrants in the communities they shared at both ends of the move. Their ties were not to places but to the migrating community itself" (1990, p. 234). Such ties in snowbird residences and parks are symbolically fortified through the availability of Canadian TV and newspapers such as *Canada News, The Sun Times of Canada, Le Soleil de la Floride*, and *RVTimes*. As Coates, Healy, and Morrison claim, "within these seasonal communities, unique fragment societies have emerged" (2002, p. 442). Indeed, the sense of migrational community is strong. As I learned in my field research with snowbird communities in Florida, even people who had lost their spouses return as "single" individuals to the snowbird flock. However, given the differences in health care systems between Canada and the United States, for snowbirds who become ill or need care, return to Canada is always the preferred option. For those who are ill, the health insurance costs of traveling or living (or dying) in America can be prohibitive.

On the one hand, the symbolic products, mobile groups, variety of residential places, seasonal communities, and metaphorical identities give snowbird culture its sociability, along with the age patterns of the groups themselves. On the other hand, the homogeneous narratives of group mobility and aging sociability are also crosscut by other narratives and realities about social difference as they are generated through spatial relations. For instance, in the smaller northern home communities of snowbirds in Canada, the loss of substantial numbers of residents during winter months can cause a loss of income to the communities, and possibly reduced participation in voluntarism, charitable work, recreational organizations, and the local sense of pride (Coates, Healy, and Morrison, 2002). And in the southern migrational communities, where most Canadian snowbirds are financially independent and healthier, they bring to their host economies a potentially higher level of prosperity through taxes, real estate, and consumer purchasing than local residents can maintain. This has led to concerns that wealthier snowbirds draw off the medical and service resources from local needs, although snowbird demands on geriatric services in Florida are hardly overwhelming (Marshall and Tucker, 1990; Longino et al., 1991; Radcliff, Dobalian, and Duncan, 2005).

Added to these social fissures, where class, cultural, and age differences can clash in the spatial distribution of permanent versus seasonal residents, are the implications of tense intergenerational narratives as well. In 1998, I visited Maple Leaf Estates, also called the Maple Leaf Golf and Country Club, which is a Port Charlotte resident-owned snowbird community in Florida largely inhabited by Canadians (see Katz, 2005). Before being devastated by Hurricane Charley on August 19, 2004, the park had more than 1000 mobile homes, three clubhouses, four swimming pools, five tennis courts, a library, a fitness center, a greenhouse, a golf course, and a lake stocked with fish.[3] During the winter months, the resident numbers swell and the mainly Canadian Board of Directors manages the park's affairs. Because the residents purchased the park in 1990, they have developed their own governance of it that includes regulations around driving, parking, cycling, use of facilities, and design of residences. The most important rule, however, is that the park exists for and is dedicated to people 55 or older. Children and younger people are allowed to visit, but not to stay. A note in the December 1998 issue of the park's newsletter *Accents* outlines some telling generational guidelines for Christmas visitors:

> We believe that as homeowners and residents of MLE we have an opportunity to deal both creatively and proactively with the projected influx of children into our Park during the coming Christmas Season. We are referring primarily to teenagers who are betwixt and between adults and the young children. Younger children are constantly under the supervision of parents or family members, and their use of Park facilities is largely limited to the kiddies swimming pool. Our challenge is to develop some creative recreational opportunities for teenagers during their stay in MLE. (*Accents*, 1998, p. 10)

In this sense, Maple Leaf Estates appears to embody some of the Sun City retirement characteristics pointed out by the critics: it is a privileged, leisure-oriented lifestyle enclave, built by property developers who profit by fostering fantastical and protective age-segregated communities. Therein new aging identities are bonded to post-traditional environments, where even the children who visit must submit to sunny retirement activities as elders-in-training. The age-graded, racially white and middle-class homogeneity is further expressed in the sameness of the park's houses and roads and unspoken lack of diversity. However, to Canadians the presence of surveillance and security systems at the park has less to do with a Canadian way of life than with adapting to an American way of life and its perceived risks and hazards. After all, many Canadians think America is a dangerous place where race and social inequality are violently emplaced across the country. To live as Canadians-in-America, despite the Canadian-named roads and places, the clubhouses serving Canadian beer, and the gates flying Canadian flags, means becoming temporarily socialized to an American concept of the retreat to safe haven.

As a fragment society consisting of mobile retirees from across cultures and places, Maple Leaf residents and managers noted, in my interviews with them, that the park is "in transition" between generations. They questioned whether or not younger cohorts would be interested in such an age-dedicated retirement or perhaps place new demands on the park, looking for alternative activities and seeking different residency arrangements. Would the rules disallowing younger groups from visiting or living in the park have to change? Above all, how might Charlotte County itself, where in many areas 50 percent of the population is already over 65, shift from being dominated by resident-owned, age-stratifying retirement communities to ones where future generations would experiment with new ways of aging unrelated to retirement? These questions were about generation, social space, mobility, family, identity, community, sociability, and the cultural tug of aging through time across places. They entwine the concerns of spatial gerontology and the contradictory cultural narratives about the meaning of age in spatial terms in ways that articulate their subjective dimension. Such questions also mark Canadian snowbird culture in Sunbelt Florida and their future prospects together as a rich opportunity to explore the humanistic side of aging studies. In the next parts of this chapter, Kevin McHugh continues to extend this opportunity by considering the changing spatiocultural relations between age, identity, and movement in the retirement communities of Arizona, beginning with some thoughts about the place of place itself.

Part II: "Placing" Sunbelt Retirement Communities in Arizona (by Kevin McHugh)

Place is the first and last of all things. Our entrance to, and exit from, this earthly realm is "place-ful" (Casey, 1997). Consider the opening words in Annie Dillard's homage to home place, the hills and valleys of western Pennsylvania, in her book *An American Childhood*:

When everything else has gone from my brain—the President's name, the state capitals, the neighborhoods where I lived, and then my own name and what it was on earth that I sought, and then at length the faces of my friends, and finally the faces of my family—when all this has dissolved, what will be left, I believe, is topology: the dreaming memory of land as it lay this way and that. (1987, p. 4)

Dillard's playful metaphor of subtraction in nearing death's door speaks to the plenitude of being in place—as patterned land and life among family, friends, and neighbors. Life in the singular does not place make. We enjoin and constitute place collectively, slipping and sliding into the future, generations unfolding, overlapping, and pushing forward as a fugue (McHugh, 2007). The press of everyday life and practice is scarcely noticed as the very creation and re-creation of place; we swim in place like fish in the sea. Only after the fact, when we stop and reflect, might we (re)call our lives as a journey in and through place, so that we "see" place as shifting sand bars in a coursing stream.

The places in aging that command our attention here are the senior worlds of Arizona, epicenter of Sunbelt leisure lifestyles. These enclaves are supportive, life-sustaining environments for groups of retirees and empty nesters who dance to the tune of "active aging." We pause and reflect on retirement enclaves in terms of the trilogy of place, community, and identity. En route we genuflect to active adult retirement communities as a utopian gesture of the past half century, meditate on these settings as idealizations of community, and then point to ongoing cultural shifts in aging that are sounding the death knell of age-restricted enclaves.

Immaculate Conception

Utopia has long captivated the human spirit and imagination. Sir Thomas More's neologism—whose roots ingeniously connote both "good place" and "no place"—is commonly used today as a noun to signify visionary schemes that seek idealized perfection, and pejoratively to ridicule unrealistic and flawed prescriptions for living that are deemed impracticable (Kateb, 1972; Kumar, 1987, 1991). It is no accident that the term *perfect* is deployed in advertisements promoting Sunbelt retirement places with nary a whiff of irony or satire (McHugh, 2003), and that residents themselves extol the virtues of retirement communities unabashedly. Pride in place attains lofty heights in retirement enclaves, an ongoing hyperbolic stream that originated with Del Webb's "Immaculate Conception" named Sun City, Arizona, located on the outskirts of Phoenix (Sturgeon, 1992). From this inaugural community launched in 1960 we have witnessed the great proliferation of Sun Cities and "copycat" leisure-based retirement communities across America. Testimonials expressed by Sun City, Arizona, residents in a 1995 community study are illustrative of this hyperbolic history in place boosterism:

> People love the community. I have never been in a community where people are prouder.
>
> And we definitely have pride in Sun City. Well, it's the greatest place that's ever been put together anywhere in the United States.
>
> I have some apprehension about dying, because to go to heaven won't be as good as this.
>
> I celebrate Sun City. It's a great community . . . In most cities, the elderly are not accepted as full card-carrying citizens. They're looked down upon and shuffled aside. They have gifts, you know. (McHugh and Larson-Keagy, 2005, p. 249)

These affirmations speak to salubrious lives of many citizens in Sun City–like communities. There is ample evidence that these are amenity-rich environments that foster active, healthy lifestyles (Marans, Hunt, and Vakalo, 1984), places where order, civility, and friendliness reign (Kastenbaum, 1993), and places where community means inculcating a sense of belonging, camaraderie, and identity in a society that denigrates old age (McHugh and Larson-Keagy, 2005). Sunbelt retirement communities surely have done their part in "placing" active aging and the "busy ethic" (Ekerdt, 1986; Katz, 2000) on the map of "the third age" (Laslett, 1996).

There seems something unreal or hyper-real about retirement communities, about retirees sequestered in neat and tidy settings, pursuing leisure lifestyles en masse. Russell, long-time Sun Citian, does not hesitate when asked to describe the ideal community: "Well, the ideal community would be Sun City with people not getting old" (McHugh, 2007, p. 297). The unreality of an ageless, timeless place underscores Russell's freeze-frame view of Sun City: "The city is not changing, but the people who are coming here are changing. They come and adapt to this lifestyle." This is a powerfully conservative view of place as normatively scripted, a concretized living museum of Del Webb's "modernist" utopian vision. Unlike utopia as a spatial play of imaginative possibilities, utopia when materialized in spatial form becomes rigidified, ossified, and, ultimately, "degenerate" in that this stultifies questioning of the social order and state of affairs (Marin, 1984; Harvey, 2000). This is a theme we will take up again in the concluding section, but now we turn to the questions of idealized communities.

Two Idealizations

Place is more than a backdrop or stage on which social life unfolds. In the parlance of social geography, place, self, and society are relational and mutually constituted (Sack,

1997; Entrikin, 1999). Identities are embodied and emplaced. Who am I? Who con-stitutes a "we"? How do we live? And extending to moral geographies, how *should* we live? What are *good* and *just* places (Tuan, 1989; Smith, 2000; Sack, 2003)? With place making and identity in mind, it is instructive to pass Sunbelt retirement enclaves through the lenses of two idealizations woven through political philosophy and dis-course: (1) community as the commingling of like people and (2) community as galvanizing diverse peoples in civil society.

If community entails shared values, shared territory, and a shared sense of belong-ing and togetherness (Anderson, 1991; Blakely and Synder, 1999; Delanty, 2003), enclaves of retirees and preretirees pursuing leisure lifestyles surely are deserving of the community seal. Anyone who spends time in retirement communities cannot help but be impressed by likeness and homogeneity, as these are congregations dominated by white, middle- to upper-middle-income Americans who tend toward social, cul-tural, and political conservatism (FitzGerald, 1986; Kastenbaum, 1993; McHugh, 2007). People in leisure-based enclaves identify strongly with community brethren, embrace the script of sociability and activity, and see themselves as soldiers battling against such negative stereotypes of older age as disengagement and decline (McHugh and Larson-Keagy, 2005).

Andrew Blaikie suggests that lifestyle enclaves "are not communities at all" (2005, pp. 168–69), drawing ammunition from Bellah et al. (1988, p. 72): "whereas commu-nity attempts to be an inclusive whole, celebrating the interdependence of public and private life and of the different callings of all, lifestyle is fundamentally segmental and celebrates the narcissism of similarity." Blaikie is nodding toward community as the ideal of pluralism, openness, and inclusion whereby diverse "groups dwell in the city alongside one another . . . interacting in city spaces" (Young, 1990, p. 227). Pluralists are skeptical of community as "birds of a feather flocking together" for this invites romanticized, nostalgic longings for togetherness, whether national or local, which engenders exclusionary impulses, marginalization, inequalities, and antagonism (Sen-nett, 1990; Young, 1990, 2000). On these grounds, it is not surprising that Sunbelt retirement communities have been subject to critique as symptomatic of escapism, separation, and segregation in America, problems already mentioned above (Kasten-baum, 1993; Laws, 1993, 1995; McHugh, Gober, and Borough, 2002; McHugh and Larson-Keagy, 2005).

Rather than seeing Sunbelt retirement communities in unidirectional terms—as seniors escaping to preserves with like-minded folk to fill sun-drenched days—we believe the creation and legal sanction of age-segregated settings is part of an unwrit-ten social compact and currently popular cultural narrative about aging in America: the mutual separation of generations. For example, a pervasive theme in Ralph Scho-enstein's (1986) melancholic account of retirement communities, *Every Day Is Sunday*, is that elders, removed from families, speak often about not wishing to interfere in the lives of their children, of not wanting to be a burden. Listen to the words of a Sun City gentleman who views a strong connection with one's children as problematic:

> You have another category of people, those who can't leave their children. I mean, some people, they've got their children saddled right to their hip and they go into trauma if they can't be with their kids. In other words, they're not independent of them. In some cases, the kids are crying, and they say: "You've got to come back." And so you have that problem. (McHugh, 2007, p. 300)

In conversing with residents it is easy enough to unearth vapors of escapism and what Robert Kastenbaum (1993) terms a "fortress mentality." A former editor of the *Daily News Sun* expressed these in memorable terms during an interview about community life in Sun City:

> There is a certain kind of isolation in Sun City which is—well, I guess as a group they feel as though they're aligned against the outside, and those white walls, those white walls around the community mean a great deal to them. It keeps out crime and it keeps out people they don't want. It keeps out young people and it keeps out children and it keeps out all the things that were attendant on their lives when they lived other places. And so there is a concerted feeling of splendid isolation. (McHugh and Larson-Keagy, 2005, p. 251)

In the Sun Cities in Phoenix, one need only inquire about the absence of children or ask about funding public education to tap a defensive posture; seniors are quick to defend their communities. The history of political conflict between the Sun Cities and surrounding communities over school funding measures, control of school district governing boards, and de-annexing from school districts to avoid paying local school taxes has exacted a deep cultural wound in the Northwest Valley of Phoenix. The latest flare-up occurred in the mid- to late 1990s, in which a group of seniors in a newly developed portion of Sun City West defeated school funding measures, took control of all five seats on the Dysart School District Board, and attempted to de-annex from the district (McHugh, Gober, and Borough, 2002). Since this latest battle in the "Sun City Wars," all has been quiet on the northwestern front. Residents in newer communities on the urban fringe such as Sun City Grand and Sun City Festival show no inclination to hassle about paying local school taxes or maneuver to de-annex from school districts.

Requiem for the Retirement Community

In large measure, we have been singing yesterday's song, looking back in appraising the leisure-based model of retirement living wildly popularized by Del Webb, the Sun

Cities, and more recent jazzed-up, amenity-laden versions of the same. What does the future portend? Do we hear today the opening notes in a requiem for the retirement community?

First of all, we are witnessing a decline in the age requirement for entry into existing adult-only communities in the Phoenix metropolitan region. The "55 or better" slogan is being eroded as a defining signature in the residential landscape. A few years ago, Leisure World lowered its age requirement to 45 years and Sun Lakes to 40, and in 2007, Sun City Grand followed suit with a reduction to 45 years of age for the purchase of resale homes, on the heels of a similar lowering by nearby Westbrook Village. Reducing the age requirement is a maneuver to slow the process of community aging, to try and retain a youthful image in the face of a highly competitive residential market for the hearts and pocketbooks of folks in midlife, empty nesters, and early retirees.

In one instance, a Phoenix area retirement community lost their age restrictions altogether and is now open to people of all ages, owing to a legal challenge and subsequent ruling by the attorney general of Arizona. In 1998, the attorney general ruled that age restrictions in Youngtown were invalid, as this community had not properly established age stipulations in original deeds, which, through a cascade effect, complicated and, ultimately, invalidated the age-overlay zoning ordinance established in 1986 (Fletchall, 2005). Youngtown, a modest community of small ranch-style homes and a minimalist lake, was founded in 1954, predating Del Webb's original Sun City by six years. Owing to its smaller size (3,000 residents), humble homes, and lack of amenities, few people have ever heard of Youngtown, which lies in the shadow of its giant neighbor, Sun City. Youngtown's luster as a quaint senior haven has long grown dim, as retirees look to settle in newer, more sprite communities such as Sun Lakes, Sun City West, Sun City Grand, and Sun City Festival. The legal challenge and loss of age restrictions proved the death knell in a community already waning as a retiree magnet. In wake of the loss of age restrictions in 1998, some Youngtown seniors opted to relocate to nearby Sun City or elsewhere, others have passed away, and the remaining linger. Owing to modest, affordable homes and its location in a suburban zone of population expansion, Youngtown is rapidly transitioning to a community of younger, working-class families, many of whom are Latino (Fletchall, 2005). Might other long-time retirement communities and villages in the Phoenix region follow suit?

Second, many development companies in Arizona are now marketing smaller communities with no age restrictions, upscale places promoting niche lifestyles and social distinction, not passé images of yesteryear (read ABSC: Anything But Sun City). These communities are popular among childless couples, empty nesters, and early retirees and, thus, will evolve as de facto places in post-traditional aging. Del

Webb Corporation (now part of Pulte Homes), for example, has marketed a suite of trendy communities of this genre across the Phoenix urban fringe with melodious Mediterranean-inspired names, such as Terravita, Bellasera, Corte Bella, and Solera.

Third, Del Webb Corporation has birthed what is termed the "multigenerational community" under the identity tag "Anthem." The inaugural Anthem is a large, sprawling, master-planned affair situated in the Sonora desert 32 miles north of Phoenix (Romig, 2004). Here the advantages of age diversity and mixing are touted, although, tellingly, Anthem is spatially separated into two lifestyle spheres: Anthem Country Club, "gate-guarded, resort living" (popular among empty nesters and re- tirees) and Anthem Parkside, "real neighborhood living" (for families). As of this writing, three more multigenerational Anthems are being built on the far-flung fringes of Phoenix.

Trends in community development and marketing are mold and mirror of shifting societal attitudes and wider cultural narratives about age and aging (Phillipson, 1998; Blaikie, 1999; Katz, 2005). A fascinating and far-reaching revolution underway in America is the cultural "eradication" or "death" of old age (Bauman, 1992), evident in the rampant proliferation of antiaging products and in the offing of spiritual elixirs as alternatives to growing old, as perusing the New Age section in the bookstore demon- strates. Old age is being erased, supplanted by agelessness and the endless prolongation of midlife, which is now a stand-in for the age-old desire for perpetual youth (Feather- stone and Hepworth, 1991; Kastenbaum, 1995; Andrews, 1999; McHugh, 2000), part of a process we have labeled as post-traditional aging. In a society obsessed with antiaging and agelessness, will a cultural form that explicitly inscribes and emplaces age, the *de jure* retirement community, survive long in the American landscape?

Part III: Dwelling in Movement (by Kevin McHugh)
Place and Movement

The first part of this chapter discussed the importance of the relationship between place and movement, particularly as it emerges within practices of recreational mobil- ity in retirement. In this third concluding section about age and mobility, we wish to emphasize again that place and movement are inescapable bedfellows. The cultural geographer Yi-Fu Tuan sounds this coupling with the aphorism, "place is a pause in movement" (1978, p. 14), while J. B. Jackson, the noted landscape historian, opens his essay *Roads Belong in the Landscape* with a rhetorical question, playfully pitting one against the other: "Which came first, the house or the road leading to the house?" (1994, p. 189). In the modern world we live the dialectical tension *home and away*, as people simultaneously wish to make home and leave home (Sopher, 1979; Williams and Van Patten, 2006).

In some cultural quarters and settings one, home or away, may be favored vis-à-vis the other, yet this is a necessary relation. The dialectic assumes an origin, a home place, from which one ventures forth and to which one returns, the circle completed. These sentiments perhaps ring a tad cliché in today's "Astral America," a culture of speed, circulation, and "star-blast vectors," to draw on the language of Jean Baudrillard (1988, p. 27). Can there be true home places in a culture of speed, in a world of time-space compression (Harvey, 1989), hypermobility, and roiling social and cultural change (Cresswell, 2006; Sheller and Urry, 2006)? Is the notion of home a quaint fiction, vestige of a past—real or imagined—to which we cling, an elixir that seeks to quell ontological insecurity and existential anxiety (Giddens, 1991; Sanders, 1993)?

In mulling over these questions my mind turns to folk in their retirement years who take to the highway, crisscrossing North America in recreational vehicles (Counts and Counts, 2001). Several years ago, Bob Mings and I found striking differences in life histories and sense of place and home among migratory seniors with whom we interacted while they spent all or part of the winter season in Phoenix-area RV parks and resorts (McHugh and Mings, 1996). One group exhibited deep roots and unwavering attachment to a long-term home place, such that travel and spending time elsewhere, such as Phoenix, were a "reach" from home. We described their space-time path as circular, with return home as certain as the coming of spring. Another group of snowbirds were suspended between dual homes, typically a northern abode and a winter residence in Arizona, akin to the Canadian snowbirds in Florida. Seniors suspended between dual homes expressed a pendular space-time path, swinging back and forth, neither place dominant in social or emotional terms. Finally, a third group of traveling folk with whom we engaged were footloose in that they did not demonstrate long-term attachment with any particular place. Footloose couples typically broke from home as young adults and, in pursuing education and career, moved from place to place, never establishing deep roots. Places and homes served as way stations in life. We characterized their space-time paths as linear, always pushing forward, looking toward the horizon (McHugh and Mings, 1996).

RV Nomads

An intriguing group of footloose retirees are so-called full-timers, people who sell their place-based home and live full-time on the road in their RV, dwelling in movement. Gary Hawes-Davis's documentary film, *This Is Nowhere*, captures the ironic and paradoxical nature of American culture through the prism of RV travelers who circumnavigate North America camping overnight in Wal-Mart parking lots. Using varying film speeds and a jagged, edgy musical score, the film captures the cacophony of vehicles, signs, sights, and sounds of highways and highway strip landscapes. This is

America in motion. Filmmaker Hawes-Davis elevates motion and placelessness to an art form (McHugh, 2005).

This Is Nowhere is especially rich in balderdash of peregrinating people who revel in mobility as freedom and extol the virtue of America's natural bounty, even as they seek the sameness and convenience of camping and shopping at Wal-Mart. Mobility and freedom take an escapist turn among some RV nomads. Dave Jenkins speaks of not having roots or ties; he and his wife come and go as they please. Dave remarks that if there happened to be a loud party in the Wal-Mart parking lot tonight, he would fire up his rig and move on, something not possible for people living in homes who have rowdy neighbors.

Equating movement with freedom is often draped with historical sensibilities and allusions. Steve Ohms likens his freedom in mobility to westward-trekking pioneers in covered wagons, and he comments, "Of course, there weren't any roads back then—that made it a whole lot more free." Leon North explains that most of his travels are based on wars: "We've seen just about everything to do with the wars that have been in the United States. That's basically been our history: one war after another." Garrett Covington III is reading the journals of Lewis and Clark as he travels west in his motor home equipped with multiple computers, GIS software, a GPS unit, and four satellite dishes. Garrett, a retired aerospace engineer, is a pioneer in our technological age. He wishes to know at all times where he is located on planet earth. And this technology allows Garrett to map and locate all the Wal-Marts in North America in charting his westward course.

This Is Nowhere imparts an existential flavor. Among the most poignant scenes in the film, especially for viewers attuned to age, are shots of older couples ambling about Wal-Mart parking lots, seemingly lost in the crosscurrents of America. These images whisper of loosened moorings in aging, of disconnection from place and community, reminding me of a stanza from Donald Hall's poem, *The Exile*:

> In years, and in the numbering of space
> Moving away from what we grew to know
> We stray like paper blown from place to place
> Impelled by every element to go. (1990, p. 9)

In one scene in *This Is Nowhere* we view a black dog with a slight limp, a stray I name Lucky, making her way across the Wal-Mart parking lot and, then, across a busy highway, avoiding onrushing traffic. In viewing this scene I could not help but muse, "are we not all lonely travelers making our way as best we can in the face of cultural clutter and our own infirmities" (McHugh, 2005, p. 85)? This is the journey in aging, dwelling in movement, in and through place.

Part IV: Conclusion (by Stephen Katz and Kevin McHugh)

Whether in the Sunbelt coastal regions of Florida or the desert enclaves of Arizona, or even the parking lots of Wal-Mart, we can look to these as spatial expressions of what it means to grow older in post-traditional society. By combining approaches from spatial gerontology and humanistic studies of aging, we can also discover in such spaces some of the lived practices by which people negotiate retired identities through cultural narratives of generational sociability and experimental mobility. Behind our work on retirement spaces, however, looms a larger question about utopian aging in our time. As mentioned above, the image of utopia is often evoked in advertisements about tropical and desert retirement places, despite their different environments and lifestyle activities, as small heavens on earth that promise leisure and health to hard-working elites. As Robert Kastenbaum (2008) demonstrates, this idea was also part of the fantasy of utopia as it was first articulated almost five centuries ago by Sir Thomas More in *Utopia* (1516). More characterized Utopia as an age-friendly, community-dedicated, family-oriented society where aging was a moral virtue because people lived longer as well. The problem, as Kastenbaum argues, is that the strict regulatory world of More's Utopia also marginalized or criminalized free expression and creative difference (and had a system of slavery and war). Saved from the violent Europe of More's time, the denizens of Utopia paid for their life of contentment with obeisance to its stifling codes of human control.

Kastenbaum, by way of More, asks if utopia is the best response to the prospects and problems of aging and old age, and if an idealized society unconnected to reality should be our dream for a gerontopolis. Our case studies and interpretive analyses of retirement communities have also been asking this question. Looking to Michel Foucault's work on "heterotopia" (1986) expands the question further. For Foucault, heterotopias are "counter-sites, a kind of effectively enacted utopia in which the real sites, all the other real sites, can be found within culture, are simultaneously represented, contested, and inverted" (1986, p. 24). Heterotopias are "other places" into which converge the contradictions of all places. For Foucault, these include prisons, psychiatric hospitals, and retirement homes, but also brothels, cemeteries, and museums (pp. 25–26). They are born of the need to spatialize crises, deviations, and social order, and we look at them reflexively to see how "others" are differentiated and excluded. Yet within heterotopias, even where they are idealized as utopias, people invent, subvert, recreate, and reclaim such places for themselves and in so doing present a different picture of what it means to live worthwhile lives. Perhaps retirement communities as we have described them in this chapter are like special heterotopias. They embody the social contradictions between exclusivity and diversity, the tension between the acceptance of and resistance to aging, the mediation between local place and global nonplace, and the intersection between the nomadic forces of our time and the individual journeys and biographies through which they flow. Utopia may be the destination, but it is never reached.

NOTES

1. There are parallel developments in Europe, where northern Europeans migrate to and retire in Spain and other areas of the Mediterranean (King, Warnes, and Williams, 2000; Gustafson, 2001; Huber and O'Reilly, 2004).

2. Mexico has recently become a favored destination for Canadian and American snowbirds because of the availability of inexpensive health care, cheap prescription drugs, and even cosmetic surgery (Sunil, Rojas, and Bradley, 2007). In addition, and for Canadians in particular, the Lake Chapala region combines this kind of medical tourism with a perfect climate, lower costs of living, and tax advantages not available for Canadians in the United States (Bentein, 2003; King, 2007).

3. Hurricane Charley severely damaged one-third of Maple Leaf Estates and destroyed about 450 homes and wrecked many others, leaving them without power or water. Since that time, there has been a great recovery effort; new homes were replaced and new people have come to the park.

REFERENCES

Altman, I., P. M. Lawton, and J. F. Wohlwill, eds. 1984. *Elderly People and the Environment.* New York: Plenum Press.

Anderson, B. 1991. *Imagined Communities.* London: Verso.

Anderssen, E., and H. Mick. 2007. The aging population of suburbia. *Globe and Mail,* July 18, pp. L1, L3.

Andrews, G. J., and D. R. Phillips, eds. 2004. *Ageing and Place.* London: Routledge.

Andrews, M. 1999. The seductiveness of agelessness. *Ageing and Society* 19:301–18.

Baudrillard, J. 1988. *America.* Trans. C. Turner. London: Verso.

Bauman, Z. 1992. *Mortality, Immortality and Other Life Strategies.* Cambridge: Polity Press.

Bellah, R., R. Madsen, W. Sullivan, A. Swidler, and S. Tipton. 1988. *Habits of the Heart: Middle America observed.* London: Hutchinson.

Bentein, J. 2003. Canadian snowbirds and retirees flock to Mexico. In *Seniors' Housing Update.* Vancouver: Gerontology Research Centre, Simon Fraser University at Harbour Centre.

Blaikie, A. 1999. *Ageing and Popular Culture.* Cambridge: Cambridge University Press.

———. 2005. Imagined landscapes of age and identity. In *Ageing and Place: Perspectives, policy, practice,* ed. G. Andrews and D. Phillips. London: Routledge.

Blakely, E., and M. G. Snyder. 1999. *Fortress America: Gated communities in the United States.* Washington, D.C.: Brookings Institution.

Casey, E. 1997. *The Fate of Place: A philosophical history.* Berkeley: University of California Press.

Coates, K. S., R. Healy, and W. R. Morrison. 2002. Tracking the snowbirds: Seasonal migration from Canada to the U.S.A. and Mexico. *American Review of Canadian Studies* 32:433–50.

Counts, D., and D. Counts. 2001. *Over the Next Hill: An ethnography of roving seniors in North America*. Peterborough: Broadview Press.

Cresswell, T. 2006. *On the Move: Mobility in the modern Western world*. London: Routledge.

Dannefer, D. 2003. Whose life course is it, anyway? Diversity and "linked lives." In *Invitation to the Life Course: Toward new understandings of later life*, ed. R. A. Settersten Jr. Amityville: Baywood Publishing.

Delanty, G. 2003. *Community*. London: Routledge.

Dillard, A. 1987. *An American Childhood*. New York: Harper & Row.

Ekerdt, D. 1986. The busy ethic: Moral continuity between work and retirement. *Gerontologist* 26:239–44.

Entrikin, J. N. 1999. Political community, identity and cosmopolitan place. *International Sociology* 14:269–82.

Featherstone, M., and M. Hepworth. 1991. The mask of ageing and the postmodern life course. In *The Body: Social process and cultural theory*, ed. M. Featherstone, M. Hepworth, and B. Turner. London: Sage Publications.

FitzGerald, F. 1986. *Cities on a Hill: A journey through contemporary American cultures*. New York: Simon and Schuster.

Fletchall, A. 2005. As Youngtown grows young. Master's thesis, School of Geographical Sciences, Arizona State University, Tempe.

Foucault, M. 1986. Of other spaces. *Diacritics* 16:22–27.

Furman, F. K. 1997. *Facing the Mirror: Older women and beauty shop culture*. New York: Routledge.

Gamliel, T. 2000. The lobby as an arena in the confrontation between acceptance and denial of old age. *Journal of Aging Studies* 14:251–71.

Giddens, A. 1991. *Modernity and Self-Identity*. Stanford: Stanford University Press.

Gilleard, C., and P. Higgs. 2000. *Cultures of Ageing: Self, citizen and the body*. Harlow: Prentice-Hall.

Gubrium, J. F. 1975. *Living and Dying at Murray Manor*. 1997 ed. Charlottesville: University Press of Virginia.

———. 1993. *Speaking of Life: Horizons of meaning for nursing home residents*. Hawthorne: Aldine de Gruyter.

Gustafson, P. 2001. Retirement migration and transnational lifestyles. *Ageing and Society* 21: 371–94.

Hall, D. 1990. *Old and New Poems*. Berkeley: University of California Press.

Harvey, D. 1989. *The Condition of Postmodernity*. Cambridge: Blackwell.

———. 2000. *Spaces of Hope*. Berkeley: University of California Press.

Heywood, F., C. Oldman, and R. Means. 2002. *Housing and Home in Later Life*. Buckingham: Open University Press.

Hockey, J., and A. James. 2003. *Social Identities across the Life Course*. Basingstoke: Palgrave MacMillan.

Hoyt, G. C. 1954. The life of the retired in a trailer park. *American Journal of Sociology* 59:361–70.

Huber, A., and K. O'Reilly. 2004. The construction of Heimat under conditions of individualised modernity: Swiss and British elderly migrants in Spain. *Ageing and Society* 59:327–51.

Jackson, J. B. 1994. Roads belong in the landscape. In *A Sense of Place, A Sense of Time*. New Haven: Yale University Press.

Kastenbaum, R. 1993. Encrusted elders: Arizona and the political spirit of postmodern aging. In *Voices and Visions of Aging: Toward a critical gerontology*, ed. T. R. Cole, W. A. Achenbaum, P. Jakobi, and R. Kastenbaum. New York: Springer.

———. 1995. *Dorian Graying: Is youth the only thing worth having?* Amityville: Baywood Publishing.

———. 2008. Growing old in Utopia. *Journal of Aging, Humanities, and the Arts* 2:4–22.

Kateb, G. 1972. *Utopia and Its Enemies.* New York: Schocken Books.

Katz, S. 2000. Busy bodies: Activity, aging, and the management of everyday life. *Journal of Aging Studies* 14:135–52.

———. 2005. *Cultural Aging: Life course, lifestyle, and senior worlds.* Peterborough: Broadview Press.

King, J. 2007. Living in Lake Chapala. *Canadian Snowbird News* 64:24–29.

King, R., T. M. Warnes, and A. M. Williams. 2000. *Sunset Lives: British retirement migration to the Mediterranean.* Oxford: Berg.

Kumar, K. 1987. *Utopia and Anti-Utopia in Modern Times.* Oxford: Basil Blackwell.

———. 1991. *Utopianism.* Buckingham: Open University Press.

Laslett, P. 1996. *A Fresh Map of Life: The emergence of the third age.* 2nd ed. London: Macmillan Press.

Laws, G. 1993. "The land of old age": Society's changing attitudes toward urban built environments for elderly people. *Annals of the Association of American Geographers* 83:672–93.

———. 1995. Embodiment and emplacement: Identities, representation and landscape in Sun City retirement communities. *International Journal of Aging and Human Development* 40:253–80.

———. 1996. "A shot of economic adrenalin": Reconstructing "the elderly" in the retiree-based economic development literature. *Journal of Aging Studies* 10:171–88.

Lawton, M. P., P. Windley, and T. Byerts. 1982. *Aging and the Environment: Theoretical approaches.* New York: Springer.

Longino, C. F., and V. W. Marshall. 1990. North American research on season migration. *Ageing and Society* 10:229–35.

Longino, C. F., V. W. Marshall, L. C. Mullins, and R. D. Tucker. 1991. On the nesting of snowbirds: A question about seasonal and permanent migrants. *Journal of Applied Gerontology* 10:157–68.

Marans, R., M. Hunt, and K. Vakalo. 1984. Retirement communities. In *Elderly People and the Environment*, ed. I. Altman, M. P. Lawton, and J. F. Wohlwill. New York: Plenum Press.

Marin, L. 1984. *Utopics: Spatial play.* Trans. R. Vollrath. London: Macmillan Press.

Marshall, V. W., and R. D. Tucker. 1990. Canadian seasonal migrants to the Sunbelt: Boon or burden? *Journal of Applied Gerontology* 9:420–32.

Mattelart, A. 2000. *Networking the World, 1794–2000.* Trans. L. Carey-Libbrecht and J. A. Cohen. Minneapolis: University of Minnesota Press.

McHugh, K. 2000. The "ageless self"? Emplacement of identities in Sun Belt retirement communities. *Journal of Aging Studies* 14:103–15.

———. 2003. Three faces of ageism: Society, image and place. *Ageing and Society* 23:165–85.

———. 2005. Oh, the places they'll go! Mobility, place and landscape in the film *This Is Nowhere*. *Journal of Cultural Geography* 23:71–90.

———. 2007. Generational consciousness and retirement communities. *Population, Space and Place* 13:293–306.

McHugh, K., P. Gober, and D. Borough. 2002. The Sun City wars: Chapter 3. *Urban Geography* 23:627–48.

McHugh, K., and E. M. Larson-Keagy. 2005. These white walls: The dialectic of retirement communities. *Journal of Aging Studies* 19:241–56.

McHugh, K., and R. Mings. 1996. The circle of migration: Attachment to place in aging. *Annals of the Association of American Geographers* 86:530–50.

More, T. 1516. *Utopia.* 1975 ed. New York: W. W. Norton.

Phillipson, C. 1998. *Reconstructing Old Age: New agendas in social theory and practice.* Thousand Oaks: Sage Publications.

———. 2006. Aging and globalization: Issues for critical gerontology and political economy. In *Aging, Globalization and Inequality,* ed. J. Baars, D. Dannefer, C. Phillipson, and A. Walker. Amityville: Baywood Publishing.

———. 2007. The "elected" and the "excluded": Sociological perspectives on the experience of place and community in old age. *Ageing and Society* 27:321–42.

Radcliff, T. A., A. Dobalian, and R. P. Duncan. 2005. A comparison of seasonal resident and year-round resident hospitalization in Florida. *Florida Public Health Review* 2:63–72.

Romig, K. 2004. The new urban "anthem": Neoliberal design and social fragmentation. *Critical Planning* 11:3–16.

Rowles, G. D., and H. Ravdal. 2002. Aging, place and meaning in the face of changing circumstances. In *Challenges of the Third Age: Meaning and purpose in later life,* ed. R. S. Weiss and S. A. Bass. New York: Oxford University Press.

Sack, R. 1997. *Homo Geographicus: A framework for action, awareness, and moral concern.* Baltimore: Johns Hopkins University Press.

———. 2003. *A Geographical Guide to the Real and Good.* London: Routledge.

Sanders, S. R. 1993. *Staying Put: Making a home in a restless world.* Boston: Beacon Press.

Schoenstein, R. 1986. *Every Day is Sunday.* Boston: Little, Brown and Co.

Sennett, R. 1990. *The Conscience of the Eye: The design and social life of cities.* New York: W. W. Norton & Co.

Sheller, M., and J. Urry. 2006. The new mobilities paradigm. *Environment and Planning A* 38:207–26.

Smith, D. 2000. *Moral Geographies: Ethics in a world of difference.* Edinburgh: Edinburgh University Press.

Smith, S. K., and M. House. 2006. Snowbirds, sunbirds and stayers: Seasonal migration of elderly adults in Florida. *Journals of Gerontology* 61B (5):S232–39.

Sopher, D. 1979. The landscape of home: Myth, experience, social meaning. In *The Interpretation of Ordinary Landscapes,* ed. D. Meinig. Oxford: Oxford University Press.

Sturgeon, M. 1992. "It's a paradise town": The marketing and development of Sun City, Arizona. Department of History, Arizona State University.

Sunil, T. S., V. Rojas, and D. E. Bradley. 2007. United States' international retirement migration: The reasons for retiring to the environs of Lake Chapala, Mexico. *Ageing and Society* 27:489–510.

Tuan, Y.-F. 1978. Space, time, place: A humanistic frame. In *Timing Space and Spacing Time,*

Vol. 1: *Making Sense of Time*, ed. T. Carlstein, D. Parkes, and N. Thrift. London: Edward Arnold.

———. 1989. *Morality and Imagination*. Madison: University of Wisconsin Press.

Tucker, R. D., V. W. Marshall, C. F. Longino, and L. C. Mullins. 1988. Older anglophone Canadians in Florida: A descriptive profile. *Canadian Journal on Aging* 7:218–32.

Tucker, R. D., L. C. Mullins, F. Beland, C. F. Longino, and V. W. Marshall. 1992. Older Canadians in Florida: A comparison of anglophone and francophone seasonal migrants. *Canadian Journal on Aging* 11:281–97.

Twigg, J. 2000. *Bathing: The body and community care*. London: Routledge.

Urry, J. 2000. *Sociology beyond Societies: Mobilities for the twenty-first century*. London: Routledge.

Vesperi, M. D. 1985. *City of Green Benches: Growing old in a new downtown*. Ithaca: Cornell University Press.

Wahl, H.-W., and G. D. Weisman. 2003. Environmental gerontology at the beginning of the new millennium: Reflections on its historical, empirical, and theoretical development. *Gerontologist* 43:616–27.

White, P. 2007. Welcome to Elliot Lake, Canada's most elderly community. *Globe and Mail*, July 30, pp. L1, L4.

Williams, D., and S. Van Patten. 2006. Home and away? Creating identities and sustaining places in a multi-centered world. In *Multiple Dwelling and Tourism: Negotiating place, home and identity*, ed. N. McIntyre, D. Williams, and K. McHugh. Oxfordshire: CAB International.

Young, I. A. 1990. *Justice and the Politics of Difference*. Princeton: Princeton University Press.

———. 2000. *Inclusion and Democracy*. Oxford: Oxford University Press.

CHAPTER THIRTEEN

Old Age and Globalization

RÜDIGER KUNOW, PH.D.

How have the experience and meaning of old age come to be reconfigured under the aegis of globalization? At stake in such an inquiry is nothing less than the relationship of *bios* and *kosmos*, of life, in the later stages of its course, and the world at a time when this "world" has become an inescapable context and horizon for individual and collective experience and action (Robertson, 1992). "Global" and "aging" both designate transformative processes, the former unfolding in space, the latter in time; their convergence, "global aging," however, designates not simply a seamless fit between the somatic and the economic, but rather an open-ended and conflictual correlation that requires the sustained attention of sociologists, cultural critics, and, of course, gerontologists. As globalization in our time asserts itself primarily through borderless, deregulated market exchanges, it also changes the relations between the economy and human beings, and this change affects with particular severity people in the later stages of the life course. As I hope to show, globalization transforms not only the meaning and purpose of old age itself but even more so its place inside the social manifold.

Writing from the perspective of humanistic gerontology, I seek to preserve both place and purpose for old age in the public arena of modern democracies. Both this arena and democratic nation-states themselves are going through dramatic changes under the impact of neoliberal (i.e., market-driven) globalization. For this reason, my inquiry will proceed on two levels simultaneously: one empirical and descriptive, the other ideological-critical and normative. The empirical description will reveal how differently age is perceived and constructed across the globe, while at the same time some links and overlaps can be observed. Particularly striking in this regard is how aged cohorts are often placed in a special, even symbiotic relation to nation-states: they are not only clients of a given state but also tokens of its fitness for global competition. This evokes the second, normative dimension of my argument. Here I will combine the essentially moral agenda of humanistic gerontology with the materialist critique of the Frankfurt School. The Frankfurt School's critical theory is a particularly useful tool in the present context for a number of reasons. First of all, its particular form of "historical materialism as open-ended critique" (Jay, 1973, p. 295) presents a comprehensive ideological-critical account of instrumental rationality as embodied most forcefully in economic rationalization with its ever-quicker cycles of investment and return, a rationalization that seems to have reached a new apogee in our own time in the capital-driven processes of globalization (Sklair, 1998). Second, Frankfurt School critique has similarly traced the effects of instrumental reason on the normalization and administration of the body in the social and medical sciences (Scambler, 2001; Greco, 2004). These two rationalizations, each for itself and taken together, are crucial factors in the ongoing "modernization of aging" (Cole and Winkler, 1994, p. 3) and, I might add, its "globalization." Third, critical theory has from its beginnings in pre-Nazi Germany been conceived as a contribution to a normative theory of democracy (Fraser, 2007), and "age" must find a place within such a theory in order to safeguard the meaning endowment of age, its symbolic and social significance, within the emerging new global connectivities, which overflow in many ways the traditional bounds of territorial nation-states that have so far been the principal agents in defining what "age" meant.

My argument starts from a position that understands "age" and the "global" not as generic umbrella terms but rather as tropes of disjunction, *spectral universals*—spectral because in the broad light of closer scrutiny the projected notions of ecumenical unity and sameness dissipate like an apparition to reveal important and densely structured relations of difference and hegemony. Thus, "age" is often scripted as a biological universal—"we all age"—but this purported commonality of "fate" dissembles the ways in which the actualities of senescent life are shaped by inequalities of gender, race, or class. In a related way, the "global" designates a terrain of planetary connectivity that is in reality based on operative differentiations in wealth, power, and privilege. Hence, it makes sense not to take "age" and "global" at their semantic face value, but to understand them as two powerful regulatory grids that generate descriptions, authorize interpretations, and, most important, manage and supervise diversity.

To present comprehensive definitions of "globalization" or "age" lies beyond the scope of this chapter. Both terms have complex histories of usage and refer to deeply contested concepts meaning different things to different people. Their juxtaposition within the same semantic and conceptual space—"global aging"—is a relatively recent phenomenon, a process that by and large began in the 1980s and intensified during the 1990s. It originated in the economic sector and evolved into a recurrent feature in debates about the future of the welfare state, social equity, or demographic change. The currency of the term "global aging" reflects a new historical juncture: it has now become impossible to understand the experience and meaning of old age without taking into account currently unfolding transformations in the economy, society, and culture of nation-states all over the world. Without doubt, globalization is framing and reframing social and cultural practices, including those that are age-identified. But this is not the whole story. It is not only that globalization is the framework within which contemporary experiences and interpretations of aging must necessarily unfold; inversely, "age" is also a critical horizon against which processes of "globalization" have to be analyzed and questioned.

The major stages of the ongoing conversation about "global aging" are marked by, for example, the First World Assembly on Ageing (Vienna, 1982), the 1994 World Bank paper *Averting the Old Age Crisis*, the 1999 Human Development Reports, and the 2002 Valencia Forum/Second World Assembly on Ageing (Madrid, 2002), among others. Especially the World Bank paper and related pronouncements from the International Monetary Fund (IMF), the World Trade Organization (WTO), the Organisation for Economic Co-operation and Development (OECD), and other intergovernmental organizations (IGOs) such as the United Nations or the European Union have in various ways inserted age into the force field of a deregulated global economy. More important, they have defined key terms in which "global aging" came to be viewed. These terms are primarily economic in nature, and David Korton's assertion that "the [global] system treats people as a source of inefficiency" (Korton, 1996, p. 10) is borne out by the praxis in lay and professional statements alike to view the presence of elderly populations first and foremost in terms of a problem, even a crisis, a "pressure on a country's resources and government budgets [which] increases exponentially as populations age" and that "hinder[s] economic growth" (*Averting*, 1994). In a kind of trickle-down effect, the World Bank statement (including the 2005 amendment "Old Age Income Support in the Twenty-first Century") continues to define the parameters of the popular debate, as evidenced, for example, by Petersen's enormously influential book *Gray Dawn* (1999) and a host of other scholarly and journalistic publications.

The trajectory taken in most of these pronouncements on individual and population aging highlights the symbiotic relation between aged cohorts and nation-states. It reveals that much more is at stake in the "coming of age" on a global scale than simply forging a new and worldwide understanding of the later stages of the human life course. "Global aging," in other words, is not just about finding answers to questions of how market-driven globalization affects the material and mental life prospects of aging individuals, or, inversely, how the increase in elderly populations affects the continuing evolution of globalization. Rather, the conceptual linkage of the two terms "global" and "age" designates a wholesale reconfiguration and replacement of the latter by the former, a resolute effort to take age—and the populations designated by that term—outside national denominations and to deliver them instead into the invisible hands of global markets. This reconfiguration is not just a change in the conceptual geography of senescence, nor can it be simply seen as an expression of the inexorable demands of the global market. It changes the very framework within which it is possible and reasonable to speak of "age" as a factor of our private and public lives. Any attempt to situate age inside the evolving global framework therefore involves more than repeating the message "we all age" in the echo chamber of market-driven globalization.

Attempts to develop a global perspective on individual and population aging have taken a number of paths; these include reflections on general social policy implications (Phillipson, 2006), on problems of governance (Neilson, 2003), and, most frequently, on the nexus between changing demographies and the competitiveness of national economies in the global market (Powell and Biggs, 2000; Polivka, 2001; Grimley Evans, 2008). In my own chapter, I will follow another course: I will read "global aging" as a configuration situated at the intersection of *geopolitics* and *biopolitics*. Geopolitics is generally seen as referring to the management of economic or political relations between different regions of the globe; biopolitics designates a similar such management concerning the individual body and its relation to the body politic (Neilson, 2003). When it comes to "global aging," both management regimes intersect to produce an *errant aged subject*, a subject with multiple attachments and determinations, simultaneously inside and outside the nation-state, formed by globalization's pressures while also eluding them—inside the nation-state because the meaning and material entitlements of old age have traditionally been defined here, outside because the territorial nation-state has lost some of these same defining powers. At the same time, the processes of globalization have an impact on but do not exhaust the meaning endowment of old age, if for no other reason than that the "global" has so far remained a more or less abstract and elusive cipher. While globalization is an unavoidable *horizon of reference* or can be observed as a *cause* changing the meaning and experience of age in important ways, the global itself resists representation; no empirical object or incident can be unambiguously defined as "global." In the absence of an empirical global geography of age, it is necessary to shift the terrain of discussion. "Global aging" as a configuration at the intersection of *geopolitics* and *biopolitics* can therefore be explored most comprehensively in the context of the ongoing "evolution of a global civil society" (Benhabib, 2004, p. 15), and it is to this context that I will return at the end of my argument.

Clearly, the configuration of individual and societal aging in the context of global markets is a multidimensional process that takes place in an endless variety of political, economic, social, and cultural contexts. Given the limited space of the present chapter, I will focus on three exemplary constellations: (1) demography, (2) the polity, and (3) culture.

Demography

Demography is a useful starting point for any reflection on global aging for two reasons: (1) demography is a vantage point from which the nexus of biopolitics and geopolitics in the area of population aging can be observed with particular clarity, and (2) demography provides the lion's share of the publicly available vocabulary on this phenomenon.

Biopolitics and Geopolitics

Biopolitics is commonly understood, *pace* Foucault, as expression of the state's efforts to monitor the life processes of individuals and even whole collectivities, "births and mortality, the level of health, life expectancy and longevity" (Foucault, 1978). The successful implementation of biopolitical controls is today often functionally linked to a nation-state's position in the politics and economics of the global arena. However, such successes may have their own ironies, as in the case of the People's Republic of China. The resolute monitoring by the government of the population's reproductive activities—the "one-child policy"—is being viewed by many observers as one of the preconditions of China's economic miracle that helped make the country a global power. Domestically, this policy has resulted in a situation in which China now has a severe gender imbalance and the lowest birthrate and highest life expectancy in the hemisphere (Gregg, 2000). This has put a severe strain on what social security systems there are (left) in a country that has turned into a market economy. Destitute seniors have even taken to the streets to protest against the neglect by the government and have thus produced some of the rare instances of public disaffection with the regime (Chan, 2007). To this day, China has not instituted a coordinated state policy to deal with the growing numbers of its elderly citizens, and the ruling Communist Party is confronted with the need to develop strategies matching the demands of its elderly citizens with those of the country's ambitious plans for China's role in the global economy.

It is useful to compare this situation to the one in Cuba, where biopolitical interventions by the state have also drastically changed the demographic makeup of the population. As a result of a historically unprecedented access to health care through a state-sponsored egalitarian system, Cuba today boasts the highest life expectancy of all Latin American countries; it also reports a steadily declining birth-rate. For the first time in the history of the island nation there are more grandparents in Cuba than grandchildren (Giraldo, 2007). Low mortality and low fertility rates here combine with low growth rates in the economy. Cuba's socialist system suffers from chronic shortages in almost all areas of life and is as yet outside the reach of market-driven globalization. The crucial question for the post-Castro era will be whether the current social security system (supported with about 10% of the GNP) will or will not be transformed as Cuba's socialist traditions are renegotiated in the coming years.

Demographics

Demography, broadly defined as collection of statistical data on populations, is usually credited with delivering the hard facts that enable societies to make informed policy decisions, especially in the field of social policy. At the same time, however, demographic figures are an effective and powerful representational strategy (representation here understood in both its semiotic and political senses), with data producing "objective knowledge" about segments of the population and inserting these segments in certain ways into the public space of deliberation and decision making. This is true also of the observable aging of the populations in many nation-states across the globe, "the demographic transition from high mortality and high fertility to low mortality and low fertility" (Grimley Evans, 2008). This transition is well documented and undeniable, but its critical momentum derives from the way in which statistics on aging or old age enter the public sphere.

Sanctioned by the World Bank report and a host of other documents, a recognizable new genre of predictions and projections has developed around population aging, an "apocalyptic demography" (Gee and Gutman, 2000) that not only paints a gloomy picture of the future of certain nations but consistently invokes globalization as a reference point to paint demographic profiles in even more somber colors. An example of this process is a particular demographic narrative that might be labeled the "northernization" of aging. Here, the spectral universality of both "global" and "age" reveals itself in the way the latter is often scripted as a demographic characteristic primarily of societies of the Global North.[1] Italy, Japan, and Germany routinely serve as exemplars of societies hopelessly mired in a gray doom that, "like a massive iceberg, looms ahead in the future of the largest and most affluent economies of the world" (Peterson, 1999).

Demography is a key area in which the symbiotic relation of aged populations to nation-states mentioned above plays itself out. Statistics is here a stand-in for economics as the nation-states in the Global North are projected to lose their economic competitiveness vis-à-vis the "younger" nations of the Global South. Even the enhanced mobility stimulated by globalization is regarded as doing little to offset the demographic disadvantages of the developed countries: "there can be little doubt that immigration will play only a minor role in countering population aging in the North"

(Neilson, 2003, p. 165). In the context of the "War against Terror," the perceived aging of the Euramerican nations attains an even greater geopolitical urgency as the much-vaunted "Battle of the (Youth) Bulge" (Howe and Jackson, 2008). In his comparative sketch of rise and fall of civilizations, Samuel P. Huntington makes reference to what he calls the "demographic bulge" (i.e., the relative youthfulness of some Muslim nations) to suggest that in the coming clash of civilizations the Euramerican sphere will be seriously disadvantaged because its population is older (Huntington, 1996) and hence less likely to withstand the assault from an aggressive Islam that can rely on large cohorts of young people, especially males.

The popular view of an aging Global North is as compelling as it is misleading, however, and at worst it is a showcase example of how imperial Western universals subtend contemporary discourses of global aging. This global yet lopsided perspective disregards the fact that already at this moment 60 percent of the 65+ population worldwide resides in the developing countries of the South, a margin that is expected to grow to 71 percent by 2030 and 78 percent by 2050 (Kinsella and Phillips, 2005). In many of these countries, population aging will accelerate even faster (*World Economic and Social Survey*, 2007, p. 6). In India, for example, the number of people 65 and older will have more than doubled by 2030 alone. Demographic profiles of many other Asian nations develop along similar lines: in Singapore, for example, the elderly population will grow by more than 370 percent in the next 25 years, in South Korea by 210 percent, and in China by 170 percent (Kinsella and Velkoff, 2008).

In this context it bears emphasis that alarmist demographic projections of global aging often rely on a relatively stable arsenal of rhetorical figures and cultural archives. To name just one example: the same generation whose social presence was once greeted with clarion calls of a "baby boom" is now entering old age under the auspices of a "gray bust." It is highly significant that demographic statistics should in these and other instances be clothed in the vocabulary of economic effectiveness, referencing the upward and downward turns of economic cycles of profitability.

The much-vaunted fears of "a graying world" (Featherstone and Hepworth, 1995) are the most conspicuous and possibly most effective form in which demographic knowledge affects the debate on global aging. In a more sober way, demographic knowledge on the global distribution of aging bodies can invite and sustain international and cross-cultural comparisons (Gilleard and Higgs, 2000; Neilson, 2003). Such comparisons can usefully make visible a process that is planetary in reach, but distributed unevenly across the globe. It is an interesting fact in itself that the public debate in nation-states that are most likely to be dramatically affected by population aging, most often low-income countries, is much less frenzied than in nations that will be less affected (Vaidyanathan, 2006). I read this as evidence of the necessity for humanistic gerontology to interrogate the statistical findings of demographic research and to view the field less as a producer of objective knowledge on aging and more as a site of struggles over the presence of old age in the polity.

"Age" and the Polity: From Rights to Risks

So far, humanistic and traditional gerontologies alike have looked at aging and age almost exclusively from inside the nation-state. The aged body is in this view something like "the anatomical focus and embodiment" (Hewittt, 1991, p. 231) of the polity. This reflects a particular sociopolitical constellation that is now rapidly becoming a thing of the past, the post–World War II welfare state within which both popular and academic views of age revolved around material and legal arrangements undertaken by states and state-run organizations under the banner of social rights. Within this system, material and symbolic old-age identities were configured around biopolitical institutions, "the tutelary complex" (Donzelot, 1979, p. 97), of the nation-state. This complex was commissioned to regulate its elderly population, to monitor and administer their rights and duties, and also to manage the economic relations between generations with a view to intergenerational equity. Entitlement programs for elderly people were part of an expansive (and expensive) human rights regime that recognized the "right of everyone to social security" as defined, for example, by the 1966 International Covenant on Economic, Social and Cultural Rights. In this context, the regulation of retirement, access to health care, provision of a minimum standard of social security, etc., were often regarded as rights emanating from citizenship status and as a (if not the) defining principle of citizenship and even of the "democratic substance" (Habermas, 1999) of the political order.

In our own day, all this is changing. The triumphant march of capital-driven globalization has recast the terms, and in due course also the location, of the debate about the civic meaning of old age from the political arena to the global marketplace. An important factor here is that globalization has made it possible for corporate capital to complete the process that Karl Polany described as the "disembedding" of the market from "all other modes of interaction" (Polany, 2001, p. 110). This disembedding has, in the context of market-driven globalization, created a situation in which citizenship as traditionally understood is disaggregated into a rights and a market component, with the latter progressively eclipsing the former. This means that the balance between rights and duties of aged populations has been shifting in the direction of the latter. This process goes hand in hand with the transition from a *rights-oriented* to a *risk-oriented* approach to old age and age-identified entitlements. This transition expresses itself most forcefully in two areas that are crucial for the way elderly people live: health care (including geriatric care) and pensions.

In both areas, "global" actors and factors are intervening more and more into what was once a client relationship between the tutelary nation-state and "its" clients, the aging or aged population, as something like a "third party." Health care providers and privately managed retirement funds are now in many nations worldwide the principal agents to accommodate the needs and demands of old people. This does not mean simply that issues such as health care or social security are now subjected to calculations of profitability, but also that these policy issues are now (re)negotiated in a different arena, that of global markets and capital flows.

Health Care

In countries all over the world, health care systems have for some time now come under a severe strain due to dwindling finances, growing numbers of claimants, and increased treatment costs. Given the prevailing climate of deregulation and reliance on the market, the suggested panacea for the perceived "health care crisis" has been wholesale "privatization." Privatization, commonly understood as the transfer of functions from the public to the private sector, means more than a retooling of management practices through the entry of the private agents into health and geriatric care: "This means understanding market realities and eliminating regulatory and policy barriers that impact on commercialization and business development" (Health Care, 2004, p. 14).

The actors operating in this global and increasingly deregulated health market are themselves a motley crowd, but they all come from the private (i.e., corporate) sector: among them are banks, insurance companies, and managed funds. The most momentous feature of their intervention has been to turn quondam claims made to the public sector into marketable commodities. In the process, aged populations and their needs have become functionally a part of the global market system and its imperatives. These imperatives are best met by multinational corporations that have greater expertise than traditional, often national or local health care providers in maximizing efficiency and accessing capital resources worldwide. Over the last years a "medical industrial complex" has been developing that is directed toward "the interest of increasing sales, maximizing efficiency and containing costs" (Hall, 1990) in a globalized health care economy. To cite just one example: the Coalition of Service Industries (CSI), often working in tandem with the Global Service Network (GSN), is a Washington, D.C.–based private sector advocacy organization lobbying aggressively for liberalization of the global trade in services. CSI members have so far invested approximately $110 billion worldwide into the health care market; they own hospitals and geriatric care facilities in both the developing and the developed world (Estes and Phillipson, 2002).

The framework for such global market–oriented health and geriatric care markets is currently developed under the auspices of the General Agreement on Trade in Services (GATS). This framework, to be sure, is less directed at regulating foreign direct investment in health care for elderly people than at facilitating it, for example, by (re)defining the requisite "policies affecting access to, and conditions of competition in, service markets [as] firmly rooted in the multilateral trading system" (Stern and Sauvé, 2000). GATS is a spin-off of the GATT (General Agreement on Tariffs and Trade) process, which since the 1960s has played a key role in the worldwide process of deregulation and of downsizing the role of nation-states in central policy areas.

Deregulated and market-oriented health care can be a highly profitable business, if for no other reason than because in times of economic retrenchment it is one of the few remaining growth markets. The U.S. health market accounts for about 15 percent of the GNP, valued at $0.35 trillion; the global health market is estimated at double that figure. Both markets are expected to more than double in less than a decade (Health Care, 2004). In this context "global aging" is a term designating an extremely *lucrative investment opportunity*, which for this reason is targeted by corporate investors and private equity investors worldwide. Says one venture capital analyst, "as the baby boomer generation gets older, VCs [venture capital companies] are seeing a need to put money in health care" (Cutland, 2006). And they do so in figures shading out the hitherto most favored IT or semiconductor industries: private equity investment in health care alone has risen by more than 25 percent during the last four years (Cutland, 2006; *Raymond James*, 2008).

Here again, globalization proves to be a spectral universal: it eclipses local health care practices while enabling on a worldwide scale new degrees of selectivity in market access and participation, generally working in favor of corporations that are themselves global operators. The evolving global market in health care develops in the different parts of the globe along highly uneven lines. While in the Global North the marketization of welfare states infrastructure does meet with strong resistance, from both governments and the population, and especially in the European Union, it proceeds more smoothly elsewhere, such as in the United States and in the Global South. Here, the social infrastructure of postindependence nations was never well developed to begin with, but under the impact of budget cuts ("fiscal responsibility") mandated by the IMF or the World Bank, "developing nations" have little choice but to open themselves to private investment: "The forced reductions in public expenditures in social, health and education services and the privatization of many of these services (the minimalization of the state) have created a 'crisis of care' in many developing countries, even as the populations in need of care, especially children and elderly people, continue to grow at very high rates" (Polivka, 2001, p. 154). This process can be observed at work in many countries of the Commonwealth of Independent States (CIS), where at the transition from a state socialist to a market economy, existing health systems were rearranged, often precipitously, to a highly selective health service market that excludes large proportions of the population, and especially elderly people (Ghai, 2002).

In the privatization of health care, the interrelationship between geopolitics and biopolitics makes itself felt with particular force. Population transfers from the Global South and postcommunist countries to Europe and North America, in particular the mass emigration of young workers, have in many areas brought about a collapse of existing informal systems of geriatric care provided by the extended family network. At the same time that market-driven globalization undermines the resources for such a "relations-based" system of care, the transition to a "rule-based" Western system (Vaidyanathan, 2006) is an option only for a small group of affluent people, which leaves growing numbers of old people without access to even minimum forms of care.

Access to health care innervates not only questions of intergenerational justice but also those of gender equity. Health care is in many places all over the world provided through the unpaid work of women, mostly in the domestic sector (*Human Development Report*, 1999, p. 78). The cross-hatching of biopolitical with geopolitical maneuvers in this area is particularly noticeable in countries where under the impact of globalization more women are taking up formal employment. Bangladesh shows one of the largest increases in women entering the labor force (42% in 1995, up from 5% 30 years ago), with no formal or market-based health care system in place to respond to the growing demand for care. Overall, the consequences of the marketization of health care hit women harder than men because they are overrepresented among both providers and "consumers."

The deregulation of the health care market is often paralleled by a closer regulation of the aging body. The market provides strong "incentives" for individuals to monitor their bodies carefully (Featherstone and Hepworth, 1995) to minimize their risk of ever even needing health care that would be available only at market prices. At the same time, it should also be noted that such a risk management has worked to change assumptions about the meaning or even the advent of age, which in the view of more affluent elderly people can be warded off by high-cost late-life medical treatment (see chap. 10 of this volume).

In 1983, a U.S. Presidential Commission on health care had found that "society has a moral obligation to ensure that everyone has access to adequate care without being subject to excessive burdens" (*Securing Access*, 1983, p. 22). The emerging globalized health care economy, however, is not answerable to obligations that a society imposes on itself as embodying the essence of democratic community. But who then is? Health markets, like any other markets, "cannot be democratized," and the criteria for an equitable social order "differ from those used to measure economic success" (Habermas, 1999). The gap that opens up here between the instrumental rationality of the economic sphere and the moral obligations of a democratic society highlights "the fundamental biopolitical fracture" (Agamben, 2000, p. 32) at the heart of a globalized health care market: the procedure of inclusive exclusion of population segments that are marginalized or excluded in the practice of health care provisions but are nonetheless in their very exclusion a functional part of the market that can operate only through a high degree of selectivity. Such selectivity is making access to health care for elderly people increasingly precarious, even in the developed nations of the Global North. Access to health care, however, is not only a question of access to the health care market; it also involves the larger issue of the access of elderly people to the public sphere. As Michael Walzer argued, losing access to "medical care . . . is a double loss— to one's health and to one's social standing" (Walzer, 1983, p. 89).

Social Security and "Pension Reform"

Like health care, state-sponsored social pension systems are a form of publicly mandated beneficence that is now increasingly perceived as a strain on the diminishing fiscal resources of the nation-state. As Social Security costs increase at an exponential rate and as the number of elderly people also grows, both the general public and some experts are insisting that both developments are causally related. Often the blame for the perceived pension crisis has been placed squarely before elderly people when it is argued that they unduly strain, even "eat up," fiscal resources that should rightfully be going to younger, more productive population segments: "The costs of the system [of publicly managed retirement programs] . . . make it difficult for the government to finance important public goods—another growth-inhibiting consequence" (*Securing Access*, 1983, p. 13). The Three-Pillar Model advocated by the World Bank (public pensions, private savings, employment-based contributions) is often advertised as the ultimate wisdom in solving "Old Age Security Problems around the World." While still leaving a space for residual publicly managed pensions, this model puts the emphasis on mandatory personal and additional "voluntary" saving plans. Such a three-tiered system, it is argued, provides a safety net and is "an instrument of growth" (*Averting*, 1994, p. 9).

Elderly adults who can no longer save up for their retirement because they are already in it, as well as those in "casual labor" arrangements who never make enough money to invest in their own retirement, are thus increasingly cast in the role of obstacles to prosperity or, in Mary Antin's memorable simile, "like a heavy garment that clings to your limbs when you would run" (Antin, 1997, p. xxii). The solution to problems that are, as even the World Bank admits, if not caused then at least exacerbated by market-driven globalization is more market-driven globalization, or more precisely "the internationalization of pension funds . . . Opening the door to international investments of pension funds would seem to be warranted, to diversify and thereby diminish risk" (*Averting*, 1994, p. 192).

The World Bank, the IMF, and other IGOs have consistently included age in the structural adjustment policies that they mandate as a prerequisite for participation in the globalized market. "Development" is the major ideological goal or value here (Omvelt quoted in Sklair, 1998, p. 299; Spivak, 1999, p. 390). Under the label of "Pension Reform," the World Bank, the United Nations Conference on Trade and Development (UNCTAD), and other IGOs have been actively promoting the inclusion, if not total system change, in the direction of private sector personal savings schemes in developed and developing countries alike. Latin American states and especially Chile are in this context frequently commended for having made (under General Pinochet) this transition to a system organized around the competition among private companies (*Averting*, pp. 4, 9 et passim). Critics are pointing out that this privatization of Social Security for elderly people has so far amounted to a wholesale residualization of benefits and beneficiaries: "The overall conclusion is that the privatization reforms have been disappointing and have not fulfilled the expectations of the proponents. The problems include poor coverage, high management fees charged by the private sector (half the contributions by Chilean workers . . . went to management fees) and a questionable impact on economic growth" (Minns, 2006, p. 101; Reynaud, 2006).

The insertion of old-age retirement in the global finance markets proceeds as unevenly on the global plane as globalization in general does. However, what this insertion does mean in most cases is that the beneficiaries of retirement plans, both employment-based plans and IRAs, are willy-nilly becoming actors themselves in the worldwide theater of finance markets. Labor capital morphs into venture capital. One of the most striking examples of this role change is the California State Employees Retirement System (CalPers), the largest pension fund in the United States. This fund is investing more and more of its $170 billion in assets in private equity companies or hedge funds such as the Texas Pacific Group (TPG). TPG, in turn, as critics have charged, has been buying up flourishing businesses all over the world, extricating their value, laying off employees, and ultimately driving them into bankruptcy (*Heuschrecken*, 2007). In this way, elderly people become, if only by proxy, agents in the pauperization of people in other parts of the world, among them elderly people. Such activities by agents that are called "locusts" in Europe are likely to become more intensive in the wake of the 2006 Pension Protection Act, which authorizes U.S.-based hedge funds to increase their holdings of pension plan money, allowing them then to look for lucrative investments worldwide (Graw and DeFalco, 2006).

Capital-driven globalization has, among many other things, also brought about a shift in the relationships between the young and the old. Questions of social security for elderly people are in this context often represented in terms of an impending intergenerational conflict between young and old. It bears emphasis that such a conflict is the mise-en-scène for the World Bank, the IMF, and other advocates of capital-driven "pension reform" interventions in the pension reform debate. At times, these interventions rely on obsolete cultural archives of ageist stereotypes. Figures of the "greedy geezer" variety are often used to frame discussions of social security issues, even in the 1999 *Human Development Report.* This document suggests that over "the past 30 years the elderly in the United States have received far more than the young for a simple reason—the elderly have more votes than parents with children" (*Human Development Report,* 1999, p. 80). Statements such as this provide even further evidence of how "our cultural tradition understands age in terms of a binary system. Old age is defined in relation to young," which in this way becomes the yardstick by which the acceptable properties are defined, by default, as it were (Cristofovici, 1999, p. 269). And this default notion of age as significant / signifying lack is underwriting much of the ongoing (re)construction of the meaning endowment of age in economic terms. Age is thus not only a signifier for a lack of health, mobility, good looks, etc., but also a signifier for a lack of economic usefulness.

It is one of the articles of faith concerning capital-driven globalization that the management of all social systems should and will eventually pass from nation-states to the market: "The time has come for private actors to provide what were once assumed to be public services" (Whitfield, quoted in Estes and Philippson, 2002, p. 288). However, the record so far of market-based social security schemes for elderly people suggests that the role of the state in this area is far from over. With the notable exception of the United Kingdom, where "New Labour third way" policies have installed private sector pension reforms even in advance of projected GATS regulations, nation-states in Europe, and also some in Asia or Africa, are still functioning—many of them against their will—as a protective space against the "predatory mobility of unregulated capital" (Appadurai, 2001, p. 7). China, for example, where old-age pensions until recently had relied on occupational plans underwritten by companies, is facing a major social security crisis now that during the transition to capitalism many of these companies have folded. Of the 37 million people entitled to company pension benefits, 35 million are now receiving them instead from the public sphere (*Chinese Embassy,* 2007; Yu, 2007). As in many developing countries, the extended family system in China had once also taken up some of the functions provided in the North by state-sponsored systems. Now that the younger generation is entering the job market in often faraway places, the system is falling apart and the state has to step in. A similar development is occurring in India, where "with globalization and migration, the joint family system is on a decline . . . and to that extent the challenge of caring for the elderly has become greater for society and government" (Vaidyanathan, 2006). In view of these developments, it is deeply ironic that advocates of private pension funds should continue to rely on the corporate sector and suggest that employment-based benefits could take the place of state-managed systems, while in point of fact the public sector, in India, China, and elsewhere, has to foot the bill accumulated by private enterprise.

There is, in other words, a continuing need for the "sheltering singularity" (Moreiras, 1998, p. 90) of the nation-state, and that need is growing all over the world. Clearly, this singularity cannot be understood independently of the realities of global interconnectedness, but it still comes as a surprise given customary constructions of the postnational era in which the nation-state is routinely represented as obsolete, as one of those "shell institutions" that "have become inadequate to the tasks they are called upon to perform" (Giddens, 1991, p. 19). Its resurgence, even if only by default, in those pockets of globalization where *the economic production of age identities has remained incomplete or inadequate* is a useful reminder that questions of social equity, especially for old and aging populations, need a framework in which they can be negotiated in processes of democratic deliberation and decision making. This framework, however, is nowhere to be seen, at least not in the transnational realm, where the contours of an international human rights regime that would provide an address for the legitimate claims of elderly populations or for a Habermasian "transnational solidarity among [aged] strangers" are at best only emerging.

Summing up the findings so far, I would like to point out that the encroachment of market imperatives on what was until recently a relationship between the public domain and "its" elderly population amounts to a wholesale restructuring of the social infrastructure of old age, a restructuring that I have sought to describe as a paradigm shift from claims to commodities, from rights to risks. At the same time, however, the effects of market-driven globalization on the sectors of health care and retirement, while socially upsetting, cannot be comprehended in social terms alone.

Under the conditions of market-driven globalization, the hoary ageist metonymy[2] of using frailty and dependence as stereotypical designators for life in old age now returns in economic guise as efficiency argument: aged populations are routinely viewed as falling outside or being antithetical to the productivist ethic stipulated by visions of economic "development." Against this background, old-age rights such as health care and social security are viewed as negative assets, as "pressures on a country's resources" (*Averting,* 1994) that need to be averted or minimized in the name of market efficiency and profitability. The meaning endowment of age and the mysteries and paradoxes of the latter stage of the life course do not translate easily into the instrumental reason of the market. Modifying a pithy statement by Linda Weiss in a related context, I would define a salient characteristic of the current debate on old age as "corporate construction of uselessness" (Weiss, 1998, p. 110). This not only means that routine invocations of the allegedly iron, immutable laws of capital-driven globalization and its social fallout are designed to gain the willing compliance of politicians or populations with cuts in health care and social security, but also entails a systematic shifting of the balance in senior citizen entitlement from the polity to the economy, a withdrawal of arguments about health care or social security from the polity to the market, from the arena of democratic deliberation and will formation to the imperatives of the economic reason, from the protective space of the nation-state to the everywhere and nowhere of global market interaction.

The intervention of the market as something like a "third party" into the social infrastructure has had profound effects also on the *civic agency* of elderly populations, that is, their role in the procedures and politics that make up democratic societies. The issue of civic agency is crucial, especially for humanistic gerontologists, because the reconfiguration of elderly rights and risks under the auspices of globalized markets involves questions that go way beyond the distribution of increasingly scarce resources to embrace central issues concerning the makeup of civil societies. I will return to this point at the end of this chapter.

A Global Age Culture?

From the beginning of time, old people have been active and influential participants in cultural practices. Not only were they the "subject matter" of art in all cultures that we know of, but from Praxitiles to Picasso, from Rabindranath Tagore to Doris Lessing, old men and women have themselves created great artworks that have stood the test of time. It is plausible to expect that "the intensification of consciousness of the world as a whole" (Robertson, 1992, p. 2) as a result of capital-driven globalization will have its impact also on the creativity of old people and their cultural representations. Early evidence of this impact can be found, for example, in fictions and films that explore the daunting challenges faced by elderly characters who at the end of their lives find themselves stranded on the trade routes of globalization, struggling to sustain their cultural heritage in unfamiliar settings. This is the donnée of otherwise so diverse texts as Amy Tan's *The Joy Luck Club* (1989), Zadie Smith's *White Teeth* (2000), and Marina Lewycka's *A Short History of Tractors in Ukrainian* (2005). They gesture toward the possibility of the "global" acting as catalyst for new old-age representations that counter some of the practices of cultural disenfranchisement of old age in national cultures. Thus, the "coming of age" worldwide might even raise the prospect of the emergence of an *écriture grise*, of new cultural practices, outside national traditions that are galvanized by and configured around the experience and the meaning of old age in a global context.

However, as I have insisted throughout this chapter, globalization is a spectral universal that suggests planetary equality while in fact composing relations of inequity and domination. If this is so, such a *global cultural imaginary of/by/for the aged* may be not forthcoming anytime soon, and it may even be the wrong imaginary because it embodies the risk of replicating in cultural terms the spurious universality that is subtending the global market. The pressures of market-driven globalization may be imperative, but they cannot exhaust the multiplicity of aging. For this reason, I will refrain here from looking for something like the "global content" in age-identified cultural practices and focus instead on particular old-age identities, which I regard as emblematic of the cultural dynamics affecting elderly people under the aegis of globalization, and which are located at the intersection of geopolitics and biopolitics to which I have repeatedly turned in this chapter. The contours of such *errant aged identity*, an identity with multiple attachments and determinations, simultaneously inside and outside the nation-state, can be observed, however provisionally, in two interrelated but recognizably different guises, which I call the *Gray Nomad* and the *Aged Migrant.*

The Gray Nomad and the Aged Migrant are two versions of aged mobility produced by the worldwide network of economic relations in our time. The difference between these two runs roughly parallel to the distinction originating in cultural anthropology between "globalization from above"—the flows of capital, commodities, and environmental risks—and "globalization from below"—the flows of migrants, refugees, and displaced populations (Appadurai, 2001, p. 3).

Globalization "from Above" and the Gray Nomad

Within the archives of globalization, the intense movement of peoples across the world is often cast in a schematic, binary pattern according to which the young are mobile whereas elderly people either stay behind or are left behind. In such a scheme, aging and old age are often seen as the local, the surplus, the elsewhere of global connectivities. Practices of "gray nomadism" (Onyx and Leonard, 2007), "RV-lifestyle" (Curtin, 2007), or "Ulyssean aging" (Onyx, 2007) disprove much of this scheme and suggest that the enhanced mobility made possible by globalization has created a new cultural template also for elderly people whose postwork identity can now organize itself around self-enhancing forms of voluntary mobility or nomadism that is potentially unlimited—global—in outreach.

A related aspect of this nomadism is the phenomenon of retirement migration across international borders. This new form of age-identified mobility has a tradition of its own in the United States (with regard to Mexico) and has more recently become popular across Europe, where it was facilitated by social security regulations inside the

European Union and the relative ease with which financial resources could be transferred between different member states. Nowadays, retirement migration of financially independent seniors is no longer restricted to North America or Europe but is itself becoming a global phenomenon as sending and receiving countries are promoting it. Malaysia, for example, has set up a "Malaysia, My Second Home" plan designed to attract wealthy foreign retirees; Panama has recently started a program along similar lines, while "Thailand 4Ever" offers assisted living facilities, and aged U.S. baby boomers find luxury retirement homes in Mexico (Hamilton, 2006; Thomson, 2006; Toyota, Böcker, and Guild, 2006).

Like the related phenomenon of health tourism, these forms of mobility are underwritten by a variety of motivations, among them looking for the best weather or the best value for one's dollar, euro, or yen. In addition to being expressions of personal preferences, retirement migration also has a wide-ranging significance for forms of global cultural interchange that are only now developing. Recent studies have shown that the mobility of retirees is often motivated by a "must see before I die" (Onyx, 2007) interest in different places and people, an interest that is primarily cultural. For this reason I want to read this form of aged nomadism as an emerging form of *gray cosmopolitanism.* "What cosmopolitanism popularly evokes—among other things, the thirst for another knowledge, unprejudiced striving, world travel, supple open-mindedness, broad international norms of civic equality" (Brennan, 2001, p. 659)—all of these can be said to apply to gray nomads as well. This has also made affluent ethnic elders an interesting vantage point from which to explore the transgressive dynamic of living in two cultures. In *Kabhi Alvida Naa Kehna*, for example, a 2006 Indian movie (Karan Johar, director), it is cosmopolitan detachment that allows a wealthy Indian expatriate in the United States to take a long, pragmatic view on the contested subject of arranged marriages in his own cultural tradition, which is not available to the younger cast of characters who are still immersed in that tradition.

At the same time, there are obvious limits to this brand of cosmopolitanism and its intercultural outreach. Some gray nomads living in an adopted country do so in congregated compounds, staying among themselves and, like tourists, limiting their forays into the host culture to occasional sightseeing. In this way, social and cultural enclaves are forming in the receiving countries that reflect and reinforce the inequalities of globalization (Toyota, Böcker, and Guild, 2006). What is more, because gray cosmopolitanism is a form of old-age identity that is adopted voluntarily and conditional on financial resources, it is less a stable form of age identity and more a lifestyle choice among many other possible such choices that "now form the dominant mode by which personal and social identities are expressed" (Gilleard and Higgs, 2000, p. 28).

Aged Migrant

laborers, is not a lifestyle choice, but one of the
1 globalization has come to shape the life course
t throughout the world. The first generation of
eat numbers to the Global North as unskilled
ting old.

is of the Global North of care facilities designed
ns reflects ongoing changes in the nexus between
t homes for migrant laborers are not only them-
ely, a growing niche market (Phuong, 2003), but
enclave for aging migrant populations in which
zed are yet again marginalized, only in other
annot be included in the whole of which it is a
uded—in the care regimes of the host cultures.
lvertised as ethnic enclosures, as "culture-sensi-
lding experiences of a work life away from home
do in fact reflect entrenched age biographies
such constructions of how to age properly and
y mobile" has been shown by research conducted
t-growing numbers of retirement homes in East

patial expressions of the dominant trajectory of
naster narrative of aging that reflects established
s. Into these practices aging migrants are now
neir will and almost always against their expecta-
ng in the Global North, or, rather, being aged in
to be like that of their elders. What they are
f their life course is not only totally different but
ne concept of "age." Lawrence Cohen's astute
India" previous to the advent on the subconti-
ogies" of aging (Cohen, 1998) makes a similar
ending countries. Inversely, a study of elderly
many elderly migrants feel disempowered by
t countries (Gardner, 2002), which are perceived
lity of aging in accord with their traditions.
tirement facilities such as the Paulo Agabayani
ted Farm Workers for aging Filipino field work-
ei Manor for Japanese seniors, while facilitating

interaction between chronological and cultural peers, do little more tha
construction of age in the host and not the home culture. This is not just
finding; this indicates also a cultural pathology that reminds us on
important the civic meaning of age is. Will Kymlicka (1989) argued t
cultural structure" is a primary good in democratic polyethnic societies
the evidence available at this time suggests that host societies in the
have by and large failed in providing this good. Rather, Western-style
said to contain "institutionalized patterns of cultural value [that] im
participation in social life" (Fraser, 2000, p. 107). This denial of particip
life that has been an integral part of the Western construction of
extended to another segment of the population.

A "Global Age Culture" in which globalization acts as an enabling, ev
horizon for an extended and enriched experience of aging and old
powerful and enabling vision, but at this point in time it remains just
The imbrications of aged people with globalization processes are from a
of view deeply ambivalent in nature and outcome. The Gray Cosmopc
Aging Migrant are just two (and certainly not the only) ways in which
insert themselves or are inserted in the crucible of globalization. Perhaps
before do terms such as "old age," "elderhood," "senescence," and oth
refer to a clearly recognizable cultural identity across the board and a
Hence, I have found it more appropriate to speak—as I have done repe
chapter—of forms of *errant age identity* produced, as it were, *en route*,
move along different routes and with different degrees of rootedness thr
tially global space.

Conclusion

Globalization is at this time still an incomplete project that is continuo
by capital-driven market forces. The transformations unleashed by
make a rethinking of the meanings of aging and old age both suggestive
the term "global aging" is to have any analytical purchase in this context
all to face the fact that globalization has altered the relations between *b*
by effectively disembedding life forms from their wonted local atta
identifications. Specifically, it has disembedded the later stage of life
perhaps most, of its social and symbolic entitlements. And if age has
designated "a physical, moral and spiritual frontier" (Cole and Winkler,
various cultures across the world, the advent of globalization has c
forward that frontier in new and uncertain ways.

Whether the evolving "consciousness of the world as a whole" (Rob will compensate for the losses incurred by creating and sustaining new age identities that perhaps even enrich the experience and meaning of a now globalized old age cannot be known at this moment. What is reasonably clear, however, is that the public presence and the public vocabulary of old age have already changed dramatically.

The epistemic violence contained in much of this vocabulary has repeatedly surfaced in this chapter. This epistemic violence marks also the site of intervention for a humanistic gerontology that has consistently viewed the aging body as being more than mere *fait social* or mere physicality. Its commitment to record "the lived experience of age as expressed in the words, speech, stories, and writings of older people" (Cole and Sierpina, 2007, p. 252) and to safeguard the social and cultural specificity of old-age experience makes it possible to think and write about the global coming of age in a nonappropriating, noninstrumental way. Such commitment is becoming even more urgent if we expand the focus by taking into account that old people do not age alone as private persons, but that private persons live together as part of a public. And in this public domain, the experience and meaning are "likely to be decided by political negotiations rather than by moral deliberation" (Cole and Sierpina, 2007, p. 255). This is the point where the *epistemological obligations* of a discipline such as humanistic gerontology become indistinguishable from its *ethical obligations*, where cultural critique of the (mis)representations of older people in the public image expands into a political critique of their (non)representation in policy decisions.[3]

Today, in "the chill of globalization" (Gilroy, 2005, p. 142), the cultural and political role of elderly populations has become precarious. While the "tutelary complex" (Donzelot, 1979) of the nation-state is weakening, the public sphere of communication, deliberation, and contestation is becoming a central arena, perhaps the only one, in which questions of the social integration, the rights and obligations of aged cohorts, and, more generally, the civic meaning of old age can be arbitrated with any degree of fairness.

The Frankfurt School vision of this public sphere as possessing a critical function, checking and even ameliorating the structural inequalities of the political process, may seem unduly idealistic in view of today's media politics. What remains pertinent about this vision, however, is the insight in the mutual interdependence between public voice and political clout, the "co-implication of private and public autonomy" (Habermas, 1998, p. 420). This requires from us as humanistic gerontologists to pay even more attention to the civic meaning of old age. This involves traditional advocacy work, i.e., combating specific prejudices and stereotypes (Featherstone and Wernick, 1995; Gullette, 1997) that cloud the public presence of elderly people. This involves also advocacy in the more general sense of supporting elderly people in their attempts to be or become interlocutors in the public domain of our political communities. Only if among "the din of voices in the public sphere" (Habermas, 2005) older people can be heard, in their own voice, can they hope to realize the full potential of their citizenship, and for this end, the public debate about old age must expand its scope beyond a "thin version of rights" for elderly people (i.e., life, liberty, and property) (Benhabib, 2006, p.16) to a "thick version" of such rights, a form of "achieved citizenship, based in agency and difference" (Dahlgren, 2007). This is by no means a utopian project. The public sphere has proven an effective location for negotiating "the principles and practices of incorporating aliens and strangers, immigrants and newcomers, refugees and asylum seekers, into existing polities" (Benhabib, 2004, p. 1) through processes of deliberation and the public use of good reason. These same processes can be enabling also in terms of a more effective incorporation of elderly populations into societies, safeguarding their full participation in the public life, their ability to "voic[e] their concerns and incorporate[e] their demands into the public debate and the policy agenda" (*World Economic and Social Survey*, 2007, p. 82).

This kind of civic age agency is all the more important in our own postnational moment because, as I hope to have shown, the market forces that drive globalization cannot and do not provide, let alone safeguard, such agency. While the globalized market forces respond only "to messages coded in the language of prices" (Habermas, 1999), the civic meaning of old age needs to be defined in the public sphere in its own language. What is at stake in this process is the *sustainability of old age*, the continuing commitment of societies to set aside a semantic and social space for its elderly populations. This space is endangered today, "smothered through colonization by [the] instrumental reason" of the market (Beilharz, quoted in Scambler, 2001, p. 4), and humanistic gerontology must take care that options for what I would call an "age-friendly society" will continue to exist even in the trials and tribulations of market-driven globalization.

NOTES

1. Throughout this chapter, I will use "Global North" and "Global South" not as geographical designators but as conceptual shorthand to describe the relative position of nation-states in the global economic system, as "developed" or "developing"/"underdeveloped" regions.

2. Metonymy is a figure of speech in which a part is substituted for the whole.

3. I am speaking here of humanistic gerontologists' "concern for values and meaning" vis-à-vis the counterintuitive "objective" knowledge produced by the "hard sciences." The epistemological and ethical obligations to which humanistic gerontology is committed require that the objects of its inquiries should not be reduced to mere "facts" but must be recognized as human beings whose difference and resourcefulness cannot be exhausted by scientific protocols.

REFERENCES

Agamben, G. 2000. *Means without End: Notes on politics.* Trans. V. Binetti and C. Casarino. Minneapolis: University of Minnesota Press.

Antin, M. 1997. *The Promised Land.* New York: Penguin.

Appadurai, A. 2001. Globalization and the research imagination. In *Globalization*, ed. A. Appadurai. Durham: Duke University Press.

Averting the Old Age Crisis. 1994. Washington: World Bank.

Benhabib, S. 2004. *The Rights of Others: Aliens, residents, and citizens.* Cambridge: Cambridge University Press.

———. 2006. *Another Cosmopolitanism.* Oxford: Oxford University Press.

Brennan, T. 2001. Cosmo-Theory. *South Atlantic Quarterly* 100 (3):659–91.

Chan, J. 2007. *Mass Protests in China Point to Sharp Social Tensions.* World Socialist Web Site 2004 [cited September 23, 2007]. Available from www.wsws.org/articles/2004/nov2004/chin-n01.shtml.

Chinese Embassy to Germany (Press Release April 4). 2007. 2005 [cited October 25, 2007]. Available from www.china-botschaft.de.

Cohen, L. 1998. *No Aging in India: Alzheimer's, the bad family, and other modern things.* Berkeley: University of California Press.

Cole, T. R., and M. Sierpina. 2007. Humanistic gerontology and the meaning(s) of aging. In *Gerontology: Perspectives and issues*, ed. J. M. Wilmoth and K. F. Ferraro. New York: Springer.

Cole, T. R., and M. G. Winkler, eds. 1994. *The Oxford Book of Aging.* Oxford: Oxford University Press.

Cristofovici, A. 1999. Touching surfaces: Photography, aging, and an aesthetics of change. In *Figuring Age: Women, bodies, generations*, ed. K. Woodward. Bloomington: Indiana University Press.

Curtin, R. 2007. *Reuters/University of Michigan Surveys of Consumers* 2005 [cited October 10, 2007]. Available from www.sca.isr.umich.edu/main.php.

Cutland, L. 2006. Health care investments outpacing all other industry sectors. *Silicon Valley/San José Business Journal*, March 31, 2006.

Dahlgreen, P. 2007. Civic identity and net activism: The frame of radical democracy. In *Radical Democracy and the Internet: Interrogating theory and practice*, ed. L. Dahlberg and E. Siapera. London: Palgrave.

Donzelot, Js. 1979. *The Policing of Families.* Trans. R. Hurley. Baltimore: Johns Hopkins University Press.

Estes, C. L., and C. Phillipson. 2002. The globalization of capital, the welfare state, and old age policy. *International Journal of Health Services* 32 (2):279–97.

Featherstone, M., and M. Hepworth. 1995. Images of positive aging: A case study of *Retirement Choice* magazine. In *Images of Aging: Cultural representations of later life*, ed. M. Featherstone and A. Wernick. New York: Routledge.

Featherstone, M., and A. Wernick, eds. 1995. *Images of Aging: Cultural representations of later life.* New York: Routledge.

Foucault, M. 1978. *The History of Sexuality.* Trans. R. Hurley. London: Allen Lane.

Fraser, N. 2000. Recognition without ethics? In *The Turn to Ethics*, ed. M. Garber, B. Hanssen, and R. L. Walkowitz. New York: Routledge.

———. 2007. Transnationalizing the public sphere: On the legitimacy and efficacy of public opinion in a post-Westphalian world. *Theory, Culture and Society* 24 (4):7–30.

Gardner, K. 2002. *Age, Narrative and Migration: The life course and life histories of Bengali elders in London.* Oxford: Berg.

Gee, E. M., and G. Gutman. 2000. *The Overselling of Population Aging.* Oxford: Oxford University Press.

Ghia, D. 2002. Social security priorities and patterns: A global perspective. Geneva: International Institute for Labour Studies.

Giddens, A. 1991. *The Consequences of Modernity.* Cambridge: Polity Press.

Gilleard, C., and P. Higgs. 2000. *Cultures of Ageing: Self, citizen and the body.* Harlow: Prentice-Hall.

Gilroy, P. 2005. *Postcolonial Melancholia.* New York: Columbia University Press.

Giraldo, G. 2007. *Cuba's Aging Pains (and Gains).* Cuba Health Reports 2007 [cited June 10, 2007]. Available from www.medicc.org/cubahealthreports/chr-article.php?&a=1031.

Graw, A. F., and M. T. DeFalco. 2006. Ability of hedge funds and private equity funds to attract pension investors made easier by the Pension Protection Act of 2006. *Metropolitan Corporate Counsel,* November 2006, p. 9.

Greco, M. 2004. The politics of indeterminancy and the right to health. *Theory, Culture and Society* 26 (6):1–22.

Gregg, J. 2000. Confronting an aging world. *Washington Quarterly* 23 (3):213–24.

Grimley Evans, J. 2008. *What Does the Epidemiology of Aging Tell Us Now?* 2002 [cited June 12, 2008]. Available from http://catalogue.iugm.qc.ca/GEIDEFile/13121.PDF?Archive=193687 991186&File=13121_PDF.

Gullette, M. M. 1997. *Declining to Decline: Cultural combat and the politics of the midlife.* Charlottesville: University of Virginia Press.

Habermas, J. 1998. *Between Facts and Norms: Contributions to a discourse theory of law and democracy.* Cambridge: MIT Press.

———. 1999. The European nation-state and the pressures of globalization. *New Left Review* 235:46–59.

———. 2005. Religion in der Öffentlichkeit. In *Zwischen Naturalismus und Religion.* Frankfurt: Suhrkamp.

Hall, R. H. 1990. *Health and the Global Environment.* London: Polity Press.

Hamilton, M. M. 2006. Sometimes age is a bargain. *Washington Post,* November 26, p. F01.

Health care and the innovation agenda: Advancing innovation and economic development in the life sciences sector in Atlantic Canada. 2004. In *Directions for Canadian Health Care, 7:* Life Sciences Development Association.

Heuschrecken am Wasserhahn. 2007. 2005 [cited October 30, 2007]. Available from www.tag esspiegel.de/zeitung/Die-Dritte-Seite;art705,1889399.

Hewitt, M. 1991. Bio-politics and social policy: Foucault's account of welfare. In *The Body: Social process and cultural theory,* ed. M. Featherstone, M. Hepworth, and B. S. Turner. London: Sage.

Howe, N., and D. Jackson. 2008. Battle of the (youth) bulge. *The National Interest,* July/August.

Human Development Report 1999. 1999. New York: United Nations Development Program.

Huntington, S. P. 1996. *The Clash of Civilizatons and the Remaking of the World Order*. New York: Simon & Schuster.

Jay, M. 1973. *The Dialectical Imagination: A history of the Frankfurt School and the Institute of Social Research, 1923–1950*. London: Heinemann.

Kinsella, K., and D. R. Phillips. 2005. Global aging: The challenge of success. *Population Bulletin* 60 (1).

Kinsella, K., and V. A. Velkoff. 2008. *An Aging World, 2001*. U.S. Census Bureau 2001 [cited June 16, 2008]. Available from www.census.gov/prod/2001pubs/p95–01–1.pdf.

Korton, D. 1996. *When Corporations Rule the World*. West Hartford: Berrett-Koehler.

Kymlicka, W. 1989. *Liberalism, Community and Culture*. Oxford: Oxford University Press.

Lewycka, M. 2005. *A Short History of Tractors in Ukranian*. London: Viking.

Minns, R. 2006. The future of stock market pensions. In *The Futures of Old Age*, ed. J. A. Vincent, C. Phillipson, and M. Downs. Thousand Oaks: Sage.

Moreiras, A. 1998. Global fragments: A second Latin Americanism. In *The Cultures of Globalization*, ed. F. Jameson and M. Miyoshi. Durham: Duke University Press.

Neilson, B. 2003. Globalization and the biopolitics of aging. *New Centennial Review* 3 (2):161–86.

Onyx, J. 2007. Ulyssean aging: An alternative model for the Third Age. In *Australian Social Policy Research Conference*. Sydney, Australia.

Onyx, J., and R. Leonard. 2007. The gray nomad phenomenon: Changing the script of aging. *International Journal of Aging and Human Development* 64 (4):381–98.

Peterson, P. G. 1999. *Gray Dawn: How the coming age wave will transform America and the world*. New York: Random House.

Phillipson, C. 2006. Aging and globalization. In *The Futures of Old Age*, ed. J. A. Vincent, C. Phillipson, and M. Downs. Thousand Oaks: Sage.

Phuong, L. 2003. Immigrants grapple with elderly care. *Washington Post*, July 1.

Polany, K. 2001. *The Great Transformation*. 2nd ed. Boston: Beacon Press. Original edition, 1944.

Polivka, L. 2001. Globalization, population, aging, and ethics (pt. 1). *Journal of Aging and Identity* 6 (3):147–62.

Powell, J., and S. Biggs. 2000. Managing old age: The disciplinary web of power, surveillance and normalization. *Journal of Aging and Identity* 5 (1):3–13.

Raymond James Health Care Investment Banking Group Advises Amedisys on $395 Million Acquisition of TLC Health Care Services, Inc. 2008. Business Wire 2008 [cited March 12, 2008]. Available from www.financialservicesbiz.com/Banking-Services/Raymond-James-Health-Care-Investment-Banking-Group-Advises-Amedi.html.

Reynaud, E. 2006. Social Security for all: Global trends and perspectives. *Comparative Labor Law and Policy Journal* 27:123–50.

Robertson, R. 1992. *Globalization: Social theory and global culture*. London: Sage.

Scambler, G. 2001. Introduction: Unfolding themes of an incomplete project. In *Habermas, Critical Theory and Health*, ed. G. Scambler. London: Routledge.

Securing Access to Health Care: A report on the ethical implications of differences in the availability of health services. 1983. President's Commission for the Study of Ethical Problems in Medicine and Biomedical and Behavioral Research.

Sklair, L. 1998. Social movements and global capitalism. In *The Cultures of Globalization*, ed. F. Jameson and M. Miyoshi. Durham: Duke University Press.

Smith, Z. 2000. *White Teeth*. New York: Random House.

Spivak, G. C. 1999. *A Critique of Postcolonial Reason: Toward the history of the vanishing present.* Cambridge: Harvard University Press.

Stern, R. A. M., and P. Sauvé, eds. 2000. *GATS, 2000: New directions in services trade liberalization.* Washington, D.C.: Brookings Institution Press.

Tan, A. 1989. *The Joy Luck Club*. New York: Putnam's Sons.

Thomson, A. 2006. *Retirement Homes: Americans buy into luxury.* 2006 [cited October 20, 2007]. Available from www.ft.com/cms/s/002f1632–005b-11db-8078–0000779e2340.

Toyota, M., A. Böcker, and E. Guild. 2006. Pensioners on the move: Social security and transborder retirement migration in Asia and Europe. *IIAS Newsletter* 40:30.

Vaidyanathan, R. 2006. *Declining Joint Families: Looming social security crisis.* The Hindu Business Line 2006 [cited August 20, 2007]. Available from www.thehindubusinessline .com/bline/2006/11/30/stories/2006113000450800.htm.

Walzer, M. 1983. *Spheres of Justice: A defense of pluralism and equality.* New York: Basic Books.

Weiss, L. 1998. *The Myth of the Powerless State*. Ithaca: Cornell University Press.

World Economic and Social Survey. 2007. United Nations Department of Economic and Social Affairs 2007 [cited October 20, 2007]. Available from www.un.org/esa/policy/wess/wess 2007files/wess2007.pdf.

Yu, W. K. 2007. Pension reforms in urban China and Hong Kong. *Ageing and Society* 27:249–68.

CHAPTER FOURTEEN

Ageism and Social Change

The New Regimes of Decline

MARGARET M. GULLETTE, PH.D.

> When those who have power to name and to socially construct reality
> choose not to see you or hear you . . . there is a moment of psychic
> disequilibrium, as if you looked into a mirror and saw nothing.
> —*Adrienne Rich*

Age studies is an emerging multidisciplinary field that merges humanistic, anthropo-logical, and other social science approaches, by highlighting (depending on the needs of one's topic) narrative, popular culture, especially the media, literary fiction, politi-cal economy, antiageist ethics, and/or history. Our work focuses on not only old age but also whatever age(s) or aspects of aging are relevant.[1] Age studies—also called "cultural studies of age"—arises out of a commitment to analyzing contemporary age ideology and advancing the causes of the vulnerable.

The study of "social change" in the age culture of the United States requires such an engaged eclecticism. Aging is a narrative each of us tells,[2] but with an inadequate backstory. My own aging narrative rarely becomes analytically informed about how I am being aged by ageist trends in culture. Not only my own life experiences but also societal influences move me. In the 1990s and 2000s, decline narrative leaks more and more into my head, tainting my formulations of life's events: "senior moment," "aging [sic] boomers," "dried-up old woman." I use the words they teach me, to paraphrase Samuel Beckett. Or I resist, using up tremendous energies. Even when sideswiped by social change—major developments in the corporate economy, media spin, medical-ization, Supreme Court decisions—I often don't know what hit me.

Americans don't get good information about the hit-and-run drivers on the life course. Like feminist, critical-race, and queer studies, as well as social gerontology, age studies monitors the oppressors. Herewith I offer three cases of misrepresented or

Parts of this chapter are condensed from the versions in Margaret M. Gullette's book *Agewise*.

neglected trends in U.S. ageism and middle ageism. Together, these trends do increasing violence to essential aspects of well-being: midlife employment, midlife health, and respect for life even in old age. An age studies approach, capable of dealing with all three attacks, can bring out their cumulative and overlapping decline effects on individuals and the social fabric.

The cohorts most flattered for their power, the "boomers," were in fact unlucky in their timing as they aged past youth. They ran into constructed job scarcity because of globalizing and privatizing capitalism; they smacked into the voracious multi-billion-dollar commerce in aging; and their retirement and later-life health care are being assaulted by the right-wing drive to weaken social welfare. As younger people may discover, giant forces and ideologies have been creating excess losses as each generation grows older.

Midlife Job Loss

In Donald Westlake's *The Ax*, the first-person narrator, a midlife man, starts murdering men his age, laid off as he has been—men who also possess long resumes as managers in the production of specialized polymer paper products. Before readers can quite focus on the horror, the economic issues become painfully clear. Burke Devore is too young for Social Security and knows that people his age don't get new jobs quickly: "The layoffs are too extensive, and are in every industry across the board, and the number of companies firing is much larger than the number of companies hiring. More and more of us are out here now, another thousand or so every day . . . Middle management, that's what's being winnowed now. And none of us are unionized." He sees that it's the so-called boomers who are being "shunted off the social order." One of his rivals works as a counterman in a diner. He says to Devore, "But this is the first society ever that takes its most productive people, at their prime, at the peak of their powers, and throws them away. I call that crazy" (Westlake, 1997, pp. 21, 82, 42, 104).

For these workers, their age—or, more precisely, American ageism—is the problem. They can't get rehired. Their resumes cannily avoid providing photos: "It's best . . . not to include anything at all that points specifically to the applicant's age." The "bad and faithless employer" can afford to be picky. He can find someone who is "eager to come to work . . . at lower pay and fewer benefits, just so it's a job." "I've read the same stuff we've all read, how it's going to be necessary in the brave new world of tomorrow for people to move on from job to job, learning new skills along the way, and how males older than fifty have the hardest time . . . and I was absolutely prepared to prove that particular generalization false." But what good does getting two months training fixing air conditioners do Burke when thirty guys will apply "who have had *years* of experience repairing air conditioners . . . Are you gonna hire me? Or are you not that crazy?" (Westlake, 1997, pp. 9, 23, 224).

Burke has a plan. He is killing the men competing for the one job in his narrow field. What drives him to murder are the emotional, sexual, financial, and familial consequences of being fired. "Miss a payday, and you'll feel that flutter of panic. Miss every payday, and see how *that* feels." He's worried about his mortgage, his kids losing their health insurance, family dysfunction—all the "fringe banes." There's no sex left in his marriage. "A lot of wife-beating goes on these days among the middle-class unemployed," but he's killing in part to avoid turning against his wife. He might have given in completely to despair: "some of these people have considered it and some will do it. (This world we live in began fifteen years ago, when the air traffic controllers were all given the chop, and suicide ran briskly through that group, probably because they felt more alone than we do now.)" (Westlake, 1997, pp. 13, 220, 28, 47).

Tweaking the classic populist *noir* into a savage Swiftian economic satire, Westlake got it right. Capitalism since at least the Reagan years has been eroding seniority to obtain a cheaper workforce that is demoralized and more flexible. Getting rid of midlife workers is an international trend in developed countries (Kohli et al., 1991). Louis Uchitelle notes in *The Disposable American* that layoffs first appeared as a mass phenomenon, absent a Depression, for the first time two decades ago. At least 30 million full-time workers have lost their jobs since the early 1980s (Uchitelle, 2006, pp. ix). It's still hard to find data that direct attention to *midlife* workers rather than the entire workforce, but Raymond Gregory, the foremost lawyer writing on midlife discrimination, says, "Just about every worker . . . has been or will be affected by an employment decision based on age" (Gregory, 2001, p. 14).

The typical U.S. household headed by a 47- to 64-year-old is at risk in an increasingly insecure job market. It is poorer today, in constant dollars, than a similar household was in 1983, despite women working (Porter and Walsh, 2005). Men have fared badly, historically. *Half* of male workers have lost ground economically as they aged into their forties, fifties, and sixties, a figure so big it means that the middle class and professionals are affected. (In 2003, a sizable portion—20%, or about 1.6 million of the 8 million unemployed—were white-collar professionals; Ehrenreich, 2005.) The highest rates of displacements in the 1990s occurred among midlife segments of the workforce (Hipple, 1999). Displacement among workers in their fifties and sixties often results in lasting unemployment (Chan and Stevens, 2001). Only two-thirds of men aged 55 to 65 are in the workforce at all, down from 90 percent in the early 1950s. Although we are told that baby boomers are healthy and so rich they want to retire early, this is far from the whole story. Most of the early retired, female or male, are disabled, according to the Congressional Budget Office (2008).[3] Others who need work can't find it.

Women at their midlife peak are also at risk, with gendered differences. Unlike some midlife men, they are less able to use job experience as an asset in the job interview (McMullin and Berger, 2006, p. 215). They may earn more than their mothers, but they still earn only 73 percent of what men earn. Barbara Ehrenreich, Ph.D., author of 13 books and an intrepid adventurer into the dark side of our economy, decided "well into middle age" to try anonymously to find a good white-collar job. She couldn't, despite having allocated 10 months and $5000 in up-front costs. *Bait and Switch*, the book about her search, anticipated that the first of her disadvantages was her age, which she disguised by omitting the year of her college degree and all jobs before 1989, thus trying to look 40. She concludes that at some point "age discrimination renders people unemployable for all practical purposes—unless as a people greeter at Wal-Mart" (Ehrenreich, 2005, p. 243). The presentable and articulate Ehrenreich was rarely offered an interview, however, and the only "jobs" she was offered—commissions only—came with no salary, no benefits, and no office. Men typically suffer age discrimination in their mid-fifties, women almost 10 years younger, Gregory (2001) notes.

What happens to the people downsized and outsourced? Five months of job seeking was average for the unemployed in 2004, but some people Ehrenreich ran into didn't have a job after two years (Ehrenreich, 2005, p. 12). Many outlive their unemployment insurance benefits, if they ever got them. Few get retraining, and the picture is bleak. To significantly reduce a displaced worker's losses would require, according to three experts in job dislocation, "about the equivalent of two years of college education" (Jacobson, LaLonde, and Sullivan, 1993, p. 170). In Richard Russo's novel *Nobody's Fool*, Sully, a carpenter with a badly fractured knee, is required as a condition of receiving partial disability to attend a brief community college program in—you guessed it—refrigeration and air-conditioning (Russo, 1994, p. 21; see also p. 65).

Earnings in new jobs are typically lower than before, often much lower. In 1993 three well-respected economists were puzzled to find that workers with *more* labor market experience had postdisplacement earnings as low as those of similar younger workers (Jacobson, LaLonde, and Sullivan, 2005, pp. 47–66). After getting a new job, midlife women work longer hours than men (Moen et al., 2004). One-third of workers 50 to 59 cash in their 401(k)s—potential retirement money—when they leave a job, not a good sign.[4] The level of debt for people between 50 and 64, earning in the middle of the income scale, more than doubled in the 1990s.[5]

Estimates vary, but even before the recession roughly one-third of midlife people would be able to retire with adequate income, one-third would be hard-pressed in retirement, and the bottom third would not be able to afford to stop working. Pensions disappeared during this same period; many didn't earn enough to save. More are trying to find paid work even as late as age 65 to 74, according to census data

(Ohlemacher, 2007, p. A4).[6] "The most notable trend," according to a *New York Times* article comparing 1986 to 2006, "is that men and women are both much more likely to keep working than were their parents in what used to be known as the golden years" (Norris, 2006, p. 12). Presumably they face long waits for work, many rejections, or extreme downward mobility, taking on exhausting ill-paid jobs. Many people too frail for their low-wage jobs slog on to supplement Social Security.

The discharge of a midlife worker has been described as "the industrial equivalent of capital punishment" (Gregory, 2001, p. 7). Dismissal is a trauma by itself, and prolonged unemployment is even more demoralizing.[7] Even after mass layoffs and entire plant closings, people with pink slips believe that it is their own fault. Midlife workers may lose health insurance and assets as well: they lose their homes or go into debt. Ehrenreich tells a story of a middle-aged woman who moved back in with her parents (Ehrenreich, 2005, p. 204). Suddenly people who had been growing toward midlife peaks as parents, coaches, guides, and friends become vulnerable to depression, divorce, alcoholism, and suicide. Being stripped of their identity,[8] such people lose hope. The only prospective narrative that makes sense is a decline narrative.

There has been a disturbing rise in the number of suits based on the Age Discrimination in Employment Act (ADEA, 1967), which was passed to help workers over 40: 2200 percent [sic] between 1970 and 1989. Women's complaints grew to 36 percent of all complaints lodged with the Equal Employment Opportunity Commission (EEOC) by 1997 (Gregory, 2001, pp. 9, 115, 116).[9]

There is not much legal recourse, despite the ADEA. It was meant to have the same force as antiracist or antisexist legislation, through "disparate impact," but the Supreme Court's judgments in *Hazen* and *Hicks*, Gregory shows, have made it harder to make claims. Underfunding by Congress and a meager 5 percent rate of "for-cause findings" create the impression that "the EEOC is engaged in discovering where discrimination does not exist rather than where it does." If you sue, many conservative Reagan- and Bush-appointed judges are less sympathetic to the objectives of the laws (Gregory, 2001, pp. 185, 188, 215). Neither ADEA (for older people) nor Title VII (for women) specifically grants protection to "older women," who may fall between the cracks.

"60 is the new 40"? Maybe 40 is the new 60. When journalists and pundits boast that the so-called baby boomers are changing the face of aging, they overlook the hard facts of midlife job loss. Ignorance can be tinged with blame. I invented the term *middle ageism* in 1997 and I use the term *midlife workers* to highlight the worsening impacts of premature superannuation. Economists still use the term "older workers," which disguises the fact that ageism as job loss is backing down the life course to much younger people. Boomer-bashing insinuates that midlife people—rich, powerful, greedy "deadwood"—should vanish off the stage of life to make *Lebensraum* for the young (Gullette, 2004, pp. 42–60).

When CEOs as well as state and city administrators decided to end seniority, firing employees who had the most experience and were the next most expensive, both Democratic and Republican administrations declined to intervene (Uchitelle, 2006, chaps. 6–7). The erosion of the midlife contingent of the workforce, middle class as well as working class, became TINA: a social fate for which it is believed There Is No Alternative. The social costs are high, in terms of loss of productive capacity, stagnation of wages, damaged psyches, miserable old ages, the heightened stress and longer work hours of retained workers and growing workforce insecurity even among the young, the relentless weakening of the values accompanying seniority, and a widespread reduction in the ability to tell a progress narrative about the later stages of the life course.

Hormone Nostalgia[10]

In 2002 the Women's Heath Initiative (WHI) of the National Institutes of Health announced that it was ending its vast study of so-called hormone replacement therapy (HRT) abruptly because of the risks of cancers and heart disease. Even the North American Menopause Society (NAMS), heavily funded by the pharmaceutical industry, called the WHI the "gold-standard"[11] of experiments. News outlets of all kinds carried the data and editorial warnings.[12] The conclusion was "monotonously consistent" with earlier randomized controlled studies (Fugh-Berman and Scialli, 2006, p. 120). Taking synthetic (or "exogenous") hormones also doubles the risk of developing dementias.[13] Far from being a lifetime "therapy," synthetic hormone was now to be taken *warily*—only when unavoidable, and then in low doses, for the shortest possible term.

The 2002 hormone debacle was historically significant because it was the first major dislocation in a century of menopause demonization and estrogen hype— phenomena that underpin the fantasy of "antiaging medicine" for women. At first the debacle seemed to have some effect. Almost 11 million U.S. women stopped taking hormones—56 percent of users (Ginty, 2008).[14] Breast cancer rates (which had been rising for decades) fell dramatically in 2003. Cancer researchers attributed this astonishing drop in part to the fact that millions of women had stopped taking hormones (Kowalczyk, 2006, pp. A1, A36). A total of 5000 women with breast cancer who formerly took the most used form of HRT filed suit cases against its manufacturer, Wyeth (Lattman, 2007).

Estrogen is a carcinogen. Exposure to it—even to a woman's own endogenous production—is an important determinant of the risk of cancer (Yager and Davidson, 2006, pp. 270, 271). "The link between the female hormone estrogen and cancer is hard to miss," a 1998 article in *Science* began. "It contributes to the development of three of the top five cancers of women—those of the breast, uterus, and ovaries . . . an estimated 240,000 new cancer cases a year in the U.S. alone" (Service, 1998). The International Agency for Research on Cancer (IARC), part of the World Health Organization, in 2005 moved synthetic estrogen up from the category "possibly carcinogenic to humans" to the highest risk category, "carcinogenic to humans." The current research controversy is over whether estrogen carcinogenesis means that estrogen *initiates* cancer mutations or stimulates the proliferation of existing cancerous cells in women (Yager and Davidson, 2006). Synthetic estrogen could now join drugs like thalidomide (effect: birth deformations), exogenous testosterone (prostate cancer), and Vioxx (heart attacks) as one of many "treatments" approved by the Food and Drug Administration (FDA) and hyped and prescribed without being adequately tested.

To a dispassionate observer, it is not menopause but exogenous hormones (their medical risks, weak governmental regulation, commercial manipulation, effects of biomedicalization on women of all ages) that should be the social issue, a collective public health and cultural concern. It becomes necessary to explain why menopause was ever considered newsworthy.

The end of menstruation is unremarkable to about 90 percent of the women who go through it—the vast majority of whom never seek help.[15] The ending of menstruation is universal, but the experience of menopause is biocultural: o percent of Mayan women have hot flushes, while 80 percent of Belgians do (Ussher, 2006, p. 131). In a peak year before the debacle, national rates of estrogen use varied—from a low of 8 percent in Massachusetts to 40 percent in California, the youth-cult capital of America (McNagny, Wenger, and Frank, 1997). Most women soon forget menopause.

Widespread reporting of the hormone debacle had the potential to cause cultural paradigm shifts. The precautionary principle—first, do no harm—could finally be applied to midlife women's bodies. Given that the menoboom (including enormous off-label use of estrogen for purported "rejuvenation") took off in the 1990s shortly after a heavily lobbied Congress let Big Pharma advertise directly to consumers, there should now be skepticism about direct-to-consumer advertising. Magazines and newspapers, with less marketing pressure from the companies, should find menopause less dire, even less newsworthy. The disparaging terms—*menopausal, postmenopausal, perimenopausal,* which serve to medicalize women and age them younger than men—should have disappeared. Because menopause never was like hypothyroidism, science reporters should help wither the "hormone-deficiency" myth. Journalists could encourage skepticism about future chemical or genetic "enhancements" that are not properly tested—which would make everyone safer. Menopause had signaled the early onset of midlife female decline. "The very process of aging has been widely reinterpreted as a deviation from the normal, a process against which [to] take major precautions," warns anthropologist Margaret Lock. "Living-past-menopause," according to an evolutionary argument that compares women to apes, has by itself been considered "unnatural" (Lock, 2000, p. 269). If menopause had come to seem less dangerous, less salient, and less marketable, the "Change" could have weakened as a magic marker of the female life course.

Since 2002, has our culture been offered a better—a more reliable, informative, nonsexist, and antiageist—prospective narrative? On the whole, the answer is "no." Women still have more to fear from menopause *discourse* than from menopause itself (Gullette, 1993). Men should pay attention. The drummed-up "disease" of menopause created a model for selling treatments to "andropausal" men. Having lost many female users, Big Pharma focuses on men, promoting "erectile dysfunction," selling Viagra, testosterone for women and men, and human growth hormone. The commerce in aging (not just Big Pharma, but antidepressant manufacturers, cosmetic surgeons, the fashion magazines) creates a widespread, growing need to appear young and the resultant desire for "lifestyle medicines"[16] and dangerous enhancements.

The hormone debacle, as we'll see, is a case where a major backlash, backed by science, could have happened but—because of powerful opposing forces—hasn't.

Did *anything* good occur? Yes. Before 2002, when HRT was becoming obligatory, a feminist could fear that women who refused it and subsequently acquired osteoporosis or cardiovascular disease might eventually be penalized by Medicare or Medicaid because they *had neglected their health*.[17] That no longer seems plausible. Globally, smaller percentages are *starting* on hormones than in the past. In the United States, it's better-informed women who are stopping (Ekström, 2005, pp. 11, 12).

For individual midlife women, any advance depends mainly on their practitioners. Responsible doctors or gynecologists, says historian Judith Houck, will no longer "routinely" promote estrogen to you in your forties (Houck, 2006, chap. 9). They now have to diagnose the individual who presents with relevant symptoms—"by far the difficult bit" (Genuis and Genuis, 2006, p. 6). Isolated reporting on midlife health has improved. A *Globe* article in December 2005, "Health by the Decade," brought general good sense a bit closer. The page for the 1950s highlighted osteoarthritis and sleep deprivation, which strike both genders, and, miracle of miracles, issued a warning to *men* to visit their doctors more regularly. The word *menopause* does not appear. "Hot flashes and night sweats" are mentioned under other causes of reduced sleep, including stress; in fact, "stress" is sensibly the first cause. A *Newsweek* article trumpeted "The End of the Age of Estrogen." A 330-word *Time* article on hormone treatment ended, mildly, "Many women find they do just fine without it" (Cowley and Springen, 2002, p. 38; Gorman, 2005, p. 57).

Despite pockets of good sense, my main conclusion is that since 2002 there are still too many dire media features on the topic of the "troublesome menopause." One still has to read feminist anthropologists and women's health activists to learn how slight an impact menopause has on most women's lives. Major antiestrogen evidence goes unreported. How many newspapers reported the IARC recategorization of estrogen as carcinogenic to humans? According to the Internet search engine LexisNexis, only the *Herald Sun* of Melbourne, Australia (Houlihan, 2005), not a single British, Canadian, or U.S. paper. The unspoken rule seems to be that the words *menopause, estrogen,* and *carcinogen* cannot appear in the same report.

The term *hormone debacle* is rarely seen. *Medicalization*—an indispensable concept —is rarely found in the mainstream. The term *perimenopause*—a life "stage only recently created to strike fear and anxiety into the hearts of forty-somethings and even thirty-somethings," according to philosopher Christine Overall (2003b, p. 313)—continues to be used (even in the state-of-the-art manual *Our Bodies Ourselves: Menopause*). The term backs female sickliness down the life course by construing menstrual problems as "early menopause." Women are still being aged by culture at ever younger ages.

Informational failures are not due to cultural "lag," which implies mere inertia. The forces that keep menopause looming are active players. Business as usual in America produces new estrogenic products, advertising directly to the public. Its pseudoscientific press releases create "news" for the media. Journalists, gynecologists, and doctors have continuing responsibility for maintaining female aging as a bugaboo.

Far from disappearing, "Menopause," a *Washington Post* headline of 2003 told us, "Has Become the New Hot-Button Topic in Women's Health" (Mundy, 2003). *USA Today* in 2005 headlined "Change of Life Remains Hard" (Painter, 2005). Women have to "navigate" it, in the tricky-shoals metaphor of a *Pittsburgh Post-Gazette* headline (Carpenter, 2005, p. F1). An article in *Business Week* suggested that menopause lasts from the early forties until death (Freundlich, 2004). The *Boston Globe* published another unlikely study tying depression to the "approach to menopause," although the author of the article knew that two authors had financial ties to antidepressant manufacturers (Johnson, 2006, p. A6). (Insofar as any age has a link to depression, the period of most acute female depression is during the childbearing years; Solomon, 2001, p. 174.)

Rarely do articles tell us about the *benefits* of being postmenstrual (a useful substitute term): no more bleeding, drying up of fibroids, abandoning birth control devices, wearing white suits. Nor do they report that depression, joint pain, and incontinence have nothing to do with menopause and that libido can rise. If they're responsible on the topic of estrogen, print and Web sites repeat "only in low doses for short terms" and put hormone risks before benefits or prominently feature the WHI study. If they're not responsible, writers put benefits foremost and attack these studies.

A pro-estrogen bias persists in myriad subtle ways. The *NAMS Menopause Guidebook* (North American Menopause Society, 2003) saves its overview of the WHI results for page 49 of 60 pages, and only on page 48 does it list antidotes to relieve the "side effects" of taking estrogen—possibly the first time many readers knew there were side effects. The *Washington Post* article implies that the millions who stopped treatment all had "maddeningly unanswerable" questions (Mundy, 2003). Many articles give midlife women the same implicit character: like addicts going "cold turkey," their drugs are being withheld, and they are desperate for new products. Yet a special study in the *Journal of the American Medical Association* reports that when women tapered off hormone treatment, as recommended, only 21.2 percent had a recurrence of "hot flashes" (Ockene et al., 2005, p. 192).[18]

Two worrying media trends are now at work: to fault the 2002 WHI study and to introduce untested commercial products. The main thrust—as in an article in the *Wall Street Journal*—is that the WHI "overstated the risks" and women are now *too* frightened of hormone treatments (Parker-Pope, 2005). This is the line that Wyeth, the makers of the hormone treatment on trial, pushed to medical societies and 500,000 health care providers the day the WHI report broke. The Wyeth commentary convinced 81 percent of gynecologists, according to Sheila and David Rothman in *The Pursuit of Perfection* (2003), that women's fears of HRT were overblown (Rothman and Rothman, 2003, p. 100). A 2006 article in the *St. Louis Post-Dispatch* quoted a chair of Ob/Gyn as saying "The WHI was way overdone . . . the damage has been done" (Jackson, 2006). When a *JAMA* study in 2007 confirmed most risks and found that only one small category of women would have fewer heart complications than thought, many papers deemphasized the confirmations, as in the *Boston Globe* headline, "Risk found by '02 hormone study challenged." Some journalists now say that the WHI data were "confusing," denying the original clarity. Complicit with the industry, they present its newest products—creams and gels—as if they were tested breakthroughs. A lot of news is about lower-dose versions, which are stabilizing sales, although even a Wyeth spokeswoman admits, "We do not have data evaluating those particular risks" (Berger, 2005).[19]

Many doctors cannot overcome their training, when hormone treatment was considered a magic bullet for the sickly and pathetic state of a female body wrapped around "nonfunctioning" ovaries. The program director for the National Women's Health Network worries that doctors "find reasons why the [WHI] findings shouldn't apply to their patients" (Berger, 2005). Estrogen is still, irrationally, linked not to cancer but to a youth-oriented definition of femininity.

Pharmaceutical companies are wistful about their past profits, while doctors and gynecologists are wistful about their obsolete knowledge. Wistfulness about "rejuvenation"—one outcome of age anxiety—affects the risk-benefit decisions women make. Gina Kolata (2003) begins a *New York Times* article with an anecdote about a woman who took double her prescribed dose of hormones to look younger. The effect is to keep a mad hope in circulation. Neither health writers nor fashion magazines publish former users of exogenous estrogen who declare, "I was foolish to worry more about 'youth' than 'health.'" Although sexual difficulties occur in younger women, numerous articles on female "dysfunction" overemphasize midlife "hormonal imbalance."

Estrogen is still believed to be a liquid that makes younger women *women*. In this metaphoric vein, the *Globe*'s Judy Foreman wrote a column on whether estrogen, "bathing" women's arteries, might still lower the risk of heart disease (Foreman, 2006). The implied readers are still those desperate dried-up postmenstrual women. In the same *New York Times* article, Kolata faulted the indefatigable Barbara Seaman, the author of *The Greatest Experiment Ever Performed on Women*, for holding estrogen critics to a "looser standard" than the mystic promoters, as if even-handedness were still obligatory (Kolata, 2003). Some scientists defend estrogen and trust the manufacturers. In an article in *Best Practice and Research in Clinical Endocrinology and Metabolism*, the authors state that the media caused "panic and confusion" by reporting the WHI results and argue that the data on extra cancers and heart disease do not mean that "HRT is not safe [sic] or efficacious" for symptoms (Ussher, 2006, p. 133).

The illusion that people aging into their middle years might recapture youth in a pill maintains the Estrogen-Good hypothesis of the infamous 1968 book *Feminine Forever*, in which Robert Wilson said of menopause, "no woman can be sure of escaping the horror of this living decay" (Hoberman, 2005, p. 135). All this—the promotion of untested products, the creation of muddle about WHI's test results, the ongoing construction of deprived "menopausal" women, the disregard of skeptical feminist perspectives—resurrects estrogen nostalgia and its sequelae after what should have been a debacle.

Studies commissioned by two drug companies in 2003 found that a quarter of the women who had stopped using hormones after the 2002 announcement had resumed (Ginty, 2008, p. 3).

The Emergence of the "Duty to Die"

When Prof. Carolyn Heilbrun committed suicide in 2003, she was a writer of detective fiction who was also celebrated as a feminist literary critic, subject to depression but otherwise healthy, married, with children and grandchildren, money, and admiring friends. She was only 77. Heilbrun's death profoundly disturbed many people for whom she was a role model, because of the reason she published in advance for wanting to do it—to "quit while you're ahead," thus avoiding becoming "too weak, or powerless, or ill" (Heilbrun, 1997, pp. 7, 9). She called this kind of suicide "rational." Her final act, at a time when she was apparently not ill, and despite her history of feminist antiageism, can leave people who hear this story—especially women, but all younger people—with the idea that despair is a rational response to *normal aging*.

Suicide is rare among women, rarer yet among women in later life. Carolyn was a mentor of mine, and we had many friends in common. The more I learned about her circumstances, the more I came to believe that ageism had exacerbated her depression. From an age critic's perspective, Heilbrun's chosen death raises the general question of the power of ageism to push retired people over the edge of marginality into despair. Our thinking about suicide has to take into account not only familial, psychological, financial, and neurological factors—the usual kind of "psychological autopsy"[20]—but also the social construction of decline. The pressures brought to bear by the new regimes of ageism can cause even healthy and relatively young people to think that perhaps they should die before they can become a "burden."

Carolyn's voluntary exit from work had snowballed into a series of immense identity strippings. She resigned from Columbia University's English department because male colleagues were not advancing her protégées, denying her the influence her seniority should have brought and thwarting her ability to help the feminist movement. Carolyn thus lost a field on which she had been heroically combative.

In her last essays, Carolyn wrote about some of her losses (but not Columbia's insult) in a rhetoric of later-life flexibility: the one in the *Women's Review of Books* is titled "Taking a U-Turn." But the deprivations implied were terrible. She had lost faith in literary criticism, didn't enjoy rereading, had lost her drive for writing when she turned to science, lacked a gripping long-term project, was no longer so motivated by feminist interests, and was losing the attention of critics and her female audience.

Losing her role as a teacher left her with writing. But she had stopped writing the popular Kate Fansler mysteries. And a month before her suicide she suffered a severe publishing disappointment (according to a close friend); she had hinted at another to me earlier that year. Publishers lose faith in the audience for "aging" writers; prestige sinks, and fans drift away. Writer's block, a condition many writers know young, is worsened by such ageism. In *Darkness Visible: A Memoir of Madness*, having rejected various explanations for his suicidal depression, William Styron juxtaposes age—"I turned sixty, that hulking milestone of mortality"—and dissatisfaction with his work (Styron, 2007, p. 78). No longer being considered at the top of one's game is not "mortality"—it's a prophecy that can fulfill itself. (Being exposed to negative stereotypes weakens self-esteem and affects judgment. This is called "stereotype threat.")

There are feminist ways to fight stereotype threat and identity stripping, but Carolyn seems to have chosen an impossible ego-ideal, comparing herself to men of her age and status. Her latest book was about three famous male Columbia professors who had never chosen her (or any woman) as their protégée. With her credentials—president of the Modern Language Association, no less—she should have been able to join that coterie of top men who resist ageism through traditional patriarchal means, retaining connections, prestige, and honors. Her postretirement proved that holding on as an "honorary man" (a status men had conferred on her) was tenuous. Did her comparative disadvantage as an older woman cause her to regress into that gnawing envy of male privilege so many women endured when they were young?

The "career self"—the self identified predominantly by its work—may no longer want to go on living once its plans can no longer be carried to fruition (Overall, 2003a, p. 186). Carolyn's mistake (a common one) was to attribute her professional and emotional losses to aging, considered as an essential and unavoidable process (like a terminal illness), rather than to ageism, which is culturally induced and conferred and only then internalized.

Carolyn's situation suggests a menace pointed first at an important historical cohort: older women (including women over 40, the "boomers") whose work outside the home has been fundamental to their identity. Many struggled to change systems that had excluded women; they were among the "firsts." They had talent, energy, a movement—all the good gifts. They are probably the biggest group ever to age at the intersection of female gender, formerly male privilege, and ageism. These women have much to fear from being aged by culture in our time when they lose the identity of the career self. Whatever else they gain from retirement, many people lose income, structure, prestige, and community. Relative disadvantage is fresh humiliation; in later life it can become a gendered form of despair. Worse, the withdrawal of social capital is defined by capitalist individualism as a personal "failure." In fact, women now seem to be finding the inevitable exit from work more stressful than men do, according to Silvia Sara Canetto, who has surveyed older women's suicides (Canetto, 1995).

At all ages, men kill themselves more than women—four times as often. Men 65 or older accounted for 80 percent of suicides in this age group—even though lifelong inequities for women and for men become exacerbated in old age and women are poorer and live longer alone. Women kill themselves at the highest rate in midlife, before age 54 (Centers for Disease Control, 2008). Older women apparently have some special later-life strength. But no one can take this historical trend for granted. Will social forces cause women to start catching up to men in later-life despair, as in rates of smoking, drinking, and incarceration?

The new ageism—more devastating in combination with midlife economic super-annuation—should make men also wary of their future. Selfhood is likely to be battered by growing hostile rhetoric about the unnecessary and expendable costs of "aging America." Under U.S. capitalism, retirement—whatever its cause—unless you are classed as a rich self-sufficient consumer, moves you into the ranks of the unproductive who are bleeding society. A vile interpretation of longevity (that more people living longer produces intolerable and unnecessary medical expense) makes the long-lived a national threat rather than a matter of pride. "Alarmist demography" is Steven Katz's term for this misreading of population aging (Katz, 1992).[21]

Alarmist demography has come out of the closet of hypocrisy and flourishes in the public arena. Media discourses explicitly warn younger people that unwanted and expensive "elderly" people are becoming too numerous, nationally and globally. "Long-lived people are perceived as inevitably constituting a debilitating psychological and socioeconomic burden," writes Christine Overall. In *Aging, Death, and Human Longevity*, a carefully argued book, Overall expresses doubt that "any other group in society could be described, with acceptance and impunity, as a 'burden' " (Overall, 2003a, p. 57).

These forms of pressure on people aging are coming to a head in the "duty to die." Overall (2003a) sums up an immense and growing literature that is constructing the sense of burden. The *Atlantic Monthly*, usually considered intellectually respectable, published an essay on "The Coming Death Shortage: Why the Longevity Boom Will Make Us Sorry to Be Alive," which demonstrates the extravagance of what can get published. The essay, whose transhuman world suspiciously resembles that depicted in Bruce Stirling's sci-fi novel *Holy Fire*, pits "us"—younger people who need careers and families—against "rich oldsters . . . expending their disposable income" on "longevity treatments" like heart bypass operations or implanted defibrillators (Mann, 2005, p. 94). Treating elders, many desperately poor, as "greedy geezers"—a term that also began life in a magazine article (in the *New Republic*)—accompanies right-wing calls for reducing safety nets like Social Security and limiting hospice care. Even the *New York Times* published an article titled "How to Save Medicare? Die Sooner" (Altman, 2005). Some bioethicists, scientists, lawyers, and historians collude with the mainstream media in pushing this bias.

The mean-spirited final solution—the injunction to "die sooner"—is becoming hauntingly clear. Pundits—starting with ex-governor Richard Lamm and bioethicist John Hardwig—escalate this notion by arguing that there is a "duty to die," by which Hardwig includes "a duty [incumbent on older people] to refuse life-prolonging medical treatment and also a duty to complete advance directives refusing life-prolonging treatment" (Hardwig, 1997). Because women live longer than men by eight years and are (wrongly) considered to be sicker in old age, the two trends—longevity and alarmist demography—converge on women. They never die, they just cost more. Women who are old now may be more likely than male peers to be coerced into dying under this new regime, because they are less assertive than men, more submissive to authorities, Norah Martin suggests in *Recognition, Responsibility and Rights: Feminist Ethics and Social Theory* (2003).

Exposure to positive stereotypes makes older research subjects likelier to choose life-saving measures, as experiments in psychology indicate. In the same way, vicious stereotypes can reduce their will to live (Levy, Ashman, and Dror, 1999–2000). "Concerns about [being] a family burden are a principal reason that patients reject life-sustaining treatments," write Dr. Kenneth Rosenfeld and colleagues in a study of "End-of-Life Decision Making" (Rosenfeld, Wenger, and Kagawa-Singer, 2000). Those of us in our middle years are already being scolded by some media into abandoning our future claims on such treatments. Will the retired in general start believing that they are trapped—too old to live, but too young to die?

The rhetoric already influences medical systems, in a way distinct from legislatively defined assisted suicide. The British, who can boast a system of national health care, already ration dialysis, quietly letting people die of end-stage renal failure, according to Stephen Harrison and Michael Moran (2000). In the United States, at the very time when presidential candidates are seriously discussing national health care for all, debates are beginning about whether there should be an age limit after which not to provide "heroic" care. In a nation that does not provide long-term care, in which few can afford long-term care insurance, the media talk constantly about how expensive late-life care is. Adult children are certainly told the costs.

Despite the label "geriatric depression," depression is far from inevitable in later life. "Failing strength, isolation, and the fear of death, all of which are associated with aging, though formidable, do not inevitably cause depression," notes Rachel Josefowitz Siegel in "Ageism in Psychiatric Diagnosis" (Siegel, 2004, p. 91). Even among terminally ill patients, a majority "discuss their wish to die, to be free of sickness or to have the dying process end," according to the researcher John Linder, but "many of these references are oblique or symbolic and only a few are overtly suicidal" (Linder, 2004, p. 704).

When suicide occurs, however, it is often related to underlying major depression. The goal of age studies here is to know not just the proximate causes (e.g., job loss, widowhood). The link between depression and suicidality (perhaps also the passive acceptance of death) is the sense that life has become irreversibly intolerable. In *Declining to Decline*, I called being forced to tell a decline narrative "a stressor, a depressant . . . a psychocultural illness." Alarmist demography has effects like midlife unemployment and dismissal of "menopausal women." Corrosive forms of ageism, sexism, and ableism can make those aging toward old age or chronically ill likelier to feel unwanted—unloved, sad, outcast, isolated, ashamed, helpless, and depressed.

Anxiety and depression, although as treatable in old age, may be ignored. Or, it may be noticed but go untreated because of younger people's fatalism about the ills of old age. A report by the Alliance for Ageing Research found that "too many physicians and psychologists believe that late-stage depression and suicidal statements are normal and acceptable" in older patients (Dembner, 2005). Suicide is a possible cultural outcome of believing that the state, doctors, and your children find you a burden. "Could the idea of a duty to die become one of the proverbial last straws that could precipitate that act?" Prof. Overall asks (Overall, 2003b, p. 66).

A number of philosophers now feel the need to justify the desire for longevity. Louise Antony writes, " 'being able to live to the end of a complete human life . . . not dying prematurely' is a level of function that is necessary for a good human life, a life that we would be satisfied to have" (Antony, 2005, p. 137). That such arguments against "the duty to die" need to be made would be shocking if ageism mattered. Felicia Nimue Ackerman, a philosopher at Brown, believes that we should hear much more about *the duty to care* for the vulnerable, which she opposes to the duty to die (Ackerman, 2002, pp. 426–34).

An op-ed writer in the *Washington Post* said, "Nor, *given the aging of the population*, is the topic of rational suicide likely to disappear" (Lerner, 2004).[22] It is not aging but urging suicide on the vulnerable that keeps the topic alive: discourses about "burden," "population-based medicine," "the futility of care," and "distributive ethics" are arguments for policies that may quietly result in age-based medical rationing. They are in the driver's seat.[23] The public policy response should be to socialize our caregiving to sick aging people (as to sick younger people) so that it is more adequate to their needs. But under the best political circumstances, can America do this so that the word *burden* never comes up?

Because younger people have a duty to live, suicide may sound "rational" only when elderly people do it. "Rational" elder suicide may become far less of a choice than proponents of the right-to-die think. Perhaps it will seem sensible to go through much of the life course fearing "aging" and holding the idea of suicide in conscious reserve, as Heilbrun did. Already people at parties tell me how they are planning to do it. (In *this* context, death, not to mention suicide, is no longer taboo.)

Might American decline ideology prove so harsh that suicide becomes a rational response to normal aging? At what age should pining for voluntary death begin? At 60? At 40? Even if age anxiety never turns to suicidal ideation, it is dreadful to think how much energy is sapped by having to fend off age-linked decline discourse and internalization year after year without the support of a movement.

Conclusion

"Aging is increasingly constructed as a problem" (Slevin, 2006, p. 248)[24]—this is the dire trend that many age critics observe. Yet the media incessantly and some gerontologists present aging as a miracle of longevity and better health, at least for "the aging boomers": in breathless language, an incredible opportunity for personal growth and cultural change. In this view, biotech and cosmetic surgery will morph elderly consumers into active and youthful-looking cyborgs; computers and leisurely travel will expand their contracted spaces. Discrimination is somehow behind us.[25]

Positive-aging messages like these often attempt to combat ageism without naming its sources or estimating their power, a feeble strategy. Most gains touted depend on privilege. Individual "enhancements" cannot counteract decline ideology, and some, like cosmetic surgery, worsen it by convincing others that normal aging is ugly. Maybe to healthy, privileged older people, physiological aging seems the only dangerous driver in sight.

But by analyzing contemporary ageism and dividing it into its component parts—such as midlife job discrimination, the trauma of dismissal, forced retirement, the erosion of seniority, menopause deficiency discourse, estrogen nostalgia, medicalization of men and women, the cult of youth, stereotype bias, fatalism about old age and "geriatric depression," alarmist demography, age anxiety, the duty to die—critical age studies demonstrates how much of so-called aging, on inspection, reveals the ageist and middle-ageist dynamics of social changes. To make a space for discovery and armor ourselves for cultural combat, whenever we find ourselves using the term *aging* we could try substituting *ageism* instead.

Ageism and middle ageism hurt even more than the three cases presented here suggest. They threaten self-esteem, the oxygen of selfhood. By devaluing the entire later life course, decline ideology is changing what it means to be human. What good would it do if everyone lived healthily to 120 and hated the last 60 years of their lives?

Although aging cannot be fought (despite the promises of "antiaging" products), ageism can be. Americans need a vital multigenerational antiageist movement, the antidote to the perpetual drip-drip of cultural poison. If all the people who were lied to about their bodies joined all the people anxious about their jobs and all those furious about being pressured to die prematurely, a joint war against the regimes of decline could prove heartening. Political anger may help heal the rift between the full person as accrued over the life course and the wizened, self-deprecating person who absorbs decline. If a larger collective embraces resistance, then the harsher aspects of American decline ideology might not become more cruelly influential.[26] The task is urgent.

In Nicole Hollander's cartoon, Sylvia, the Woman Who's Easily Irritated, notes about stereotype threat, "When I'm in charge, there will be severe consequences if someone refers to an older person as a crone, old geezer, old biddy or the like." An off-stage voice asks, "Honey, how severe will those consequences be?" (Hollander, 2006).

NOTES

1. For descriptions of age studies, see Gullette (2004, chap. 6 et passim). Some age critics and critical gerontologists I read with profit are quoted in this chapter; others include Carroll Estes, Martha Holstein, Andrew Blaikie, Tom Cole, Andrew Achenbaum, Chris Phillipson, and Sara Arber.

2. Aging as a narrative and "critical age autobiography" are discussed in Gullette (2004). The first chapter suggests how young children learn the decline narrative of aging.

3. For a study of people 50 to 61 not in the labor force, see Congressional Budget Office (2004).

4. For the 401(k) data, see Opiela (2004, p. 18).

5. On midlife debt, see Gist and Figueiredo (2008).

6. A total of 23.2% of this group was either still in the labor force or looking for a job in 2006, up from 19.6% in 2000 (Ohlemacher, 2007, p. A4).

7. Uchitelle is excellent on the trauma of dismissal. See Uchitelle (2006, pp. x, 179–81).

8. I first called this identity stripping in *Declining to Decline* (Gullette, 1997a).

9. For a summary of evidence of differential treatment of midlife workers before the ADEA, see Neumark (2003, pp. 304–5).

10. This section is a version of a longer essay (Gullette, 2008).

11. The North American Menopause Society calls it the "gold standard" in a fat brochure, *Menopause Guidelines*, that was given out by my HMO in 2005.

12. Reports of declining use of HRT in various populations appeared in such specialized journals as *Obstetrics and Gynecology, Annals of Internal Medicine, British Medical Journal, Journal of the American Medical Association*, etc. See Ekström (2005, p. 3, nn. 10–14).

13. Articles about it from 2004 are cited in Fugh-Berman and Scialli (2006, p. 120).

14. Data differ on what percentage of women dropped hormone treatments.

15. Only 10% visit a health care provider. See Woods and Mitchell (2005, p. 14), which cites a 1992 study by McKinlay, Brambilla, and Posner on the typical menopause. A total of 15% have no problems at all. Many traditional and poor women—immigrants, African-Americans, Latinas—never hear hormone promises. Presumably some women can't afford medical attention. Most problems disappear by themselves.

16. This term was first used, to my knowledge, in Gullette (1997b).

17. Bettina Leysen is quoted to this effect in Hoberman (2005, pp. 7–8).

18. The study was of 8400 women who had stopped eight months before.

19. Quoting Amy Allina.

20. The "psychological autopsy" was named by Edwin S. Shneidman, the inventor of the term "suicidology" and the editor of *Autopsy of a Suicidal Mind* (Shneidman, 2004), whom I interviewed a number of times for this chapter.

21. For a thoughtful examination of population aging, see Jackson (1998).

22. Emphasis mine.

23. Faria lists these in Faria (2007, p. 1). Mullin casts doubts on alarmist demography in Mullin (2005).

24. Mullin (2005, p. 3) says there is "little left in political economy into which the aging/problem [sic] does not intrude."

25. In her column "Second Acts," Ellen Goodman (2007) writes as if discrimination had ended: "sixty-somethings . . . were prodded by discrimination. Now we are drawing blueprints for people who see themselves more as citizens than seniors."

26. I build on Kathleen Woodward's view of the function of anger in her powerful essay "Against Wisdom" (Woodward, 2002).

REFERENCES

Ackerman, F. N. 2002. For now have I my death: The "duty to die" versus the duty to help the ill stay alive. In *Ethical Issues in Modern Medicine*, ed. B. Steinbock. New York: McGraw Hill.

Altman, D. 2005. How to save Medicare? Die sooner. *New York Times*, February 27, p. (3)1.

Antony, L. M. 2005. Natures and norms. In *Feminist Theory: A philosophical anthology*, ed. A. E. Cudd and R. O. Andreasen. Oxford: Blackwell.

Berger, L. 2005. Two years after, on hormone therapy, the dust is still settling. *New York Times*, June 6.

Canetto, S. S. 1995. Elderly women and suicidal behavior. In *Women and Suicidal Behavior*, ed. S. S. Canetto and D. Lester. New York: Springer.

Carpenter, M. 2005. Choosing different paths: Three years out from blockbuster HRT findings, women are navigating menopause in increasingly personal ways. *Pittsburgh Post-Gazette*, December 21, p. F1.

Centers for Disease Control. 2008. *Suicide Data Sheet.* Available from www.cdc.gov/Violen cePrevention/pdf/Suicide-DataSheet-a.pdf.

Chan, S., and A. H. Stevens. 2001. Job loss and employment patterns of older workers. *Journal of Labor Economics* 19 (2):484–521.

Congressional Budget Office. 2008. Disability and retirement: The early exit of baby boomers from the labor force, November 2004 [cited June 19, 2008]. Available from http://cbo.gov/doc.cfm?index=6018&type=0.

Cowley, G., and K. Springen. 2002. The end of the age of estrogen. *Newsweek*, July 22, pp. 38–45.

Dembner, A. 2005. Ageism said to erode care given to elders. *Boston Globe*, March 7.

Ehrenreich, B. 2005. *Bait and Switch: The (futile) pursuit of the American dream.* New York: Henry Holt.

Ekström, H. 2005. Trends in middle-aged women's reports of symptoms, use of hormone therapy, and attitudes towards it. *Maturitas* 52 (2):154–64.

Faria, M. A. 2007. Slouching towards a duty to die. 1999 [cited October 14, 2007]. Available from www.Haciendapub.com/article29.html.

Foreman, J. 2006. Hormones: Does timing make a difference? *Boston Globe*, February 20.

Freundlich, N. 2004. Menopause: What every woman—and man—needs to know. *Business-Week*, August 30.

Fugh-Berman, A., and A. R. Scialli. 2006. Gynecologists and estrogen: An affair of the heart. *Perspectives in Biology and Medicine* 49 (1):115–30.

Genuis, S. K., and S. J. Genuis. 2006. Exploring the continuum: Medical information to effective clinical practice. *Journal of Evaluation in Clinical Practice* 12 (1):63–75.

Ginty, M. 2008. After health scare, menopause treatment matures. *Women's e-News 2005* [cited June 19, 2008]. Available from www.womensenews.org/article.cfm/dyn/aid/2367/context/cover/.

Gist, J., and C. Figueiredo. 2008. Deeper in debt: Trends among midlife and older Americans. AARP Public Policy Institute, April 2002 [cited June 19, 2008]. Available from www.aarp.org/research/credit-debt/debt/aresearch-import-339-DD70.html.

Goodman, E. 2007. Second acts. *Boston Globe*, October 19, p. A17.

Gorman, C. 2005. Menopause: A healthy view. *Time*, May 16, p. 57.

Gregory, R. F. 2001. *Age Discrimination in the American Workplace: Old at a young age.* New Brunswick: Rutgers University Press.

Gullette, M. M. 1993. What, menopause again?! *Ms.*, July/August, pp. 34–37.

———. 1997a. *Declining to Decline: Cultural combat and the politics of the midlife.* Charlottesville: University of Virginia Press.

———. 1997b. Menopause as magic marker. In *Reinterpreting Menopause: Cultural and philosophical issues,* ed. P. A. Komesaroff, P. Rothfield, and J. Daley. New York: Routledge.

———. 2004. *Aged by Culture.* Chicago: University of Chicago Press.

———. 2008. Hormone nostalgia. In *Women, Wellness, and the Media,* ed. M. Wiley. Cambridge, UK: Cambridge Scholars Publishing.

Hardwig, J. 1997. Is there a duty to die? *Hastings Center Report* 27 (2):34–42.

Harrison, S., and M. Moran. 2000. Resources and rationing: Managing supply and demand in health care. In *Handbook of Social Studies in Health and Medicine,* ed. G. L. Albrecht, R. Fitzpatrick, and S. C. Scrimshaw. London: Sage.

Heilbrun, C. 1997. *The Last Gift of Time: Life beyond sixty.* New York: Dial Press.

Hipple, S. 1999. Worker displacement in the mid-1990's. *Monthly Labor Review* 122 (7):15–32.

Hoberman, J. 2005. *Testosterone Dreams: Rejuvenation, aphrodisia, doping.* Berkeley: University of California Press.

Hollander, N. 2006. *Sylvia* (comic strip). *Boston Globe,* October 31.

Houck, J. A. 2006. *Hot and Bothered: Women, medicine, and menopause in modern America.* Cambridge: Harvard University Press.

Houlihan, L. 2005. HRT cancer link found. *Herald Sun* (Australia), August 1, p. 8.

Jackson, H. 2006. Trouble connecting? *St. Louis Post-Dispatch,* September 4, p. H1.

Jackson, W. 1998. *The Political Economy of Population Ageing.* Cheltenham: Edward Elgar.

Jacobson, L., R. LaLonde, and D. Sullivan. 1993. *The Costs of Worker Dislocation.* Kalamazoo: W. E. Upjohn Institute of Employment Research.

———. 2005. Is retraining displaced workers a good investment? *Economic Perspectives* 2005 (2):47–66.

Johnson, C. K. 2006. Studies tie depression risk to approach of menopause. *Boston Globe,* April 4, p. A6.

Katz, S. 1992. Alarmist demography: Power, knowledge and the elderly population. *Journal of Aging Studies* 6 (3):203–25.

Kohli, M., et al., eds. 1991. *Time for Retirement: Comparative studies of early exit from the labor force.* Cambridge: Cambridge University Press.

Kolata, G. 2003. Books of the times: On the trail of estrogen and a mirage of youth. *New York Times,* July 5.

Kowalczyk, L. 2006. Breast cancer diagnoses took sudden drop in '03. *Boston Globe,* December 15, pp. A1, A36.

Lattman, P. 2007. Hot Flash: $134.5 million Prempro verdict. *Wall Street Journal* Law Blog 2007 [cited October 15, 2007]. Available from http://blogs.wsj.com/law/2007/10/11/hot-flash-1345-prempro-verdict-in-nevada/.

Lerner, B. H. 2004. A calculated departure: For someone in good health, can suicide ever be a rational choice? *Washington Post,* March 2, p. F1.

Levy, R., O. Ashman, and I. Dror. 1999–2000. To be or not to be: The effects of aging stereotypes on the will to live. *Omega: Journal of Death and Dying* 40 (3):409–20.

Linder, J. 2004. Oncology. In *Living with Dying: A handbook for end-of-life healthcare practitioners*, ed. J. Berzoff and P. R. Silverman. New York: Columbia University Press.

Lock, M. 2000. Accounting for disease and distress: Morals of the normal and abnormal. In *Handbook of Social Studies in Health and Medicine*, ed. G. L. Albrecht, R. Fitzpatrick, and S. C. Scrimshaw. London: Sage.

Mann, C. C. 2005. The coming death shortage: Why the longevity boom will make us sorry to be alive. *Atlantic Monthly*, May, pp. 92–104.

Martin, N. 2003. Physician-assisted suicide and euthanasia: Weighing feminist concerns. In *Recognition, Responsibility and Rights: Feminist ethics and social theory*, ed. R. N. Fiore and H. L. Nelson. Lanham: Rowman and Littlefield.

McMullin, J., and E. D. Berger. 2006. Gendered ageism/age(ed) sexism: The case of unemployable older workers. In *Age Matters: Realigning feminist thinking*, ed. T. M. Calasanti and K. F. Slevin. New York: Routledge.

McNagny, S. E., N. K. Wenger, and E. Frank. 1997. Personal use of postmenopausal hormone replacement therapy by women physicians in the United States. *Annals of Internal Medicine* 127 (12):1093–96.

Miller, J. 2006. Reading into old age. *Raritan* 26 (1):14–30.

Moen, P., et al. 2004. *The New "Middle" Work Force*. Minneapolis: The Life Course Center at the University of Minnesota and the Bronfenbrenner Life Course Center (and Cornell Careers Institute) at Cornell University.

Mullin, P. 2005. *The Imaginary Time Bomb: Why an ageing population is not a social problem*. London: I. B. Tauris.

Mundy, L. 2003. Better living through chemistry: How menopause has become the new hot-button topic in women's health. *Washington Post*, October 5.

Neumark, D. 2003. Age discrimination legislation in the United States. *Contemporary Economic Policy* 21 (3):297–317.

Norris, F. 2006. She works, her grandson doesn't. *New York Times*, September 3, p. (4)12.

North American Menopause Society. 2003. *NAMS Menopause Guidebook*. Cleveland, OH: North American Menopause Society.

Ockene, J. K., et al. 2005. Symptom experience after discontinuing use of estrogen plus progestin. *Journal of the American Medical Association* 294 (2):183–93.

Ohlemacher, S. 2007. Immigrant number hits record 37.5m. *Boston Globe*, September 12, p. A4.

Opiela, N. 2004. Hitting the home stretch. *Fidelity Focus*, February.

Overall, C. 2003a. *Aging, Death, and Human Longevity*. Berkeley: University of California Press.

———. 2003b. Concepts of life span and life stages: Implications for ethics. In *Feminist Moral Philosophy*, ed. S. Brennan. Calgary: University of Calgary Press.

Painter, K. 2005. Change of life remains hard. *USA Today*, September 26.

Parker-Pope, T. 2005. The fear factor: Women continue to shy away from hormone therapy. *Wall Street Journal*, October 11.

Porter, E., and M. W. Walsh. 2005. Retirement becomes a rest stop as pensions and benefits shrink. *New York Times*, February 9, p. A1.

Rosenfeld, K. E., N. S. Wenger, and M. Kagawa-Singer. 2000. End-of-life decision making: A qualitative study of elderly individuals. *Journal of General Internal Medicine* 15 (9):620–25.

Rothman, S. M., and D. J. Rothman. 2003. *The Pursuit of Perfection: The promise and perils of medical enhancement*. New York: Pantheon.

Russo, R. 1994. *Nobody's Fool.* New York: Vintage.

Service, R. F. 1998. New role for estrogen in cancer? *Science* 279 (5357):1631–33.

Shneidman, E. S., ed. 2004. *Autopsy of a Suicidal Mind.* Oxford: Oxford University Press.

Siegel, R. J. 2004. Ageism in psychiatric diagnosis. In *Bias in Psychiatric Diagnosis,* ed. P. J. Caplan and L. Cosgrove. New York: Jason Aronson.

Slevin, K. F. 2006. The embodied experiences of older lesbians. In *Age Matters: Realigning feminist thinking,* ed. T. M. Calasanti and K. F. Slevin. New York: Routledge.

Solomon, A. 2001. *The Noonday Demon: An atlas of depression.* New York: Scribner.

Styron, W. 2007. *Darkness Visible: A memoir of madness.* New York: Random House.

Uchitelle, L. 2006. *The Disposable American: Layoffs and their consequences.* New York: Knopf.

Ussher, J. M. 2006. *Managing the Monstrous Feminine: Regulating the reproductive body.* London: Routledge.

Westlake, D. 1997. *The Ax.* New York: Time Warner.

Woods, N. F., and E. Mitchell. 2005. Symptoms during the perimenopause: Prevalence, severity, trajectory, and significance in women's lives. *American Journal of Medicine* 118 (12, Suppl. 2):14–24.

Woodward, K. 2002. Against wisdom: The social politics of anger and aging. *Cultural Critique* 51:186–218.

Yager, J. D., and N. E. Davidson. 2006. Mechanisms of disease: Estrogen carcinogenesis in breast cancer. *New England Journal of Medicine* 354 (3):270–82.

PERSONAL PERSPECTIVES

CHAPTER FIFTEEN

Treadmilling to the Far Side

An Informal Guide to Coming of Age with Mortality

ROBERT KASTENBAUM, PH.D.

Who will guide the guide? Who can instruct an author who has been instructed to offer a tour of death and dying at the far side of the life course? We might patch together a literature review from standard sources. Instead, let's begin where endings are postponed until further notice and borrowed time is repaid at compound interest three days a week. That would be Monday, Wednesday, and Friday, up one level at the Arizona Heart Institute's rehab center. We bring our stents, bypass scars, pacemakers, oxygen canisters, and other tokens from affairs of the heart. Crossing the threshold, we join others who have been proven immortal until further notice.

As your guide *du jour*, I have a touch of both the *emic* and the *etic* (Pike, 1969) orientations. I gained access to the rehabilitation program when my cardiac apparatus became sufficiently dysfunctional. After my rookie period, I became a fledged participant in the group's verbal and nonverbal patterns, implicit rules, and unscripted encounters with mortality. Like the other members, I could then process group knowledge from the "emic" or insider's perspective. Once I became "emic," it was hard to restrain my outsider's ("etic") side. But the dual roles of participant and observer seldom have been at cross-purpose in this setting. I have just gone about my business while minding everybody else's business along with my own.

It is time now to meet some of the several dozen people who are regulars at the cardiac rehabilitation center. Later I will turn to the larger picture.

What Say? Dreadmill Discourse
"Barely"

Immobility, thy name is Walter. He is a dignified, strongly built man with a shock of silver hair that Robert Frost might have envied. The treadmill is next on his agenda. At the moment, however, Walter has the look of a man who has gone as far as he can go.

One hesitates to inflict a conversation on him. But—and this is one of the unspoken rules—one also hesitates to ignore a fellow rehabber who is trapped in a moment of potential dissolve. And so one asks the most banal of questions: "How's it going?"

"Barely." This is barely a response, but sufficient. The lights switch back on in Walter's eyes, and his slow smile signals a perceptible upgrade in color, respiration, and energy. "Barely" is precisely how it had been going for Walter that morning. Most of us have had a similar feeling from time to time. The regulars here speak realistically and succinctly about their conditions. Who would they be fooling to pretend otherwise? A detailed organ recital or a rage against fate is conspicuously absent. The implicit rules at the rehab center, if posted, might read like this:

- We are at a time in life when honest communication is a good idea. It conserves energy otherwise expended on circumlocutions. But it is also a mark of respect: the people here appreciate candor. Bonds are strengthened when we level with each other.
- It is right to approach—thoughtfully—a person who seems unapproachable at the moment. Chances are that a staff member will already have noticed the participant who seems confused, withdrawn, inert, or despairing. But the staff cannot be everywhere all the time. Often a little companionship and a word or two will assure the troubled one that he or she is not alone. We don't have to be told that immediate call for professional assistance is in order if the troubled participant looks to be in the vicinity of a catastrophic event.
- Nevertheless, be sure you are ready to deal with the door you are opening. The sailor, the produce salesman, the engineer, the teacher might have had experiences that will now haunt you as well. Many of their bad dreams are not dreams.
- It is right to respond to others when you have drifted into that hollow and slippery place. You know that they know something of what you are going through. No need to apologize for a bad day; no need to get stuck in it.
- Be yourself. You have all inhabited the role of generic obedient patient. You have performed within normative bounds in social and work situations. Here, however, distinctive personality is welcome. Your inner grouch (Charles! Jacob!) will have entertainment value, and there will be ovations for you (Emma!) as you outsprint us on the treadmill while exalting a politician most of us would like to see do the penitentiary walk. Differences are savory. They juice up the sessions for the aching creatures making their way through still another set of repetitions.

"He will let me live until September."

Spencer is the newbie on the next bike. He has completed his basic recovery from medical procedures and is now going at the physical rehab with rather too much gusto. (Am I supposed to keep up with him?) Spencer shares good news. His cardiologist told him yesterday that there were no more procedures to go through. No changes in medication. Just do what you do. "Doesn't need to see me for three months. He's going on vacation—and he's letting me live until September."

What a sweet interlude, I thought. Perhaps I should not mention the physician who assured operetta composer Victor Herbert that he need have no concern about his health. About five minutes later, Herbert had no concerns at all, felled by a massive heart attack as he labored down the staircase he had laboriously ascended just a short time before. No, I won't mention that. Nice for Spencer to have a survival guarantee, though, a break from trying to outmuscle or out-luck death. That very afternoon I saw "my" cardiologist, who suggested we tweak one med. Other than that, I was good to go until, yes, September! He was off to Manhattan, quite possibly to see *Spamalot* for a third (or was that a fourth?) time. Death does not really take a holiday, but cardiologists do. Spencer and I believe in the transcendent power of our physicians, a concession to wishful thinking. "September," muses Spencer. "He could have picked a month with 31 days."

"It will pass, or I will."

Della is matriarch of a colossal brood. Sixty people for dinner is not a family reunion; it's just dinner. She is compassionate and tough-minded, fun-loving and fatalistic, an adored presence in our midst. Della has pulled through several near-fatal episodes and received just about every treatment option in the book. At the moment, she is sharing her chili recipe with an appreciative cluster gathered around her oxygen canister while she is also completing her turn at the cross-trainer device. These missions accomplished, Della looks weary and uncharacteristically distressed. She is ever ready to inquire when one of us is having an off day, so it is fair to ask, "OK, what's with Della?"

Della explains. The problem with today is tomorrow. Her birthday. But why is that a problem? Some years ago, her mother had decided to act her advanced age. She would leave the hustle and bustle to the younger echelons. Della persuaded her mother to enjoy a just-the-two-of-us lunch at a favorite restaurant. The family birthday celebration would be in the evening. Mother entered the car, turned pale, and asked for her nitro pills. Della quickly provided them and suggested they drive immediately to a hospital. Mother waved off the suggestion. "It will pass, or I will," she said. And without another breath, she died in Della's arms.

Every birthday has been a pained reminder of her mother's passing. It is, however, only one part of a long life's experience that has imbued Della with the sense that she is carrying both death and life with her, inseparably. Her own death has been there all along, intertwined with ongoing life. With every health crisis, she has told herself, "It will pass, or I will." Della has faith but not certainty regarding an afterlife. "My family and friends, they are on both sides of death. I have plenty of company now, and I'll have plenty of company later. "Della's eyes light up as she sees another participant approaching. "I'm teaching Herman Spanish. He's a good learner. He's teaching me Yiddish and deli!"

"Ten Cents. That was my nickname."

It's my turn with the free weights, but Drummond has also started. Pure comedy, and the joke's on me. Drummond hoists the heaviest weights on the rack with less effort than my struggles with lesser irons. Fellow exercisers in the area politely keep their amusement to themselves. Drummond brings a slow, fierce intensity to all his work-out stations. It is all the more impressive, knowing that he left an eye, a knee, half a finger, and at least half his youth in Vietnam. He shares his experiences in a calm, whispery voice several sizes too small for such a behemoth.

His memories are mostly the stuff of nightmares and, unfortunately, altogether too credible. Drummond has seen and done things that are not enshrined in over-the-counter models of the life course. The "Ten Cents" episode was not as messy as most of the others and so can be described in fewer words. He had come into possession of an elite Soviet rifle and was appointed sniper-in-chief for his unit that shared the jungle with Vietcong detachments.

"What was that like?" I asked him. "I've never had an experience anything like that."

Drummond squinted into a memory scene, speaking even slower and more whis-pery than usual.

"I'd lie on the top of a ridge. You could see everything that moved if it wasn't behind a tree. Just lie there and wait. Then wait some more."

Drummond now had his hunter's eyes engaged.

"A Charlie puts his head up. I blow it off. You could see it pop off."

"Pop off?"

"Pop off. Charlie'd think twice about attacking us any time soon."

"Where did the 'Ten Cents' part come in?"

"That's what a bullet cost. The G.I. bullets. We lucked into the Russian. They said they would take a dime out of your pay if you wasted a bullet." [He interjects one such incident.]

"How many bullets did you waste?"

"I never missed a shot. One head, one shot."

"What was the distance?"

"Three hundred yards."

I thought I had probably asked as many questions as we both could tolerate at the moment. Nevertheless: "How did you feel about it?"

"I felt good! I did what I was there to do. Get Charlie before Charlie gets us. Life was cheap in Nam. Sometimes only ten cents."

Most of Drummond's military service involved close combat, with induction into the realm of atrocities. Returning from these experiences, he married, earned a living, and raised a family. His ongoing relationships are harmonious. Drummond is neither belligerent nor impulsive. As another participant noted, "He's actually kind of sweet." Drummond has conventional tastes for his generation, and now and then he contributes striking insight or crafty humor to the mix.

Like Della, he brings death with him. Unlike Della, he has himself been a proficient agent of violent death, wholesale as well as retail. His killing days were also the prime days of his youth, to which he brought enthusiasm and not too many doubts or questions. Drummond cannot wash the blood from his hands without also rejecting his youth and the cause for which it was spent.

His amiability is authentic, but so is the laser beam of cold rage that he restricts to those he perceives as playing with war. "They don't know what war *is,* and they don't know how to finish what they start." He would fight again to save his country—especially the children and the women—but has more contempt than he can put into words for the politicians who send people to their death and never really know what they are doing.

How will Drummond's engagement with violent death influence his own end-of-life experience? Is he suited for today's muted deathbed scene, a medicated fading away? That is one of many questions we cannot answer with any confidence. Drummond does not live now as he did then. Well, sometimes he does. Flashbacks continue to invade the perimeters of security he has so diligently established. Drummond, who will you be as your reclaimed yet harrowing life comes to its end?

"Let me tell you something: I don't like dementing! I hate it!"

Ellis and I had limited interactions for the first few weeks after he joined us. He was concentrating hard on basic activities. His wife and designated driver kept an anxious eye on him. Ellis seemed a little confused around the edges, although, as time passed, he settled well into the routines.

It was surprising, then, when he approached me as I was levering and pedaling away in a cross-trainer. Ellis proclaimed his dementia without preamble. "Tell me more," I said, and he did. "I hate it. I am furious and I have nobody to be furious at. It's hard to draw a blank. It's hard not to be sure of—Something I am sure of now I might not be sure of tomorrow. It's hard and it's getting harder."

Why did Ellis feel the need to share his plight at that moment? Perhaps he had to say something while he still could. He then delivered a lucid and vehement critique of the current political regime. What made it worse: "I voted for those monsters!" He had believed they were right for his country. "I was wrong. They [naming names] are destroying America with their stupidity, their greed. Their evil! Unbelievable! Did I say "stupidity?" I'll say it again. Evil is so shallow it *is* stupidity! Nobody wins!" He paused, then added: "I am dementing. I know that damn well. But I'm still entitled to my opinion!"

Ellis was a highly successful business entrepreneur who was well acquainted with the political process. He is outraged that his mind and his nation appear to be failing at the same time. Ellis retains substantial command over his knowledge base and language skills. Ellis still possesses a strong personality. He can construct a compelling life-course narrative but occasionally loses focus regarding the just-then and the just-next. His *Now* is afloat, drifting between the indistinct shores of *then* and *next*.

Ellis does not lack for self-pride. He likes to think things through in his own way and stay in command of his life. Continued decline in cognitive function would reduce the awareness of self-loss as he nears the end of life. But what if his last days should come while he is still of two minds: the one alert and teeming with thought and feelings, and the other wandering in a disconnected haze? "Coming to terms" with life and death is contingent on having a mind that can still reason. Or is it?

Dare we wonder if dementia is nature's parting gift? Dare we feel tempted by the offer to avoid the hollows of loss, the stings of regret, and the snares of overmatched reason? Just asking.

"It's called, 'Going on.'"

The sad thing about making a chocolate pudding pie is when nobody cares if you eat the whole thing yourself.

The triumphant thing about making a chocolate pudding pie is when you can eat the whole thing yourself.

Jacob became a widower and a candidate for cardiac rehabilitation at around the same time. He was our slow-pokiest participant, spending much of his time doing nothing in particular. When finally at exercise, Jake made it through his routines with a "see-I'm-doing-it-are-you-happy-now!" defiance. He favored staff members and fellow participants with morose jibes. These remarks could be taken as either stay-away signals or cries for companionship. Jacob was a pill. Jacob was the village grouch. Everybody liked him.

Jacob could have been arrested for violating every known dress code, not excepting the last call at Mardi Gras. He would arrive in a dazzling mishmash of color, design, and material. Nobody would say anything. Nobody knew what to say. Unshaven and inattentive to the few loyal strands of hair on his head, Jacob stomped about with a furtively inquisitive look. What he hoped or feared to see was anybody's guess.

There were moments when light came through, however, and we glimpsed a prebereft Jacob. One such occasion occurred during the group's concerted effort to recall the lyrics to "Chattanooga Choo Choo." There was often something that somebody wanted to remember, and equanimity could not be restored until the elusive bit was recalled. "Track twenty-nine!" Jacob shouted out from his perch on a stationary bike. Track twenty-nine, indeed! Jacob was acclaimed hero. He followed up this triumph a few days later when another favorite topic was afoot—Arizona, what it was like, back in the day. Jacob disclosed that he had bombed Arizona—repeatedly. Got paid for it, too, and loved every minute. He was responsible for evaluating the test flights, and often given the honor of deciding where to drop the load. "Arizona was a big empty with nothing in it. I'd pick the spot and I'd say, 'Bombs away!' We really said that! Because that's what they said in the movies."

He now enjoyed the enhanced status of mad bombardier. This uptick in self-esteem allowed him to share his feelings without the usual defensive permutations. Jacob currently lived with only himself for company, and that was no treat. A drab and monotonous diet was the rule even though he considered himself a pretty good cook. Life had been empty since his wife passed. He could dress any which way. What did it matter? Why shave? Who for? He dismissed himself as "a dead weight" and seemed to expect other people to agree. Yet, strangely, the others liked him despite it all. He was respected by people he had come to respect, people who had plenty of bumps of their own along their road of life.

Jacob rescinded his harsh verdict. Of course, life could not be the same with the absence of his wife and the misbehavior of his heart. But it was time to make amends with himself. Perhaps he still had some deserves coming. "Who would that hurt?"

Hence the chocolate pudding pie. Hence the stylish garb he now sported at the clinic. Hence that hint of swagger in his step. Hence a reactivated social life with children and other family members, and a more spirited approach to the exercise rotation. "It's called, 'going on!'" Jacob explains. "Kid, if you're not dead, you should be living!"

Who We Are Not

We represent only one subset of the millions who are engaged with that larger treadmill known as life. Demographers should dismiss our credentials without hesitation. Here, for example, are more men than women, perversely reversing the situation that obtains for the general senior adult population. Here also are people from several cohorts and therefore with divergent historical time experiences. Even within this minuscule sample, there is a generous sprinkling of people who were shaped by varying ethnic and racial traditions. Our personality types are no less diverse. Most of us share only a few commonalities, such as growing old or older in Arizona, surviving cardiac adventures, choosing to grind through exercise routines several days a week, and pretending we despise the recycled television game shows that somebody thinks are just right for dully flickering Medicared minds. Nevertheless, there are more aging men and women in rehabilitation and fitness programs than ever before. It is probable that peer support groups have evolved elsewhere as well.

There is no established template for traveling companies, so it might be useful to consider who we are not, in the hope of approaching an understanding of who we are. Obvious possibilities for comparison are nomads, pilgrims, and family. We then touch on another possibility that is wide open for conjecture: are we privileged to live the life and die the death of good citizens?

Not Nomads

Traditional nomads traversed a seasonal circuit and did little to sustain and develop their sites. Their footsteps literally vanished on the shifting sands of time. Although their lives embodied challenge, risk, and painfully acquired knowledge, they bequeathed scant literature to instruct or puzzle historians. By contrast, we have been traversing a paper and digital trail even before we could toddle. Our past is marked by birth certificates, school and employment records, marriage consecrations, divorce settlements, credit reports, driver's licenses, speeding tickets, medical data, online "cookies," and, not improbably, entries in the surveillance lists of benevolent organizations with initials known or unknown to us. More of the same will shadow us into the future until our exit permit is stamped. Our subtle souls perhaps remain *terra incognita* throughout this transit, but the public side of our being is readily available with a few clicks of the mouse.

We also are disqualified as nomads because we have been on the clock and the calendar since childhood. The *Journey of Life* (Cole, 1992) from the halting steps of early childhood to the halting steps of advanced age has been recognized for centuries. Specific conditions have changed, however, and are still changing. Members of our little traveling company have been measured against time-and-achievement criteria since we "finally!" sputtered our first word, rejoiced in our first potty triumph, and achieved such other normative markers as you might care to stipulate. The immigrant generations from which we were spawned had a mighty impulse toward better and better. As youth we sensed time as an arrow in flight from an oppressive past to a resplendent future if we worked hard, fast, and long enough. We measured ourselves against expectations as we moved deeper into adulthood—Had we hit the mark? Or had time's arrow blunted and lost its way? We were supposed to get some place and become somebody. True nomads could take satisfaction in having arduously negotiated still another circuit, to have survived. But shame on us if we have traded the exuberant arrow of hope for the drudge of a repetitive cycle.

Does Any of This Impinge on Deathward Thoughts?

The Wheel of Death (Kapleau, 1971) is a salient image within the Buddhist perspective and can also be discerned in other faith traditions. "Life" and "death" are positions on a curve of illusory change that brings all things around and about. The transition from life to death is significant, but only part of the long and weary game of being. Nomads do not necessarily share the belief in a universe that cycles through death and rebirth, but they also have the template of repetitive journeying. Their not-so-merry-go-round has no certified finish line, only riders who fade slowly into the blur.

By contrast, Western culture has been motivated by a linear, directional image of time. Although the hours adhere to their allotments throughout the life course, time is not experienced in the same way. In youth, time has a way of dawdling, of taking its time, but given to sudden accelerations as we race into the future that holds everything we hope and fear (Kastenbaum, 1959). The prospect of death in adolescence and early adulthood is a threat to all one might become. Time becomes ever more a scarce resource with aging, yet death anxiety tends to be less salient. The first wave of baby boomers shows signs of a difficult transition: not quite through with the surge of youth, not quite ready to accommodate age. Time, I thought you were my friend! Death, do you really mean to take everything away?

Not nomads are we, then. We are on the clock and on the road to somewhere, shadowed by the intimation that nowhere just might be our somewhere.

Not Pilgrims

Should we suppose ourselves pilgrims? Devout seekers are we, seeking salvation, spiritual enlightenment, or, at least, a bask in the vicinity of the sacred! The journey should be arduous and not without risk, the better to test our piety. We persevere along the true path toward an authentic destination. Aging is our modality of passage. This is who we are! This is what we do!

Unfortunately, perhaps, our little traveling company is not well qualified for pilgrim status. Our spiritual temper is only sufficiently religious. Most feel comfortable with their custom blend of habit and faith, enhanced by a trace of doubt. We do not bewail our fate in an inconvenient universe, but neither are we zealots who itch for our date with eternity. In short, we are pragmatists by the inch. Our cognitive range has adjusted to the road just ahead. It is not that we lack the ability to envision heavens, hells, and everything in between. It is just that ultimate things were conveniently prepackaged for us in our generation's childhood and keep well if left undisturbed.

The default setting for a literal pilgrimage features a palpable destination. Della has obediently visited worship sites in Latin America, but she reports that it did not make her a pilgrim:

> I see a dusty old church and I think, "So, there's a dusty old church!" I think of all the people who prayed and what hard lives they had, but it's not any more holy than any place where people live and die. That happens everywhere. You know what I think? Some people can't deal with where they are, who they are. They think, "Oh, I'll get out of here. I'll go *there,* wherever." They'll go empty and come back empty. I am not a pilgrim! (Laughs.) I'll take my home and family any time.

Her perspective resonates with the group's basic take on contemplation of death and the sacred:

> I think about *people* who are dead, people I loved. I don't think about death that much. What's there to think about? You think about it, and where does it get you? I'm not smart enough to live for the next life. I've got all I can do with this one. [?] Sure, sure. I believe everything. But that doesn't have to do with every day. What do they say? "One day at a time." Thank God for that!

Della understands that pilgrimage is essentially an inward quest. Nevertheless, there still needs to be a destination and a mission accomplished. History and literature offer limited options for the purpose-driven aged (Kastenbaum, 1994). We can each strive to become a saint who merges with the divine mysteries or a sage whose wisdom encompasses both life and death. Alas, not only do few achieve either status, but society tolerates only a few. There is an implicit quota system. People tend to be nervous around the holier-than or wiser-than thou. What makes numinous elders special also separates them from the comfort zone of ordinary folk. Not infrequently, elders are caught in a squeeze by societal expectations: be saintly or sagacious, or get out of our way. Those are your proper roles. These options do not suit some personalities. Furthermore, surplus elders with claims for superior sanctity or wisdom are not dealt with kindly.

There is a third and reprehensible option. The crusty SOB is a maverick character encountered frequently on the pages of history and literature. (Yes, even the term is politically incorrect. "Son of a bitch" is a backhanded tribute to the powerful goddesses who were being shunted aside as males empowered themselves in heaven and earth.) SOBs earn no congeniality awards but are grudgingly envied for their unapologetic self-devotion and dismissive attitude toward others. What is a bad mood for genial people like ourselves is a perfected way of life for the SOB. Charon excelled in making misery even more miserable as he operated his franchise on the banks of the Styx. The Struldbrugs encountered by Captain Gulliver (Swift, 1973) converted the ordinary stubborn and self-centered follies of their youth into a purified and powerful concentrate as they aged and aged. Mission accomplished for an SOB is the transformation of humiliating physical and societal entropy into a force with which others must reckon. Admittedly, some of my favorite geriatric residents were demonic SOBs, and they were also cherished by the other staff members who daily endured their abuse.

The inner pilgrimage is known to us through the lives of saints, deathbed conversions, and the transcendent finales of tormented symphonies, among many other sources. Here we recall Tolstoy's *The Death of Ivan Ilych* (1960). Ilych is dying in agony, social isolation, and despair within a network of superficial relationships and mutual hypocrisy. His transformation at the very end of life can be interpreted as a pilgrimage of return to the fresh and vibrant person he had once been, while at the same time signaling his arrival at the threshold of spiritual enlightenment. In desperation, Ilych completes an intense delayed pilgrimage through the self-inflicted ruins of his life.

The members of our traveling company, however, would not serve as characters in that particular Russian novel. We have not been artificial people in an artificial society. We are weathered, worn, and bruised, but it is this world and the lives we have lived with other people that give and at times threaten to snatch away meaning. Moments of exceptional intimacy, clarity, or cosmic consciousness are appreciated. However, as already observed, we are pragmatists by the inch and not inclined to invest all we have in the prospect of a glorious death.

Not Family

That we might be understood as "family" is a possibility that should be raised in order to be properly dismissed. There are interactions that resemble family patterns. Nonverbals can be subtle, and Drummond's telegraphic or dangling. We can fill in the blanks. We sometimes fall into quasi-familial roles (e.g., the feuding siblings), but these have limited resonance and staying power. Routines are formed and transformed. We know how to get each other going with a remark or tone of voice taken as performance cue. Like a secure family, members do not have to prove themselves every day.

But family we are not. There are no goods to fuss over and distribute. No debts or legal complications. No long-standing antagonisms and quarrels. No official obligations to each other. No pattern of indelible experiences and memories shared since childhood's hour. Furthermore, our relationships are generally confined to the task-oriented fitness center. We have not been in each other's lives 24/7, and there is little prospect that will change in the future.

Perhaps, in an odd way, we parallel the growing numbers of people who share experiences and projects with others through computerized mediation. Online networks form on the basis of shared interests. Conventional demographics (age, gender, race, etc.) do not matter nearly so much as what a participant can contribute to the dialogue. Lively interactions and even a sense of deep bonding can develop. It is not unusual for a person to feel closer to a geographically distant network partner than to family and neighbors who do not share one's most salient hopes and concerns. Our little traveling company is old school in that we move through real time and have not yet been digitalized or equipped with a reliable rebooting program when the system crashes. Nevertheless, we might have something in common with a great many other people whose passage through life is made more companionable on the basis of shared interest or predicament.

Who Dies and Who Cares?

Where are shelf-life markers when we really need them? Our prevailing assumptions about the life course of death should bear the advisory, "best if used by . . . " Death was once the scourge of infants, young children, and their mothers (Gee, 2003). Bringing a new life into the world jeopardized a woman's health and survival. That sexual intercourse could be a life-threatening activity was for many years a hidden anxiety that complicated intimate relationships. Despite this risk, breeding large families was a common strategy: perhaps death would spare a few of the young. Then, a miracle, or rather a series of advances, occurred in medical science and public health. Average life expectancy in developed nations has doubled since the seventeenth century. Unfortunately, little of this benefit has been achieved in struggling Third World countries, where high rates of infant/child and maternal mortality continue to afflict generation after generation.

Who died, then? The young, all too often. Who cared? Everybody except the most hard-hearted. The response to loss was complex: a volatile mix of grief and anger, tempered but not anesthetized by fatalism. Periodic episodes of megadeath intensified the stress on survivors (Kastenbaum, 2004). During plague years, for example, there were too few willing and able to bury the dead. Realistic fear of contagion separated the living from their stricken family members. At times this developed into a perfect storm of death. Familiar surroundings became a necroscape. Dying was agonizing to experience and to witness. "So many people dying so horribly—is that what will happen to me?" became a common fear.

Furthermore, social disorganization interfered with providing honorable burial and memorial rituals. This led to an even more devastating thought: "I will suffer an eternity of hellish torment because I failed to see to the safe passage of my loved one to the next life." This potent combination of fear and guilt contributed to mass violence such as flagellation and massacre. Overwhelmed, some became killers through a deranged identification with death.

Death has now grown more patient and less obtrusive. In this tamed form (Aries, 1981), death administers a quiet "last tag" within sequestered chambers. More of us live and die longer. There is more time for life review, if we are that kind of person, and more time to affirm our relationships—but also more time to stew in suffering, anxiety, and despair. In fact, neither "dying" nor "terminal illness" seems quite accurate. The deathbed scene often is no scene at all as an aged person succumbs quietly after a long period of decline. It is not unusual for the long-lived and long-dying person to be alone at the last breath. Sedation stifles last words that, in any event, would have had no listener.

The changing life course of death includes facets such as the following:

- That death now more often harvests the aged bolsters the prevailing view that this is their proper developmental task. Life-course theorists have tended to run out of more exhilarating tasks by the time they reach the advanced adult years, and they assign us the obligation of doing death right. The members of our little traveling company do not seem to have received that memo. Ageism (Palmore, Branch, and Harris, 2005) still permeates society. Elders have only peripheral social value, so their little deaths require little mourning.
- Older adults often have experienced multiple losses. In a society that remains uncomfortable with mortality, elders learn to keep their sorrows to themselves. Try not to remember? But those deaths were so much a part of their lives. How can one go forward as a whole person if so much of the past is off limits? Who grieves for the old widow's grief?
- With each succeeding generation, the world is losing more of its dedicated mourners and, therefore, losing one of the life supports that keep a traditional people viable. For example, Gamliel (2007) describes the compelling lamentation performance by aged women in a Yemenite-Jewish Israeli community.

Gamliel observes that "wailing cultures" around the world are vanishing with the deaths of older women who were deeply steeped in tradition. Fewer and fewer replacements are available. Furthermore, "those still alive are sometimes silenced by members of their community on behalf of 'modern' emotional values that consecrate self-control and affective autonomy." Fewer people mourn for elderly people, and fewer will be mourned by elders whose lamentations have affirmed the integrity of a people through the years.

- "Back in the day," most people were born at home, married from the neighborhood, slotted into expected occupations, and learned to act as though they believed in whatever the authority figures acted as though they believed. They lived in place. When the time came, they also died in place (i.e., within a familiar, predictable network of relationships). Books such as *Bowling Alone* (Putnam, 2001) have described how much this pattern has disintegrated. There is far less continuity in the lives of most of us today (Kastenbaum, 2008a). Place has given way to flux. We rely increasingly on computer-mediated images and transactions for a sense of belonging to a larger and coherent whole. As compared with many traditional cultures, we are less likely to die from a familiar and coherent world.

- The world will somehow manage to get along without us. Summoning our postdeath self, we can retroprospect on who as well as what will have continued in our absence. Grandchildren playing with puppies? Bases loaded in the ninth? Our favorite music still being played? Solace can be found in the hope that the people we care for and the values we cherish will thrive after we are gone. A sense of accomplishment might also be ours if we can believe that we are contributing to coming generations.

These obvious reflections are offered here because planet earth is becoming less supportive of life. Yes, we are aware of the ongoing loss of habitat and extinction of species. It has not quite struck home yet; still less has the cosmologist's doomsday scenario for the universe become a live issue. But how will people move through the life course if there is consensus that generations will not continue to generate? That all that is, was, and might be is as though it never had been? Neither the members of our little traveling company nor gerontologists and humanists seem to be losing sleep over this scenario. No, no, no, we are not in denial! Perhaps we are simply taking the advice of the old tentmaker (Omar Khayyam, eleventh century):

Aye, take the cash, and let the credit go
Nor heed the rumbling of distant drums. (Khayyam, 1990)

Who wants to grieve for everybody and everything?

Utopia—Are We There Yet?

The first time my wife was called "Ma'am." The first time I was offered a senior discount. That was about as far as the formalities went in our coming-of-age initiations. Traditional societies are usually more definitive in marking status changes through the life course. By definition, rites of passage require a departure, a journey, and an arrival (Gennep, 1960; Bloch, 1991; Kastenbaum, 2004). We must then pass whatever tests and ordeals await us if we are to become one of *them* at the far side of our itinerary. In *Deeply into the Bone: Re-inventing Rites of Passage*, Grimes (2000) urges that rituals be updated to serve streaming pluralistic societies that stumble about in the absence of well-marked paths. Grimes is not alone in that advocacy. Yet, ritual generally draws its power from the imagined past, while we have barely learned to use our latest electronic device before rushing to purchase its successor. Ritual also presupposes a credible ruling structure stocked with priestly characters who mediate with the divinities. These requisites might be in short supply with us. I have yet to see an "Obey authority!" bumper sticker. And we might be hard-pressed to choose among the clangorous claims of authority that yammer at us through all species of media.

Perhaps what we need is a society that integrates the best of the traditional and the progressive spirit within the embrace of a compassionate rationality. Thomas More's *Utopia* (1975; written in 1519), a vigorous makeover of Plato's *Republic* (1942; written in 370 BC), is the obvious model to consider. More described a commonwealth that contrasted sharply with the brutal and oppressive realms of early modern Europe. He knew well the follies and vices of his time and was especially pained by the church's hypocrisy. *Utopia* was a sly poke at the establishment, in the hope that the establishment would not poke back too savagely. In this concise volume, More offered an alternative vision of society that inspired centuries of further thought and real-life experiments. At the same time, he deftly discredited his own creation. Give people the opportunity to flourish in a just, rational, productive, and amiable society and, sooner or later, they will find a way to make the usual mess of it. He tips his hand in the title. Eutopia would have signified an ideal realm. Utopia signifies that there is one troublesome little flaw: it could never exist, or, certainly, not for long—people being what we are.

Utopia was not intended as a gerontopolis, but attention is given to the life course of the Utopian and the status of its elders, and so we have given attention as well (Kastenbaum, 2005, 2008b). The fundamental point is that many Utopians do enjoy long lives; it is the expectation, not the exception. Into their advanced years both women and men bring educated minds and useful skills that have been enriched throughout the life course. They have had the satisfaction of contributing their efforts to a robust economy and have received benefits from the technological innovations that keep Utopia ahead of other realms.

Young women, as well as men, were free to select their own mates—after a careful examination of each other's natural assets. Having made their own beds, they were expected to enjoy the associated amenities, although not to the extent of neglecting their civic duties. The commonwealth valued pleasure, excluding the decadent sort (boozing, gambling, whoring). The joy of marital sex, sports, and healthful exercising was encouraged, but even more so was the cultivation of mind and spirit.

Moving into their later years, most Utopians would never have wanted for the basics of life or strained for riches and power. They would also have been spared entanglements with a hyperactive legal system. More, one of the great barristers of his time, was pleased to report that Utopia had no lawyers and few laws. Religious belief was taken for granted, but the form of worship was not dictated by the state. Well— one exception. Christian missionaries who had recently arrived and were making evangelical pests of themselves were deported, and good riddance!

Perhaps best of all, the aging Utopian had never felt out of it: he or she had always belonged and would continue to belong. One was first and foremost a citizen of the commonwealth. This was not oppressive, because what else would one want to be? As an elder, one would not be self-hating or self-pitying because one had grown up to respect the fine old silvery heads. Elders were appreciated in the many communal events and were, of course, a reliable pool of talent for the diligent surveillance agents who were everywhere, watching everything and everyone.

Should a good life conclude with a good death (Kastenbaum, 2009)? From the commonwealth's perspective, the contented death of a completed elder is testament to the nonpareil virtues of the realm. Perhaps More could be faulted for devoting only two paragraphs to this event, but this is a more detailed treatment of natural death than in any of the early modern utopias that followed. (War deaths are given far more coverage.)

The dying elder knows what is expected: acceptance. (The first four stages of Kubler-Ross's [1969] theory are not in play.) One should be grateful for the superb medical and comfort care that has been provided in this time of need. One should also rejoice in the prospect of graduating from Utopia to Heaven. This rite of passage is so much easier for those who have evolved their earthly selves in the incomparable commonwealth. Some are fortunate enough to receive a parting gift: swift, easeful death. If function has faltered and pain persisted with no hope of remedy, then priest and physician will recommend prompt termination. Life that is no longer pleasurable is not worth keeping: "We can help you." The good citizen will choose this good death and all will end as it should. The commonwealth will be disappointed if this option is declined, but comfort care will continue.

Is Utopia Too Good for Us?

I am trying to picture our little traveling company in Utopia. It is not fair to say that Utopia would be too good for us, because we might have turned out as proper citizens if raised there. Nevertheless, there could be something to learn from this thought experiment. In all likelihood, we would be regarded as a deplorable crew of eccentrics. Each of us has his or her own ideas about the world. Worse, we sometimes share our questions, doubts, and opinions with others, thereby threatening the faith that unites. Instead of promptly reporting nonstandard behavior to the authorities, we might choose to befriend the suspects and relish their idiosyncrasies. We also have idle curiosities and drifting daydreams that are not welded to productive purposes. Although we have worked hard throughout much of our lives, we feel guiltless about lazing around at times.

Even when things go well, we are inclined toward apprehension: when is the next bad thing going to happen? Unlike Utopians, we have participated in confused and dysfunctional endeavors and encountered too many instances of ignorance, indifference, and injustice to invest our trust completely in any corporate scheme. And, again unlike Utopians, we have often been on our own in difficult situations. Accordingly, we are a more damaged and anxious crew, but also perhaps more streetwise and creative. What else? We are alternatively oblivious to and vain about our appearance. Some of us have no doubt tasted liquor while flirting in a casino.

This partial catalog of our flaws includes three capital offenses in Utopia: tarting up our appearance, sexual adventuring, and failing to eliminate threats to homeland security. It is true that there are few laws in Utopia and that executions are much less frequent than in other realms, but those who violate fundamental rules have made themselves dead to the commonwealth and are doomed by their own intransigence.

Even death does not necessarily escape the reach of Utopian justice. As noted, our natural death in old age can be accelerated with honor if it is at the recommendation of officialdom. But what if one of us chooses to self-terminate on personal volition? The offending body will be dumped unceremoniously into the nearest bog. The commonwealth shows its rational and compassionate face most of the time, but it tolerates no doubt about who controls the death system (Kastenbaum, 2009).

Whose Death?

Utopia is replete with benefits and privileges. In exchange, one traverses the life course primarily as citizen rather than individual. There is no place for probing life reviews, transformed relationships, or deathbed confessions and revelations. The elder who breaks character by starting to think afresh about life and death will probably bring this misadventure to a halt with self-censorship. By contrast, members of our little traveling company will bring more varied selves to the end of their days. They will probably also have more constructive or reconstructive work to do and accomplish this in their own distinctive ways.

The traveling companions introduced earlier all have demonstrated a keen if at times flickering observing ego. Who it is that dies depends on the dominance among rival observing egos. For example, as a proxy for the younger self, the "I" of the observing ego might belittle the elder's faltering "me." If the post-self's observing ego is in charge, it is likely to retroprospect what this life will have been when it is over. "Me" is still vertical and exchanging gases with the environment, but already dead in the observing ego's "I." Observing egos of any sort can have a magical function: "Hah! I am still here observing, so I have survived and will survive! I am not to be confused with that residue 'me.'" The split-screen self phenomenon is perhaps best known from spectacular appearances in near-death experiences and other altered states of consciousness. However, it can also operate in everyday life to offer a subtle escape hatch from total identification with mortality.

It is not all magic, however. The ego observer position can be occupied by various voices from the past that arise to have their say about the life that is soon to expire. These can be preparations instead of evasions. The hearkening voice might belong to a frightened child awakened at midnight or a voice that gave comfort to such a child many years ago. The voices of awaiting ancestors might speak through the observing ego—or one might hear a voice absolutely one's own that quietly advises, "Well done. Now, time to go."

REFERENCES

Aries, P. 1981. *The Hour of Our Death.* New York: Alfred A. Knopf.

Bloch, M. 1991. *Prey into Hunter.* Cambridge: Cambridge University Press.

Cole, T. R. 1992. *The Journey of Life.* Cambridge: Cambridge University Press.

Gamliel, T. 2007. "Wailing lore" in a Yeminite-Jewish community: Bereavement, expertise, and therapy. *Social Science and Medicine* 65:1501–15.

Gee, E. 2003. Life expectancy. In *Macmillan Encyclopedia of Death and Dying,* ed. R. Kastenbaum. New York: Macmillan.

Gennep, A. V. 1960. *The Rites of Passage.* London: Routledge and Kegan Paul. Original edition, 1909.

Grimes, R. L. 2000. *Deeply into the Bone: Re-inventing rites of passage.* Berkeley: University of California Press.

Kapleau, P. 1971. *The Wheel of Death.* New York: Harper & Row.

Kastenbaum, R. 1959. Time and death in adolescence. In *The Meaning of Death,* ed. H. Feifel. New York: McGraw Hill.

———. 1994. Saints, sages, and sons of bitches. *Journal of Geriatric Psychiatry* 27:61–78.

———. 2004. *On Our Way: The final passage through life and death*. Berkeley: University of California Press.

———. 2005. Is death better in Utopia? *Illness, Grief, and Loss* 13:31–48.

———. 2008a. Grieving in contemporary society. In *Handbook of Bereavement Research and Practice: 21st century perspectives*, ed. M. Stroebe, R. O. Hansson, H. Schut, and W. Stroebe. Washington, D.C.: American Psychological Association.

———. 2008b. Growing up in Utopia. *Journal of Aging, Humanities, and the Arts* 2:4–22.

———. 2009. *Death, Society, and Human Experience*. 10th ed. Boston: Allyn & Bacon.

Khayyam, O. 1990. *The Rubaiyat of Omar Khayyam*. Trans. E. Fitzgerald. New York: Dover.

Kubler-Ross, E. 1969. *On Death and Dying*. New York: Macmillan.

More, T. 1975. *Utopia*. New York: W. W. Norton. Original edition, 1516.

Palmore, E. B., L. Branch, and D. K. Harris. 2005. *Encyclopedia of Ageism*. New York: Routledge.

Pike, K. L. 1969. Language as behavior and etic and emic standpoints for the description of behavior. In *Social Psychology: Readings and perspective*, ed. E. F. Borgatta. Chicago: Rand McNally.

Plato. 1942. *Republic*. Trans. B. Jowett. New York: Walter J. Black.

Putnam, R. D. 2001. *Bowling Alone*. New York: Simon & Schuster.

Swift, J. 1973. *Gulliver's Travels*. Boston: Beacon Press. Original edition, 1726.

Tolstoy, L. 1960. *The Death of Ivan Ilych*. New York: New American Library. Original edition, 1886.

The Experience of Aging in Feature-Length Films
A Selected and Annotated Filmography

ROBERT E. YAHNKE, PH.D.

The experience of aging, as portrayed in feature-length films, usually emphasizes the affirming and redemptive qualities of old age. In the majority of films the essential characteristics are intergeneration and regeneration (Yahnke, 2000). The former refers to all aspects of meaningful relationships between the young and the old—including family bonds, grandparenting, friendships across the generations, and mentoring. Films that incorporate intergeneration usually emphasize the mutual benefits of intergenerational relationships. Although the old often serve as problem solvers or role models for the young, the young also function to help elders deal with unfinished tasks. Thus, what the old bring to the young in intergeneration is reciprocated by what the young contribute to elders. Regeneration refers to elder characters finding closure in their lives, resolving significant conflicts, and restoring their lives to a metaphoric wholeness emotionally and sometimes spiritually. Something significant happens to the elders in these films: they gain a sense of redemption or freedom from former emotional constraints, an acceptance of the new terms of their lives and what is required of them now that they have survived a variety of conflicts, an awareness of their capacity for love and even forgiveness, an acceptance of the new basis of relationships within the sphere of family or society, feelings of well-being or serenity based on a sense of their accomplishments, an awareness that they have broken down long-standing barriers that separated them from others, the satisfaction of knowing that they have made a difference in the lives of the young as well as the lives of other elders, and a sense that their lives have not ended—but that a new chapter has begun that promises new adventures, new friends, and perhaps new intimacy.

Thus, the art of aging is derived from the art of living when it comes to the experience of elders in these films. Despite the constraints of finitude and approaching mortality, these elders utilize their wisdom, serenity, humor, capacity for mentoring, coping skills, and courage to maintain critical engagements with others and overcome the negative characteristics of old age, such as alienation, loneliness, grief, and depression.

Almost all the films annotated below incorporate both themes of intergeneration and regeneration. The elders in these films are, in most respects, exemplars of active aging. They are tough, able-bodied, free of dementias, and engaged in their communities (Yahnke, 2005). They are survivors, like the elders in *Antonia's Line, Harry and Tonto, Since Otar Left, Solas,* and *The Trip to Bountiful.* They are wise, articulate, and forceful. Some have the strength to make long and difficult journeys, as in *About Schmidt, Central Station,*

Harry and Tonto, The Trip to Bountiful, and *Wild Strawberries.* Some struggle to control or dominate others. The old man in *The Grandfather* learns to make peace by yielding control to others, whereas the old man in *Saraband* is unremitting in his desire to control members of his family. Only three films annotated below do not incorporate fully both themes of intergeneration and regeneration: *About Schmidt, The Dresser,* and *Saraband.* The eponymous hero in *About Schmidt* returns from a long journey feeling like a failure, but he is on the verge of regeneration when he acknowledges the potential for the mutual benefits of an unusual intergenerational relationship. In *The Dresser* the main character is left bereft of his companionship and love for an aging actor when the latter dies at the end of the film. In *Saraband,* one of two major characters fails to regenerate because he remains mired in self-loathing, filled with vitriol toward his son, and trapped in an idealized love for his son's late wife. But his former wife Marianne, the other major character in the film, has the last word about the meaning of her journey and perceives a recent breakthrough with her mentally disabled adult daughter, thus suggesting that she has made progress toward regeneration.

The 22 films annotated below were selected from a review of 130 feature-length films that were produced from 1951 to 2006. More than 38 percent (38.5%) of those 130 films were produced in the 1990s, about 20 percent of the films were produced in the 1980s and the 2000s (21% and 22%, respectively), 10 percent were produced in the 1970s, and only 8.5 percent of the films were produced in the 1950s and 1960s. The intent of this filmography is to provide readers with a list of the best films available for study and use in the service of gerontology education. One starting point might be to consider what films have become classics over the years. Although only four of the 130 films reviewed were produced in the 1950s, three of those films—*Ikiru, Tokyo Story,* and *Wild Strawberries*—are annotated below. Those three films have achieved the status of classics because they create three-dimensional—even archetypal—characters and elicit timeless themes of intergeneration and regeneration. Those films have lasted through the decades and still offer gerontologists new perspectives on the meaning of old age. One searches in vain for classic films on aging from the 1960s—and no films from that decade are included in this filmography. Two films from the 1970s, *Harry and Tonto* (1973) and *Going in Style* (1979), introduce viewers to playful elders who have the capacity to gain insights into their own aging and engage in intergenerational relationships. *Harry and Tonto* is the first film that incorporates the *elder journey,* a plot device that brings closure to the elder's experiences. Three films from the 1980s are listed: *The Dresser* (1985), *Driving Miss Daisy* (1985), and *The Trip to Bountiful* (1985). These three films are on their way to becoming classics: readers familiar with them may wish to review them and become acquainted with resilient and sometimes fierce elders—the bombastic old actor in *The Dresser* know only as "Sir"; the irascible and irrepressible Daisy and her long-suffering chauffeur and eventual companion and best friend, Hoke; and the old woman in *The Trip to Bountiful* who embarks on another *elder journey* meant to provide closure in her life, as well as perspectives on the family past that will help her middle-aged son better cope with his marriage (Cole, 1991). Two-thirds of the films annotated below were produced in the 1990s and 2000s. The emphasis on contemporary films is meant to complement the component of classic films noted earlier. Yet only one of those 14 films (*About Schmidt,* 2002) was an American production—an indication that contemporary cinema represents a renaissance of elder stories from a variety of cultures. Gerontologists need to acknowledge and address the increasingly international contexts provided in contemporary feature-length films (Yahnke, 2005).

Of course, there are always more films that one might wish to include in any selection of films meant to inspire and educate gerontologists. A listing of 15 additional recommended films is added at the end of the list of annotated films. In each case, some of the essential themes of those films are listed as well—for instance, aging in place, elder journeys, and intergeneration. Most of those films were produced in the 1980s and 1990s. Two recent films from the list are worthy of note: *The Three Burials of Melquiades Estrada* (2005), a compelling meditation on mortality and intergeneration; and *The Human Stain* (2003), a film about repressed identity, intergeneration, and love in old age. In total, then, this article provides a listing of 37 significant films that address a variety of themes relevant to the study of aging.

Although old age often is associated with mortality, the films annotated below are not usually about the death of the main characters. Some of the films end with the death of the elder: *Antonia's Line*, *The Dresser*, *Iris*, *The Man on the Train*, and *Solas*. Other films incorporate the death of one of the elder characters earlier in the film, such as *Going in Style*; *Spring, Summer, Fall, Winter . . . and Spring*; and *Tokyo Story*. But in all of these films death is portrayed as having a meaning or purpose that affects the lives of friends, family, or others inspired by and/or mentored by that elder. In these films, then, what an elder accomplishes in life is the subject of the film. In fact, another metaphor appropriate for many elders in these films is their sense of *not being fully alive* in their lives—a kind of *death in life* that makes them feel vulnerable, helpless, and captured by tiresome routines. Elders in *About Schmidt*, *Going in Style*, *Man on the Train*, *Red*, and *Wild Strawberries* share similar feelings of uselessness and despair because they feel that they have not *lived*. The best example of that theme is *Ikiru*, a film about an old man who realizes he has been *dead* in *life* as an overworked bureaucrat. Only when he is diagnosed with a terminal cancer does he find a way to make meaning with his life and contribute to the improvement of a Tokyo neighborhood. *Ikiru*, which means "to live," is a fitting metaphor for all these films about old age because in them elders are alive, restless, engaged, creative, and doing everything they can to make meaning out of their lived experience. Thus, most of the films listed below are about elders starting life over again on a variety of terms. Some elders, after completing journeys, learn that they have just begun the process of regeneration, as in *About Schmidt*, *Central Station*, *Harry and Tonto*, and *Since Otar Left*. Others find resolution in establishing renewed family ties or even a new family, as in *The Grandfather*; *Last Orders*; *Solas*; *Spring, Summer, Fall, Winter . . . and Spring*; and *Tokyo Story*. Whatever the outcome, the films annotated below suggest that aging is a time of engagement, self-reflection, and resolution.

Selected and Annotated Filmography

ABOUT SCHMIDT (2002). DIRECTED BY ALEXANDER PAYNE.

The title character (played by Jack Nicholson) spends his last day on the job at an insurance agency, survives a stereotypical retirement party at a steakhouse, and settles into the first weeks of his retirement. But after his wife dies suddenly, Schmidt descends into severe grief and depression. His sudden decision to begin a road trip from Omaha to Denver in a motor home (which the couple had purchased for use after his retirement) suggests his desire to address his grief, reconnect with family, conduct a meaningful life review, and return refreshed and reinvigorated. But he accomplishes none of the above. He meddles in his daughter's marriage plans, gains only a few sentimental insights into his past, and returns more befuddled than he was when he began his journey. Early in the film he responds to a random television advertisement about the need to sponsor poor children in Africa. He decides to sponsor a six-year-old Tanzanian boy named Ndugu, and throughout the film he works out his grief, his response to widowhood, and his frustrations with his daughter by writing long and rambling letters to Ndugu—even though he knows the boy won't read them. But the letters are therapy for Schmidt, and when he returns from his aimless and unregenerative journey, he finds a letter waiting for him from one of the nuns at the mission where Ndugu lives. He reads the letter, and he examines the simple page of artwork drawn by the boy to honor his sponsor—and at that moment Schmidt's life begins anew.

ANTONIA'S LINE (HOLLAND, 1995). DIRECTED BY MARLEEN GORRIS. Antonia, a self-confident and strong woman, returns to her childhood farm in Holland after World War II and establishes a matriarchal line that challenges the prevalent patriarchy. But Antonia's matriarchy is characterized by nontraditional elements of family life. Widowed in the war, she never remarries. The first two members of her "family" are mentally disabled adults who are drawn to her because of her compassion and kindness. When her daughter announces that she wants to have a baby, Antonia helps her find a suitable partner—but his only role is to help her become pregnant. Later, her daughter falls in love with her child's tutor, another woman. To Antonia, everyone is accepted as an equal member of the family line. The film is about the predictable and continuous rounds of the seasons and the years. Children are born and grow up, love reigns, and people die of old age or accidents. As Antonia ages, her extended matriarchal line expands with new arrivals, many of them castoffs of society. A recurrent visual motif in the film is Antonia's family eating outdoors at a long table, with Antonia at the head. Later in life, Antonia begins a conjugal relationship with an old widower, who joined her family years earlier and patiently waited for her to warm to his proposals. The power of the matriarchy is exemplified in the ways Antonia is able to root out injustice, hypocrisy, and hatred in this village. Her daughter becomes an artist, her granddaughter becomes a scientist, and her great-granddaughter Sarah becomes a synthesis of her forebears—a witness, a record, and a storyteller. At the end of the film, Sarah has an extraordinary vision of the dead and the living all together at one of the outdoor meals. Sarah inherits Antonia's legacy and will carry on Antonia's vision of the family line.

CENTRAL STATION (BRAZIL, 1998). DIRECTED BY WALTER SALLES. When a boy is orphaned in Rio de Janeiro, a retired schoolteacher and letter writer for illiterate people who pass through the railway station decides to help the boy rather than take advantage of him. The old woman, Dora, and the boy, Josuè, leave on a journey into the interior of Brazil. Initially, the purpose of her journey appears to be reuniting the boy with his father, who abandoned him when he was a baby. Along the way, Dora helps the young boy resolve his grief over his mother's death and reunites him with his elder brothers, who are living in the new settlements. Dora is tempted to live with them, but then it becomes evident that Dora's journey has been for herself even more than it has been for the boy. She gains a powerful insight into her own unresolved past—specifically her unresolved anger toward her father, who abandoned her family (just as the boy's father had abandoned his family). In the climactic scene of this film, while leaving the new settlements, she is able finally to address these feelings in a poignant letter she writes to the boy. Now another journey begins for Dora—one that will focus on resolving the pain from her past as well as discerning the potential for a new life alone.

THE DRESSER (UNITED KINGDOM, 1983). DIRECTED BY PETER YATES.

The crux of this film is the relationship between two colleagues of the stage, a larger-than-life old actor known only as "Sir" (Albert Finney), and his dresser, Norman (Tom Courtenay), members of a small Shakespearean troupe performing during World War II throughout England. Based on Ronald Harwood's play, the events of the film take place primarily over the course of a day, during which Sir is hospitalized briefly, returns to the theater, is dressed by Norman for a performance of *King Lear,* completes the performance, returns to his dressing room, and dies. Sir has acted the role of Lear 227 times in his career, and Norman has been with him for 16 years. The moments of intimacy between these two men are extraordinary. Norman sees the old man when he is vulnerable, when he is brilliant, and when he is mad. He bathes the old man, motivates him, teases him, and understands his foibles and weaknesses, and in some respects he knows him better than his own long-suffering wife. The irony of Norman's devotion is that he is a middle-aged gay man who has sublimated his identity—for his own safety and for the sake of having a well-defined and respected place in the theater. In one memorable scene we watch Sir apply his makeup as he sits in front of his dressing room mirror; and as he draws accent lines and attaches his eyebrows and wig, he *becomes* King Lear—an amazing transformation. After the final act, Sir collapses backstage. Norman tries to revive him, and then unleashes a tirade that underscores his frustration that after years of devotion to—and love for—this old man, he is now devastated and bereft of the object of his devotion.

DRIVING MISS DAISY (1989). DIRECTED BY BRUCE BERESFORD.

Based on the play by Alfred Uhry, this film illustrates the ways in which the barriers of race and class can be overcome—as expressed in the evolving relationship between an upper-class Jewish widow who lives in Atlanta in the late 1940s and her middle-aged African-American chauffeur (Morgan Freeman), hired by her son. Daisy (Jessica Tandy), 72, is excitable, cantankerous, and petty. Hoke serves as an antidote to her fragile ego; he is calm, patient, and generous. As their quarter-century relationship passes, Daisy makes progress and begins to yield to Hoke's gentle loyalty. Together they experience racial discrimination and intolerance, the Civil Rights Movement, family celebrations, and finally a sudden onset of dementia that terrifies the old woman. In the climactic scene Hoke's comforting presence seems to shock her into lucidity. She sits in her nightgown, her thin hair down around her face, and acknowledges, "Hoke? You're my best friend." In the last scene, when Hoke and Daisy's son visit her in a nursing home, Hoke feeds her a piece of pumpkin pie. Throughout her life Daisy was fearful of embracing life and yielding to intimacy. Now she finally tastes and savors the sweetness of life thanks to the kindness of her longtime friend and companion. In the last scene, as the two sit across from one another, the shot dissolves to reveal the old Cadillac Hoke drove for Daisy, moving down a highway many years ago.

Once again Hoke is driving Miss Daisy, and the visual metaphor makes permanent the intimacy of their bond.

49-UP (UNITED KINGDOM, 2005). DIRECTED BY MICHAEL APTED.

The director began this documentary series in 1964 by filming several lower- and upper-class English children and letting them share their hopes and dreams for the future. Apted revisited his subjects every seven years; thus, *49-Up* is the seventh film in the series. Some of his subjects dropped out; others dropped out occasionally and resurfaced later. In each film Apted combines interviews of the subjects with direct cinema footage showing each subject engaged in a variety of activities (e.g., family life, working, recreation). Often the director incorporates voice-over narration (by the subject) as a means of commenting on the action in specific scenes. In each segment Apted also interweaves scenes of that individual from previous films (when he or she was 7, 14, 21, 28, etc.) in order to provide a multilayered record of that person's aging.

Viewers have followed these subjects' lives as they went to school, married, had children, explored careers, experienced divorces, and experienced grief at the deaths of parents. Twelve of the subjects (eight men, four women) have appeared in the majority of the segments. Five of the men have working-class roots: one emigrated to Australia; a son of Yorkshire farmers got his Ph.D. at an English university and then became a professor at an American university; one has been a laborer most of his life and married twice; one is an East Ender and former taxicab driver who moved out of the city with his family; and the last has battled mental-health concerns, been an itinerant laborer, and now volunteers for local government in a suburb of London. Three of the men are from the upper class: one was a secondary school instructor and now is a school administrator, and the other two are Oxford educated and became successful lawyers. One of the women is a daughter of the upper class who married a lawyer, and the other three are working-class women who attended the same state-supported school. Two of these three women are now single parents. Apted's project represents an authentic and groundbreaking longitudinal study of aging (focused on life in England over almost the past half century). Although Apted was interested in examining the variable of class (for instance, the effect of public school vs. private school backgrounds on an individual's future prospects), American viewers will be engaged more so by identifying and comparing the recurring patterns in the lives of these individuals as they navigate the twists and turns in their aging process.

GOING IN STYLE (1979). DIRECTED BY MARTIN BREST.

Three old men, bored with life in retirement, stick up a New York City bank. But that summary of the film misses the meanings that are at the core of the relationships in this intriguing film. The film is actually the story of one old man, Joe (George Burns), who—despite his enduring friendship with Al (Art Carney) and Willie (Lee Strassberg)—faces an emotional crisis when the daily grind of sitting for hours on a park bench moves past boredom and begins to feel like desperation. In the early scenes the director stays with Joe's point of view as he experiences this old-age crisis. The secret to Joe's character is that he had experiences in World War II regarding *procurement*, a fancy word for stealing things. Joe was always the go-to guy in his company, and now he draws on those skills in his old age as he plans the perfect robbery. He realizes, for instance, that if they are caught, they will be put in prison for only a few years (and have room and board provided). When they are released they will cash in years of unopened Social Security checks. He sums it up this way: "Either we get the money or we get caught. We're winners either way." The other key to this film is that Joe makes his two friends come alive in unexpected ways. The shyest of the three, Willie, is rejuvenated just by choosing to participate in the robbery. For the first time in years, he is alive and thinking about the future. Unfortunately, Willie dies of a heart attack a few days after the robbery, and Joe and Al are dropped into grief. In a memorable scene, Joe sits alone in his apartment, thumbing through a box of old family photographs. He cries, and then he realizes that he has been incontinent—adding a personal indignity to grief. The film then focuses on Joe and Al—as Al takes Joe to Las Vegas and becomes a mentor as well as a friend. In that scene, Al comes alive as an old man. He enjoys life, he plays craps, he realizes that he can still take chances, and he blossoms under Joe's tutelage. But Al dies shortly upon their return home. Now three is down to one—and Joe realizes that the game is up. Although he is arrested and imprisoned, he faces his time optimistically and makes sure that the Las Vegas winnings are safely stowed away for his nephew—one more example of the older generation caring for the needs of the younger generation.

THE GRANDFATHER (SPAIN, 1998). DIRECTED BY JOSÉ LUIS GARCI.
A rich old nineteenth-century nobleman, after years spent in America, returns to Spain, visits his daughter-in-law, Doña Lucretia, and makes an extraordinary demand: because he has proof that one of his two granddaughters was born of an illicit affair between the daughter-in-law and an artist, he insists that Doña Lucretia hand over the daughter that is a direct descendant of his late son. Don Rodrigo's values are bound up in the idea of honor and the "ancestry and splendor of our lineage." But Doña Lucretia refuses the old man's request, and the old man is left to find other ways of having his demand met. He spends time with his granddaughters, Dolly and Nelly, as he attempts to discern which of the two young women shares his royal blood. They love the old man, and in one scene, he acknowledges the joy he has experienced being with them. Twice in the film Doña Lucretia's chief counselor and some of the town's leaders plot to subvert the old man's intentions, first by conspiring to have him removed to a monastery, and second by committing him to an asylum because he must be mad. But the old man foils both plots with his cunning, defiance, and wit—all done with great rhetorical flourish. A secondary theme in the film is Don Rodrigo's evolving friendship with the girls' tutor, Don Pío, a shy man intimidated by his wife and daughters. Friendship with Don Pío softens the rough edges of Don Rodrigo's menacing ego and stubbornness. The climactic scene of the film takes place along a cliff, where Don Pío has long considered jumping to his death to end what has become for him a meaningless life. Don Rodrigo, having learned the identity of his natural heir after having been told again by Doña Lucretia that she will not give up even one of her daughters to him, joins the old tutor at the cliff side and tells him, "First, I'll throw you off. And then myself." But at that very moment *one* of the two granddaughters, released by her mother, cries out and approaches the two old men. Her mother's decision is deserving of the Biblical wisdom of Solomon. The old man accepts her decision and lets go of his

enmity toward her. And as for Don Pío? Don Rodrigo tells him, "I declare from this moment we are friends. Our friendship means a new agreement—that of waiting to die of old age." And thus Don Rodrigo, Don Pío, and the granddaughter become a new family.

HARRY AND TONTO (1973). DIRECTED BY PAUL MAZURSKY.

The gregarious Harry Coombs (Art Carney), a longtime widower, lives a settled retirement in New York City with a small network of friends. As he says early in the film, "You know people—that's home." So it's a shock to see him spouting lines from *King Lear* ("thunderbolts singe my white head!") as he is carried out of his apartment by the police, executing the eviction order. His son Bert shows up and takes him back to his house, but his son and daughter-in-law are of two minds about his staying there. Bert wants to use this time to grow closer to his father, but his wife sees Harry as an imposition. So old Harry begins a compelling cross-country odyssey and visits his other two children, a daughter in Chicago and a son in Los Angeles. Along the way he has numerous adventures, as Harry brings his intellect and curiosity to bear on every encounter with other people. He is a good listener, a connoisseur of the human condition. He "gets personal" with young people—but he never lectures them. His motto: "The times change, and we change with it." There are journeys within journeys here, too, and these contribute to the overall impact of the primary journey outlined above. Harry's visits to his children remind him of what he always knew—that they have serious personal and familial problems that they can barely manage by themselves. Two of them are still growing up, and they have some discernibly rough edges. But Harry is a good father to them still—even though he knows he must move on. Harry's journey ends on the West Coast, where his beloved cat Tonto dies. Harry ends by looking forward to a new life with new friends and new opportunities to affirm others.

IKIRU (JAPAN, 1951). DIRECTED BY AKIRU KUROSAWA.

What makes a human being alive, rather than dead in life? This film is about a low-level bureaucrat, a functionary, in post–World War II Japan, who finally realizes that *to live* (the translation of the film's title) requires having a meaning to one's life. The old man, Watanabe, receives a diagnosis of a fatal stomach cancer—although the doctors are careful not to tell him of the severity of the illness. But the old man knows it will be fatal, and at first he is plunged into life review and recalls the many lost opportunities to foster a close relationship with his son after his wife died when the boy was only five. He regrets never remarrying. Although Watanabe's son and daughter-in-law live with him, they are not close emotionally to the old man, and Watanabe gives no thought of sharing his diagnosis with them. Chance meetings with a writer in a bar and then with a young employee from his branch of the civil service inspire Watanabe to share his feelings for the first time. He tells the writer, "I don't know what I've been doing with my life all of these years." But time spent drinking sake and visiting nightclubs with the young man does little to help Watanabe discover a purpose for his life. He is attracted to the young woman because, as he tells her, "When I look at you, you warm me up." Although he wasted his time with her, and bored her, he finally has a revelation: "It's not too late." Here part one of the film ends. Part two consists of the old man's wake (five months later), arranged in the traditional Buddhist style of people visiting the house, sharing food, and telling stories about the dead person's life. First the mayor and other city officials pay their respects, and they offer their thanks for his part in the completion of a new city park. But they have no insight into what this old man accomplished in the last five months of his life. Then one of his coworkers offers the theory that Watanabe single-handedly organized the establishment of that park in a neighborhood that had been plagued with pollution. In fact, in one of the first scenes of the film Watanabe, as well as others in his civil service branch, ignored the demands of the neighborhood women to clean up that mess. Now Watanabe is a hero to those women. His coworker recalls that the old man went to every office, begged for assistance, and waited for hours to be seen by officials. He persevered when others gave up. A policeman reports that he saw Watanabe sitting on a swing in the park the night before—just hours before he died of exposure. "He seemed to be perfectly happy." At the end of the evening, many of the guests vow to live their lives like Watanabe—taking on the bureaucracy. But the next day at the civil service office, everything returns to normal, and the workers are overwhelmed by the paperwork.

IRIS (UNITED KINGDOM, 2001). DIRECTED BY RICHARD EYRE.

Based on two memoirs by John Bayley, this film charts the progress of Iris Murdoch's experience with Alzheimer's disease from its onset (when she was still working on her last novel) to the advanced stages, when she began to lose control of her mind and body, and to the end of her life in a nursing home. The film emphasizes the vitality of Iris Murdoch's life by comparing scenes in the present to those in the past, when John Bayley and she first met at Oxford and fell in love. John was profoundly shy, and yet she was patient with him and taught him how to enjoy new experiences and embrace life. John was always in awe of Iris, and he was surprised that she always drew him back toward her. The ongoing comparison of life in the present versus life in the past reveals the depth of their intimacy. They were soul mates when young and lived together into old age as equal partners. Iris was a great author. As John says, "Words mean everything to her." But the disease slowly robs her of words, the capacity to write more novels, and even the capacity to engage in simple conversations. John bears the burden of caregiving in old age when Iris (Judi Dench) declines physically and mentally. John has to deal with her incontinence, her wandering, her repetitive behaviors, and her vacant stares. John also has to grapple with his long-standing fear that he was never a part of Iris's world—that mysterious world of her imagination, where she was most vital and most alluring. This festering resentment and his frustration that he may as well be a caregiver to a stranger come together when he lashes out at Iris after a particularly difficult time: "I hate you! All your friends are finished with you now! I've got you now! Nobody else has you anymore! I've got you now, and I don't want you!" Despite this emotional eruption, John realizes that when they were young lovers, Iris did share the details of her life with him. John accepts his fate. He places Iris in a nursing home, and she dies soon thereafter.

LADIES IN LAVENDER (UNITED KINGDOM, 2004).
DIRECTED BY CHARLES DANCE.

Elderly sisters living on the coast of Cornwall before World War II have an adventure when they rescue a young Polish émigré swept up after a storm on the shore below their cottage. They tend to him until he recovers, marvel at his skills as a violinist, and gradually introduce him to members of their small community before a young woman, an artist, spirits him away to England—not for romance, but so that he can study with a famous violinist. The adventure for Ursula, the younger sister (Judi Dench), is more complicated and life changing, because she falls in love with the young man, Andrea, at first sight. He is her first great love. When her sister (Maggie Smith) reminds her that Andrea is a young man, Ursula blurts out, "Yes, and I'm an old woman—silly, and ridiculous, and foolish!" But she never becomes an object of ridicule, and the folly of her emotional state is softened by her sister Janet's empathy (Janet allows her to suffer her emotional loss in private) and by Andrea's sensitivity and compassion toward her (Fisher, 2006). In fact, the film's climax reveals the mutual benefits of intergenerational ties. The young man sends a message to the sisters: "You gave me life, and now I have a chance to use it." The sisters become patrons of the arts, in effect, and even journey to London in order to see Andrea perform with a symphony orchestra. Ursula discovers the means for letting go of her first love, and she feels enriched by her part in saving Andrea and nursing him back to health. Meanwhile, the members of the village that metaphorically *raised* this young man all gather at the sisters' cottage and listen to the performance on the radio. But the film also ends with a message about another dimension of the shared experiences of the elderly sisters. Janet lost her fiancé in World War I, and his photograph hangs on her bedroom wall. At the end of the film Ursula now possesses her own icon of loss, Andrea's portrait, which he sent to her from London. She hangs it in Andrea's room as a reminder of her first great love and how it changed her life.

LAST ORDERS (UNITED KINGDOM, 2001). DIRECTED BY FRED SCHEPISI. When an old friend dies, three of his friends and the man's adult son carry his ashes from London to Margate, on the east coast of England, so that his ashes can be scattered in the sea. In keeping this promise to Jack (Michael Caine), each of the four men on this symbolic journey discovers new meanings in his life based on episodes of life review and their interactions with the others. The film's structure is organized around four types of scenes: the four men on their auto journey to Margate; a journey taken by Jack's wife (Helen Mirren) that same day to visit their mentally disabled daughter for the last time; a series of flashbacks that show Jack, his wife, and his friends interacting in various locations; and a scene showing a long conversation between Jack's wife Amy and his friend Ray—a scene that takes place just after Jack's death. On the auto journey Vince makes a detour to a location symbolic to his childhood and to his identity, and afterward he begins to embrace a father-son relationship free of anger and old resentments. He honors his father by scattering some of the ashes in this field. Amy's journey also leads to regeneration. She has visited her daughter June every week for almost 50 years, and when she leaves this time, she knows she will not need to return. The most important segments of the film are the scenes showing the conversation between the two after Jack died. Throughout the film it becomes evident that Ray loved Amy ever since Jack introduced him to her after the war. Amy knew that Ray loved her, and the two only acted on that love for a brief period 20 years ago. But they broke off their romance because they could not continue to hurt Jack. Thus, the penultimate scene in the film is the end of the conversation between Ray and Amy, and Ray leaves on the journey with the other three men knowing that Amy has agreed to begin a new life with him. In the last scene the four men arrive at the quay in Margate. Each man digs into the urn filled with Jack's ashes and then casts handfuls out into the sea. Having fulfilled their promises (and Jack's *last orders*), now the men are able to resume their social interaction in a familiar locale and resume the thread of friendship that has sustained them for so long.

MAN ON THE TRAIN (FRANCE, 2003). DIRECTED BY PATRICE LECONTE.
The film portrays the evolving friendship between the unlikeliest of acquaintances—one an old man who has lived alone in his parent's house in a small French city for 15 years, and the other a handsome, middle-aged man in town to meet his accomplices in advance of a planned bank robbery. The film is a refreshing take on the mutual benefits of intergenerational relationships. The arrival of the stranger, Milan, awakens in the old man, Manisquer, the dreams of being young and virile and desired again. But Milan's life is also changed by the time he spends staying in the old man's house and reflecting on the security, the predictability, and the comfort of a life in old age. Both men are dreaming dreams, in one sense, and yet the timing of their meeting is perfect for releasing the power of their imaginations and their yearnings to become something they cannot become in real life. One of the joys of this film is the evolving camaraderie between the two men over a one-week period. The old man has a Friday appointment at his local hospital—for repair of his heart valve; Milan awaits the reunion of his robbery team for a Friday heist. The progress of their relationship allows each man to imagine what it would be like to be the other. Manisquer's time with Milan teaches him that his life has little meaning now. He wants it to be genuine, rather than simply safe and predictable. He admits, "I stopped living before I grew old." Near the end of the film, Milan addresses the old man's lack of self-confidence by urging him to understand why women don't look at him: "They don't see you—because they are dazzled by you! Can't you see how fantastic you are?" At the same time Manisquer works his magic on Milan, as the latter begins to relax and enjoy this respite from a troubled life. Both men keep their date with destiny; and in the film's climax everything goes wrong for them: one dies on the operating table, the other dies in a police ambush because one of the gang betrayed the others. The last scene exists in a kind of parallel universe, where it is possible to imagine what it would have been like if the two men could have exchanged identities—the tough guy giving way to the quiet homebody, and the old man assuming a life of high adventure.

RED (FRANCE, 1994). DIRECTED BY KRZYSZTOF KIESLOWSKI.
A young woman befriends an old man, a retired judge, and discovers ultimately that their lives are interconnected in extraordinary ways. *Red* is the third film in a trilogy (*Blue, White, Red*) by this director. *Red* explores *fraternity* (one of three symbols in the French tricolor) from the perspective of a compassionate young model, Valentine, someone who is all "heart." When Valentine runs into the old man's dog, loose on the streets, she takes the dog to a vet and then drops him off at the old man's house. Thus begins a bizarre friendship. The two are drawn to one another, they listen to each other, and they learn from each other. Their relationship also fosters a regeneration in both of their lives. The film raises the question of why certain lives intersect but other lives never intersect. Throughout the film Valentine and another character, a young man (and a frustrated lover of another woman), never meet, even though they *almost* meet on numerous occasions. They seem to exist in parallel universes; and in a different sense, the lives of Valentine and

the old judge have also existed in parallel universes. What the old man has experienced is being experienced now by the young man Valentine never meets. Both were in law school, both became judges, and both lost their lovers to infidelity. This film is about Valentine *meeting* the old man in a different generational universe. Although they share intimate details of each other's lives, they do not fall in love. But in knowing each other, the stage is set for Valentine to fall in love with the right man—something that failed to happen in the judge's experience many years ago. In a long conversation between the two, the old man tells his story and helps her understand how much she has helped him recover from his depression and alienation in old age. At the same time, the old man has helped her resolve her ambivalence about her drug-addicted brother and her responsibility for his care. They part amicably, and the stage is set for the inevitable meeting between Valentine and the jilted lover—in the most unusual of meetings; Valentine's future emotional fulfillment is mirrored by the old man's sense of serenity as he faces old age anew.

SARABAND (SWEDEN, 2003). DIRECTED BY INGMAR BERGMAN.

After an absence of more than 30 years, Marianne, 63, visits her former husband and spends several weeks at his lakeside retreat. Marianne enters a closed world of family tensions. Johan, 86, now rich from an inheritance, has retired to a remote cabin in the wilderness. And nearby, in a cottage, his 61-year-old son, a widower for two years, tutors his 19-year-old daughter Karin on the cello. These three coexist in a tenuous balance. The father despises his son Henrik as weak and unstable; Henrik resents his father for not ever having accepted or affirmed him. Henrik has devoted himself absolutely to his daughter's talent as an artist, but Karin feels trapped in a cloying, stifling, and near-incestuous relationship with her father. Liv Ullmann and Erland Josephson reprise their roles from the 1973 film *Scenes from a Marriage*, also written and directed by Bergman. The film is organized into ten chapters with a prologue and epilogue. In the latter two segments Marianne sits in a studio and speaks directly to the audience. *Saraband* was Bergman's last film. There is one other character Marianne discovers that has an all-encompassing power over all three of these family members. That person is Anna, Henrik's wife, dead two years now. Viewers first meet Anna through a photograph of her on the nightstand in Henrik's bedroom. Anna is like a silent and omnipresent judge, observing the follies of those still in life and marveling at how tangled their lives have become. That image of Anna reappears at climactic moments in the film, as if commenting on the lives of the characters. To Henrik, Anna was his alpha and omega—and now that she is gone, he cannot bear to give up Karin. But to Johan, Anna was something ephemeral and indescribable; Henrik did not deserve her. Johan is that type of man who cannot brook another man's judgment being superior to his own. As a father, he can only humiliate his son, because that will prove that his son is inferior to himself. "Honest hate should be respected," he says, and Johan acts on that belief. All of these characters are trapped in one way or the other. Karin escapes being a surrogate for Anna (for both her father and her grandfather) by deciding to leave home on her own terms, and Marianne has to break free from this stifling atmosphere in order to make sense of her journey. She learns that there is no hope of her reestablishing a relationship of love and trust with Johan. He is irredeemable and unregenerate. But Marianne has the last word, in the epilogue, and even Marianne admits that she, too, has been touched by Anna's powerful capacity for love.

SINCE OTAR LEFT (FRANCE, 2004). DIRECTED BY JULIE BERTOLUCCI.

Otar is the favorite child of Eka, an old woman who lives with her daughter and her granddaughter Ada in Tblisi, the capitol of the former Soviet Socialist Republic of Georgia. Life in Tblisi is bleak and hopeless more than a decade after the breakup of the Soviet Empire. The destiny of the family revolves around the fortunes of Otar, who moved to Paris several years ago in order to study medicine. Eka's middle-aged daughter, Marina, has few prospects. Her husband was killed in the Soviet occupation of Afghanistan. Eka's granddaughter Ada is in school, but she seems destined to waste her life by marrying the wrong man and remaining trapped in poverty. When news comes to Marina and Ada that Otar has died in an accident, the two women cannot bring themselves to tell Eka. So Ada writes fake letters from Otar and reads them to her grandmother. Eventually, the balance of relationships shifts in the film. Eka and her daughter become closer. Ada seems to move to the periphery of the family, especially when the pressures of her deception overwhelm her and she threatens to tell her grandmother the truth. The resolution to this family's emotional distress is triggered when another journey occurs near the end of the film—a journey that in some respects mirrors Otar's original journey to Paris. This second journey is precipitated by Eka's commitment to her granddaughter's future. She knows that it is too late for her daughter, a child of the former Soviet Union. But it is not too late for Ada, who speaks French fluently and needs an opportunity to live on her own. So the old woman sells her father's French library (her most prized possession) in order to finance a trip to Paris. By this time in the film she knows, at one level, that her son Otar is dead. But she must know firsthand to confirm her suspicions. In Paris the old woman tracks down someone in the apartment building where Otar once lived, and this man tells her that her son is dead. She faces her grief alone, with quiet dignity and courage. Reunited with the others, Eka practices a deception that mirrors Marina and Ada's earlier deception, and then she declares that she is ready to tour the City of Lights. The film ends with Eka's last surprise—another deception, aimed at reestablishing, for this family, a basis for hope in the future.

SOLAS (SPAIN, 1999). DIRECTED BY BENITO ZAMBRANO.

The title of the film means "alone" in Spanish. Rosa, an elderly rural woman, stays with her estranged daughter in the city to be closer to the hospital, where her husband is a patient. The daughter Maria, 35, is unmarried and regards her mother with anger and resentment for living all these years with an abusive and alcoholic husband. That old man is an uncaring, possessive man and even calls his wife a "stupid old woman." Never once does he affirm her. While Rosa spends her days at the hospital, knitting to pass the time, her daughter tries to resolve her crises—her own alcoholism and an unexpected pregnancy. The saving grace for the mother is her relationship with an old man, a neighbor in Maria's apartment building. They meet by chance at a grocery store, where he helps her pay for her groceries, and soon he insinuates himself into her life by asking for advice on cooking. One day, the old woman returns to the apartment and hears the neighbor's dog, Achilles, whining just inside his apartment. She goes inside and finds the old man, Vecino, unable to get up from the bed and suffering from an attack of diarrhea. She helps him into the shower. When he resists her help, she says, "Enough of this foolishness! Seeing a naked man won't kill me!" The unforced intimacy between two elders in this scene is memorable.

Perhaps their warmth and affection for each other will save the old woman from her broken relationship with her mean-spirited and self-loathing wreck of a husband. But that is not the direction of this plot. Rosa will return to her village with her husband, but there are hints that she has freed herself of the burden of being the dutiful wife to this unworthy man. She will stay with him, but she will no longer be intimidated by him. She says goodbye to Vecino, after introducing him to her daughter. This scene is rich with subtle and evocative dialogue, suggesting their deeply felt intimacy, and yet emphasizing her decision to return home. But her introduction of Maria to Vecino leads to the unfolding of a remarkable if unlikely intergenerational relationship. The old man and Maria spend an evening preparing dinner, playing cards, and drinking wine. Maria tells him the details of her father's brutality and dishonesty. Vecino refuses to be judgmental when she tells him she is pregnant. They work out a resolution for her emotional crisis. He becomes an unofficial grandfather to her baby, which she names *Rosa* after her mother dies.

SPRING, SUMMER, FALL, WINTER . . . AND SPRING (SOUTH KOREA, 2003). DIRECTED BY KI-DUK KIM.

This film, about the experiences that take place on a floating Buddhist temple in a remote mountain lake, compares the metaphor of returning to a special place from one's past with the wisdom of elders that age in place. Each segment of the film is based on life on that temple in a different season. In *Spring* an old monk and a small boy live in the temple, and in *Summer* the monk (older now) resides in the temple with the same boy—now a teenager. In that segment a mother brings her daughter to live in the temple to be healed by herbal remedies known only to the old monk. But during her stay there the two young people fall in love. When the mother returns to take her daughter home, the young man runs off later in order to marry her. In *Fall* the monk, now a very old man, is startled to learn that his former disciple murdered his wife. Soon the man, now in his thirties, returns to the temple a fugitive, having escaped prison. *Fall* is the crucial section in the film because the old man, having failed the young man in his earlier years, now brings all of his wisdom to bear on the redemption of the escaped convict—even after two police officers arrive to apprehend him. In this segment the young man finally learns the significance of *place* in his life. He grasps the special quality of spirituality and sanctuary that this floating temple represents. But there is more suffering in store for him. He has to leave in order to resume serving his prison sentence. In *Winter*, he returns to the temple in middle age, having served his time, and finds the monk long dead. Now the cycle of generations requires that the middle-aged man study the *sutras*, gain insight into the role that desire and suffering play in this life, and replace the former monk. It should be no surprise that in this section of the film a baby turns up (brought by its mother who cannot care for him), and that in the last segment of the film the middle-aged monk will be raising that baby just as the former old monk had raised him—another reminder of the cyclical nature of life in the Mahayana Buddhist tradition.

TOKYO STORY (1953, JAPAN). DIRECTED BY YASUJIRO OZU.

Tokyo Story is a deceptively simple film about an old couple visiting their children in Tokyo. They live in the country with a daughter, and their visit appears to be a plan by members of the family to invite the old couple to live with their children for an extended period of time. Before long, that plan runs up against the reality of self-centered children who decide that they have no room for the elders in their homes. But the director has no intention of condemning their children for their inflexibility, intolerance, and lack of filial piety. There are really no villains in the film. The old couple tries to stay with a son and his family, but they discover that they are alone in their son's house. Life goes on, and they are not part of that life. Even their grandchildren have little interest in forming an intergenerational bond. The film incorporates three separate journeys taken by these elders. The first is to Tokyo, the second is to a resort (they are sent there by their children—so that the children won't have to deal with them), and finally their journey home once their visit is finished. Each journey-within-the-overall-journey has separate functions and reveals separate meanings for the old couple. The visit to the resort is even more awkward for them because they are surrounded by lively and noisy young people. "This place is meant for the younger generation," the old woman concludes. But she could have said the same about their visit to Tokyo. Their final journey home is ruined by the sudden illness of the old woman, and she dies at home while surrounded by most of her children. The meanings of that journey resonate with the grief responses of the children and with her husband's realization that now he must face life alone. Thus, the father's journey has been a circular one: he returns to the place where he began his journey, but now he faces the changed prospects of a new life in widowhood.

THE TRIP TO BOUNTIFUL (1985). DIRECTED BY PETER MASTERSON.

Old Mrs. Watts sneaks away from her son and her insufferable daughter-in-law, cashes her Social Security check, and buys a bus ticket—hoping to reach the town of Bountiful, Texas, where she was born and raised. Her journey is a symbolic return to her roots, a search for closure, and a means of accepting the constraints of her new life. Along the way, she finds two guides, a young woman who reminds her of the passions of her own youth and a tactful middle-aged sheriff who is kind enough to drive her out to what is left of the town of Bountiful when she reaches the end of the bus line at a nearby town. Mrs. Watts's struggle reminds us of the values associated with aging in place. Her journey is meaningful to her. She revisits her old house, takes stock of her life, and when her son arrives to take her back to town, she seems at peace with what she has found in Bountiful. Something has been restored to her now that she can stand in this field near the old house. She realizes that both her son and she are bound to this place and to the cycle of generations that planted cotton on this land, then left for the cities, then returned to farm again, and then left the land behind again. She will resume her life with her son and daughter-in-law, but when they return home she will be a changed woman, whose *escape* from that stifling multigenerational household has changed everyone in the family and promises a stronger bond between generations.

WILD STRAWBERRIES (SWEDEN, 1957). DIRECTED BY INGMAR BERGMAN.

Retired physician Isak Borg, 78, makes a journey to Lund, Sweden, to receive an honorary degree. Despite the honors, Borg is the most ordinary of men, lonely in his old age, and not one to be warm to human interactions. In fact, Isak Borg is an *iceberg* of a man. His wife, appearing in a dream sequence later in the film, will refer to him as being "as cold as ice." On his journey he is accompanied by his daughter-in-law, unhappy in her marriage.

They are hostile toward each other, but as the trip continues Borg learns the extent to which she has suffered emotional duress in her relationship and becomes sympathetic to her. For Borg, the trip is a combination of intimate moments of life review; disabling dreams about failure, guilt, and fear of his mortality; an unhappy encounter with his elderly mother; and more hopeful encounters with the variety of people he meets along the way. He and Marianne meet an interesting assortment of characters on the motor trip: a young woman, Sara (the same name as Borg's first great love), who enjoys teasing the old man; an unhappily married couple; two young men competing for the modern Sara's affection; and a man who never forgot Borg's kindness to him many years ago. Being with the modern Sara and the other young people seems to lighten Borg's mood. He revisits his family's summer home, where he spent his first 20 years of life. He observes—as if he were an onlooker witnessing his past—his first love, Sara, picking wild strawberries and flirting with Borg's older brother. Later he witnesses Sara confiding in a cousin and reporting on the drawbacks of choosing Borg as her lover. Borg tells the modern version of Sara that his first great love married his brother and lived happily with him. He experiences another vision near the end of the film, when he observes his wife Karin flirting with another man and being seduced by him. So at every turn Borg's life review reminds him of his limitations, his lack of intimacy with others, and his feelings of inadequacy. Finally, he confesses to Marianne, "I'm dead although I'm alive." But when he reaches Lund and is reunited with his son, all goes well during the ceremony and he is celebrated by the young people who accompanied him on his journey. The film ends with an idealized image of contentment, as we observe Borg in another waking dream, revisiting his youth and observing his parents in an idyllic moment. In that moment he finds bliss that otherwise has been denied him during the entirety of his life.

Additional Recommended Films

After Life (Japan, 1998). Intergeneration, love in old age.

Babette's Feast (Denmark, 1987). Aging in place, intergeneration, religion.

Cinema Paradiso (Italy, 1988). Aging in place, intergeneration, mentors.

Harold and Maude (1973). Vital aging, intergeneration, death.

The Human Stain (2003). Friendship and love in old age, intergeneration, widowhood.

The King of Masks (China, 1999). Aging and the arts, intergeneration.

Little Dieter Needs to Fly (documentary, Germany, 1997). Elder journeys, redemption, Vietnam War.

Martha and Ethel (documentary, 1995). Aging and ethnicity, intergeneration.

Pelle the Conqueror (Denmark, 1987). Father-son relationships, poverty in old age.

The Remains of the Day (United Kingdom, 1993). Failure of love in old age, unregenerative elders.

Shower (China, 1999). Aging in place, father-son relationships, redemption.

The Straight Story (1999). Aging in place, elder journeys, family dynamics.

A Sunday in the Country (France, 1984). Aging and the arts, intergeneration.

The Three Burials of Melquiades Estrada (2005). Elder journeys, friendship in old age.

Waking Ned Devine (United Kingdom, 1998). Aging in place, friendship in old age.

REFERENCES

Cole, T. R. 1991. Aging, home, and Hollywood in the 1980s. *Gerontologist* 31 (3): 427–30.

Fisher, B. 2006. Old age in feature-length films: "Ladies in Lavender." *Gerontologist* 46 (3): 418–21.

Grabinski, C. J., J. Vanden Bosch, and R. E. Yahnke. 2003. Old age and loss in feature-length films. *Gerontologist* 43 (3):136–41.

Yahnke, R. E. 2000. Intergeneration and regeneration: Old age in films and videos. In *Handbook of the Humanities and Aging*, 2nd ed., ed. T. R. Cole and R. Kastenbaum, 293–323. New York: Springer.

———. 2005. Heroes of their own stories: Expressions of aging in international cinema. In *Aging Education in a Global Context*, ed. D. Shenk and L. Groger, 57–76. New York: Haworth Press.